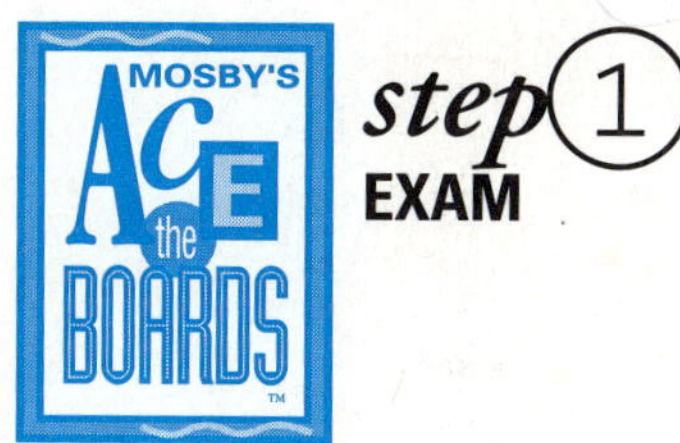

Basic Sciences

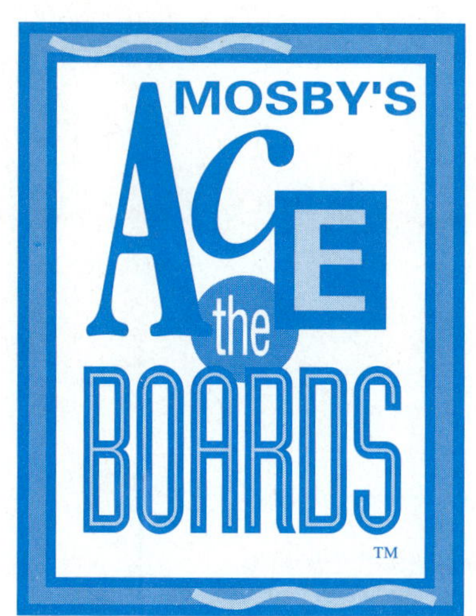

step ①
EXAM

Basic Sciences

Mosby

St. Louis   Baltimore   Boston   Carlsbad   Chicago   Naples   New York   Philadelphia   Portland
London   Madrid   Mexico City   Singapore   Sydney   Tokyo   Toronto   Wiesbaden

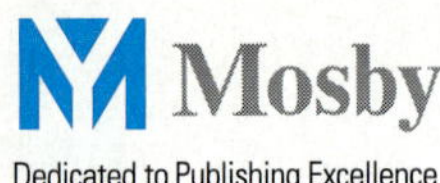

Mosby

Dedicated to Publishing Excellence

A Times Mirror
Company

Vice President & Publisher *Anne S. Patterson*
Editor *Emma D. Underdown*
Developmental Editor *Christy Wells*
Editorial Assistant *Alicia E. Moten*
Project Manager *Dana Peick*
Production Editor *Jeffrey Patterson*
Book Designer *Amy Buxton*
Manufacturing Supervisor *Tony McAllister*
Cover Designer *Stacy Lanier/AKA Design*

Printed in the United States of America
Composition by Graphic World, Inc.
Printing/binding by R.R. Donnelley

Mosby-Year Book, Inc.
11830 Westline Industrial Drive
St. Louis, Missouri 63146

Library of Congress Cataloging-in-Publication Data
Ace step 1 exam : basic sciences / [editor, Emma D. Underdown].
     p. cm. -- (Ace the boards)
   Other title: Mosby's USMLE step 1 exam : basic sciences.
   ISBN 0-8151-6904-3
   1. Medicine--Examinations, questions, etc. I. Underdown, Emma D.
II. Series
   [DNLM: 1. Medicine--examination questions. WB 18.2 A173 1996]
R834.5.A26 1996
610' .76--dc20
DNLM/DLC
for Library of Congress   96-6191
                                                                 CIP

ISBN 0-8151-6904-3 (IBM)
ISBN 0-8151-8669-X (MAC)
96 97 98 99 00 / 9 8 7 6 5 4 3 2 1

Contributors

Anatomy

Richard R. Schmidt, Ph.D.
Professor of Pathology, Anatomy and
 Cell Biology,
Department of Pathology, Anatomy
 and Cell Biology,
Jefferson Medical College,
Philadelphia, Pennsylvania

Behavioral Science

Barbara Cubic, Ph.D.
Assistant Professor,
Department of Psychiatry
 and Behavioral Sciences,
Eastern Virginia Medical School,
Norfolk, Virginia

Biochemistry

John W. Pelley, Ph.D.
Associate Professor,
Department of Cell Biology
 and Biochemistry,
Texas Tech University Health Sciences
 Center,
Lubbock, Texas

Histology and Cell Biology

James A. Hightower, Ph.D.
Associate Professor,
Department of Cell Biology
 and Neuroscience,
School of Medicine,
University of South Carolina,
Columbia, South Carolina

Microbiology and Immunology

David. J. Silverman, Ph.D.
Professor of Microbiology and
 Immunology,
Department of Microbiology and
 Immunology,

University of Maryland School
 of Medicine,
Baltimore, Maryland

Neuroscience

Mary K. Vaughan, Ph.D.
Medical Neuroscience Task Force
 Chairman,
Department of Cellular and Structural
 Biology,
University of Texas Health Science
 Center,
San Antonio, Texas

Pathology

Roger L. Sopher, M.D.
Professor and Chair,
Department of Pathology,
University of North Dakota School
 of Medicine,
Grand Forks, North Dakota

Pharmacology

Laszlo Kerecsen, M.D.
Research Associate Professor,
Department of Pharmacology,
 Toxicology and Therapeutics,
University of Kansas School
 of Medicine,
Kansas City, Kansas

Physiology

Paul H. Brand, Ph.D.
Associate Professor,
Department of Physiology and
 Molecular Medicine,
Medical College of Ohio,
Toledo, Ohio

One of the best ways to prepare for exams is by taking practice questions. Mosby's USMLE Step 1 Exam gives you the opportunity to take a simulated exam, and provides feedback that will help you improve your performance on the real test.

This book and the accompanying diskette are set up just like the Step 1 exam. Typically the USMLE booklets are administered in four 3-hour sessions, with up to 200 questions per session. Our questions are also grouped into four exams, each with 200 questions. The questions on the diskette and in the book are exactly the same to give you complete flexibility in how you study. You can use the printed questions to mimic the testing conditions and the actual USMLE. Or you can use the diskette to maximize your study time. A timing module during Exam Mode on the computer diskette can help you keep track of your timing performance; and the Test-Taking Strategies on pp. x to xiv will help you make the best use of your time both before and during the exam.

There are two ways of using the questions on the diskette. The Tutorial Mode shows the answers after each question. With this Tutorial Mode, you can answer the questions as often as you wish. For the Test Mode, however, you get one chance at answering a question, and the answers are not displayed until the end of the exam. The Test Mode, then, more closely mimics the conditions of an actual test. We suggest you use the Test Mode first to establish what topics you need to study for the USMLE Step 1 Exam. Then you can use the Tutorial Mode for a more in-depth review. The Help Index on the diskette will give you the full explanations of how to use the disk.

Questions have been tested for accuracy, and unclear or otherwise faulty questions have been deleted. We have focussed on clinical questions to give you the most up-to-date preparation for the USMLE. The result is 800 high quality questions that cover all the areas tested on the Step 1 Exam: anatomy, behavioral science, biochemistry, histology & cell biology, microbiol-ogy & immunology, neuroscience, pathology, pharmacology, and physiology.

Because knowing what you *don't* know is just as important as knowing what you *do* know, all the answers— correct and incorrect— are annotated. Furthermore, all of the questions are coded to three levels:

Level 1— the discipline (microbiology, etc.)
Level 2— the general area (bacteriology, cardiovascular system)
Level 3— the specific area (epidemiology, diseases, etc.)

Thus, you can quickly see how well you know each discipline, system and area, and you can then spend more time on topics that need the most work. On the computer diskette, questions are categorized and scored in both the Tutorial and the Exam Mode. The book contains a checklist for each exam which you can also use to track what topics you need to study. The same categories are used throughout Mosby's ACE Step 1 reviews series so you can concentrate on studying just what you need. Whether you're in a traditional curriculum or a systems-based one, the categorized questions will help you focus your study time.

It is our sincere hope that Mosby's USMLE Step 1 Exam helps make you more confident and better prepared for the USMLEs. We welcome your feedback in making future versions even more responsive to your needs. Use the comment card in the back of the book to tell us how we can better serve you.

ACKNOWLEDGMENTS

We thank the University of Maryland Class of 1997 and the Office of Academic Development at the Medical School for being a field-testing site for the questions.

Test-Taking Strategies

Suzanne F. Kiewit, M.Ed.

To perform well on the USMLEs, it is imperative that you begin with a **plan**. Preparation time is at a premium, so you will want to be as efficient and effective as possible by planning well.

MONTHS AHEAD OF THE EXAM

- Sit down with a blank calendar and block in your commitments: classes, final exams, scheduled events.
- Include time for activities of daily life: eating, sleeping, exercising, socializing, banking, maintaining your home, and so forth.
- The remaining time is available for study/review.
- Determine an orderly approach to the material you need to cover that fits your particular set of needs (e.g., subject-by-subject approach, systems approach, pathologic state approach).
- Assign the remaining time to content areas. This is done in various ways: material covered freshman year first, easiest first, least comfortable material first, detailed subjects last, whatever. Your plan should reflect your goal: to maximize your score.
- Establish a warm-up, which may consist of breaking the tension in major muscle groups (neck rolls, shoulder rolls, etc.), a quick visualization of you performing successfully, or a brief meditation. Practicing this warm-up routine before each of your study sessions will make it a familiar activity that helps you learn effectively, as well as take exams effectively.
- Designate time at the end of your study period for panoramic review. Depending on your needs, that might be a week or just several days before the exam.
- Plan for feedback on your efforts. Schedule time for answering questions on the material you are reviewing and for taking at least one mock comprehensive exam.
- Do the comprehensive exam midway through your study period so that you can refine your efforts to reflect the degree of your performance.

DAYS AHEAD OF THE EXAM

- Divide each day into thirds: morning block, afternoon block, and evening block.
- Consider the time of day that is most productive for you and do the most difficult or least favorite material at that time.
- Assign more blocks of study to those areas requiring the most review to reach a comfortable knowledge level.

- A popular way to use blocks is to pair subjects or materials. For instance, pair strong content with weaker content so that you are not always in the position of not knowing material (which would invite negative feelings or ineffectiveness). Or pair a conceptual subject with a detail subject, such as physiology with anatomy, so that you are not always doing the same kind of thinking (this invites positive effort).
- Use your most productive blocks of time for actual study/review. Use the nonpeak times for reinforcement of material covered or feedback by answering questions on material that you have covered.

Planning the blocks

- Once you determine time allocations for each content area and an orderly approach that fits your needs and goals, you want to specify what you plan to do during each block.
- Be specific as to content area, material to study, and task; for example, MICRO: review chart on viruses; PHYS: answer questions on renal; and so forth.
- Each study block will last approximately 3 to 4 hours. To be most efficient and effective, plan to take a 5- or 10-minute break every hour. If you are having difficulty getting into the study mode, plan to study for 25 minutes, then take a 5-minute break. Reserve longer breaks for switches between subjects. Get up and move around on breaks.

BEFORE THE EXAM

Knowing about the USMLEs helps demystify them. In general, the USMLE exams are a 2-day, four-book examination. Approximately 3 hours are allotted per exam book. Each day you will complete one book of about 200 items in the morning and another book in the afternoon.

In each exam book, questions are organized by question type, not content. Specific directions precede each set of questions. Only two question formats are used: one-best-answer multiple choice items (which typically come first on the exam) and matching items (toward the end of the exam). Students have reported that one-best-answer items make up the bulk of the exam (70% to 75%) and negatively stemmed items make up only 10% to 15% of the questions (Bushan, Le, and Amin, 1995). Matching sets, which make up about 15% to 20% of the items, may include short leading lists or long leading lists of up to 26 items from which to choose.

From year to year there may be variations in the organization and presentation of both content and item formats. It would be wise to read the National Board of Medical Examiners' *General Instructions* booklet, which you will receive when you register. This booklet contains descriptions of content, item format, and even a set of practice items. Be certain you read this booklet and familiarize yourself with the questions.

You can further maximize exam performance by taking control. Adults tend to perform better when the feel that they have a measure of control. For the USMLE it is easy to feel out of control. You are told what time to arrive, where to go, what writing instrument to use, when to break the seal, and so on. You want to assume control of as many aspects as possible to maximize your performance:

STUDY Follow the sage advice of planning your work and working your plan to maintain satisfactory preparation with regard to study.

SLEEP Get a good night's rest. Sleep needs vary, but 6 hours is usually minimum. Try to get the appropriate amount of sleep that you require.

NUTRITION Maintain proper nutrition during both study time and exam time. Eat breakfast. Choose foods that help keep you on an even energy level. Eat light lunches on exam days. If you have a favorite food and can take it with you, treat yourself.

MEDICATION It may be cold, flu, or allergy season. Take no medications that may make you drowsy.

CLOTHING Heating and cooling systems are rarely balanced enough to suit everyone. Wear articles of clothing that can be added or removed as necessary. Strive for personal comfort.

READINESS Develop physical, mental, emotional, and psychologic readiness for the exam. Keep your thoughts about the exam and your preparation efforts running positively. You must believe that *you can do this!*

ARRIVAL Plan to arrive as close to the designated time as possible and still allow yourself sufficient time to check in. Keep to yourself so that other people's anxieties will not affect you. Take care of personal needs. Find your seat.

ACCLIMATION Settle in and get comfortable. Take several deep breaths . . . RELAX. A relaxed mind thinks better than a tense one—it's that old "fight-or-flight" syndrome. Do your warm-up routine to help you relax.

ATTENTION Pay attention to the proctor. Complete all identification material as required. Read all instructions carefully. Ask for clarification as needed. Do not open your booklet until told to do so. After you are told to break the seal, quickly glance through the whole test to see how it is set up and how questions are organized. Again, you want to take control of the situation. A quick purview eliminates surprises and allows you to develop a plan.

DURING THE EXAM
Plan your approach

There are numerous approaches to answering questions. Answer questions in the order that appeals to you. Doing the easier ones first may give a psychologic boost; however, the ones you skip may stay on your mind and cloud your thinking.

Another approach is to answer each question in sequence. Start with the first one in the section with which you begin and fill in an answer for each question. Do not leave any blanks! The theory behind this is that if you spend any time at all on an item, you should mark your best response at that time and go on. If you are not certain of your choice, mark "R" in the test booklet for review and return to it later as you have time.

Some students plan to do the matching items first. Matching items are the last set of questions in the booklets. If you prefer matching items, this is a reasonable plan because it helps you get started with items about which you feel confident. It is also reasonable because matching items are not good items on which to guess if you run short of time. **You** must decide the order in which you want to do the questions.

Complete the bubble sheet or answer card carefully

There are two schools of thought on this matter. One is to fill in the bubble sheet **item by item** as you go. This method minimizes transcription errors. The other method is **block transfer.** Complete a logical chunk of questions in the test booklet (one or two pages) and then transfer responses to the bubble sheet. Be sure that the last question number of the page is the last numeral you blacken. This method saves time and offers a mini–mental break at the end of each block. Such mini-breaks help decrease fatigue during a long exam. Choose the method that will work for you and *practice* it as you take prep questions.

Budget your time

If only the allotted time and the number of questions were considered, you would have approximately 54 seconds per question. Obviously, some questions may go more quickly and balance out the ones that take longer. To keep track, you need a pacing strategy. A good strategy is to establish checkpoints at 30-minute intervals. When you overview the booklet, circle the numerals corresponding to where you should be at 30 minutes, 60, 90, 120, and so on. For example, if you have 200 questions on a 3-hour exam, you should be at question number 33 at 30 minutes. As you complete the exam, check your time at the circled items. This technique keeps you from watching the clock too much, yet permits multiple opportunities to adjust your pacing.

If you find yourself spending too much time on any one question, select your best choice at that time, mark an answer, and "R" it for later review. The point is to keep going. Laboring too long on one question limits you from responding to other items you may know well. Remember, controlling your time helps you maximize your points.

ANSWERING THE QUESTIONS

- **Read and *understand* the stems and alternatives.**

The most frequent error made on exams is misreading or misinterpreting the various aspects of a question. The **stem** is the introductory question or statement. The **alternatives** are the options from which you select the one best response. To encourage reading and understanding, use a process.

- **Follow a process to answer questions.**
  1. Quickly read the stem.
  2. Quickly read the options. (Combined, the first two steps create a preview of the item.)
  3. Carefully read, underline, and mark the stem in a timely fashion.
    - Selectively underline key words and phrases. Pay attention to nouns, verbs, and modifiers.
    - Circle age and gender.
    - Note data in telescopic form (e.g., $\uparrow$ BP).
    - Graphically represent material if it helps you to understand (e.g., diagram the renal tubule to answer a question about reabsorption).
  4. Carefully read each alternative. Mark as appropriate.
- **Consider each alternative as one in a series of true, false, or not sure (?) statements.**

Read each alternative. Rather than slashing out the ones you eliminate, work with each one and designate it as **true, false,** or varying degrees of **true/false/?**. This marking strategy requires you to make judicious decisions about alternatives relative to the stem. It also provides a record of your original thinking, which will save you rethinking time if you need to reconsider a question. Practice this strategy on preparation questions so it becomes second nature.

- **Avoid premature closure.**

Sometimes you may read a question and anticipate a response. Such a reaction helps focus your attention. However, be sure to read *all* the options so that you are selecting the *best* response. In one-best-answer multiple choice questions, there is one *best* and several *likely* responses. Avoid being misled; consider all the alternatives.

- **Be leery of negative stems.**

Negative stems require shifting to a negative thinking mode to determine which alternatives are not correct. You can avoid this shift by using this strategy:

- Circle such words as *except, least, false, incorrect, not true* to raise your awareness of them.
- Cross out the negative and read the stem as though it were a positive.

- Mark each option as T/F/?. The F option will then be the appropriate choice.
- **Keep your original answers.**

To change or not to change answers is a difficult decision. The answer depends on a person's previous history. If you are the kind of student who, if you change answers, changes them from wrong to right, then selectively changing answers may be worthwhile. If, on the other hand, your past experience has been to change right answers to wrong answers, selectively changing answers is probably not a good idea. Good performers change answers, but only if they have reason, such as acquired insight or discovery of misreading or misinterpretation.

- **Maintain an even emotional keel.**

If a question upsets you, calm yourself. Take several deep breaths. Tell yourself, "I can do this!" Give yourself a mental or physical break. Pay special attention to the next two or three questions after a bout of emotional uneasiness. It is possible to miss items when attention is diffused.

THINKING THROUGH QUESTIONS

- **Use logical reasoning and sound thinking.**
  - Read the item carefully. After careful reading, ask "What is this question really asking?" Restate it so that you know what is being asked.
  - Engage in a mental dialogue with the question. Talk to yourself about what you do know. Always start with what **you** know. Verbalize your thinking.
  - If a diagram or graphic representation is included, orient yourself to it **first** so that the options do not lead your thinking.
- **Use information found within the questions themselves to help you answer others.**

There will not be "gimmes" on a nationally standardized exam. However, there may be items or graphics that trigger remembrances.

- **Create a diagram, chart, map, or graphic representation of given information.**

Material that is visually presented usually helps clarify thinking. Use selective, quick sketching as warranted.

- **Reason through information like a detective.**
  - Sift through the details (preview).
  - Determine the relevant information (selectively mark).
  - Put the clues together as in solving a puzzle (reason).
- **Read carefully and note key descriptors.**
  - Note words such as *chronic, acute, greater than, less than, adult, child.*
  - Attend to prefixes such as *hyper-, hypo-, non-, un-, pre-, post-.*
- **Analyze base words and affixes.**

Studying a question at the word level may help you remember salient information. Look for base words or related words. Determine Latin or Greek word parts and use their meanings to assist you.

- **Consider similar options equally.**

If you mark one alternative as "false" for a particular reason and another option is qualified for the same reason, it's probably "false" as well.

- **Trust the questions.**

The questions are designed to determine if you have a working knowledge of the material. They are not written to trick you. You need to believe that your medical school curriculum and your study efforts prepared you for most of the questions.

- **Meet the challenge of clinical vignettes.**

Longer, vignette items challenge you to discern the relevant from the irrelevant material. In doing so, you are given multiple clues to consider. To effectively handle the vignette item, follow this strategy:

- Scan the stem and read the first several lines.
- Skip to the end of the stem and read the last several lines.
- Check the alternatives to narrow your focus.
- Now that you know what the question is about, go back to the stem; read and mark what's important to your informed decision making.
- Make good T/F/? decisions.
- **Reread your underlines and markings when you are down to two choices, at 50/50.**

By the time you work through a stem and numerous alternatives, it is easy to lose the gist of the question. Checking your focus by rereading only the underlines ensures that you are answering the question being posed.

ANSWERING MATCHING ITEM SETS

Matching items are used to measure your ability to distinguish among closely related items. They acquire knowledge of specific sets of information. As you study, be alert to potential material that could be tested in this way.

Matching items can be formatted in two ways. **Short leading list matching** items include a set of five lettered options followed by a lead-in statement and then several numbered stems. **Long leading list matching** items include a set of up to 26 lettered options, followed by a lead-in statement and then several numbered stems.

To efficiently deal with a short leading list item, consider it as an upside-down multiple choice item with the same repeated options. To handle it effectively, do the following:

- Scan the list; determine the topic.
- Read the lead-in statement; determine the focus.
- Quickly read the stem; then read and mark key words.
- In the left margin, create a grid with A, B, C, D, E at the top.
- Make good T/F/? decisions about each stem, marking them in the grid. In this way you can see the pattern of your responses. Similarly, a grid with the item numbers can be drawn beside the leading list and responses marked there.

Handling long leading list matching items effectively requires some modifications in the process. It is not efficient to make T/F/? decisions about each option, so follow this strategy:

- Scan the list; determine the topic.
- Read the lead-in; determine the focus.
- Read a stem and generate your own response.
- Narrow the focus. Put a check mark by those related options in the long list.
- Read and mark specifics in the stem to differentiate among those alternatives you marked.
- Make good T/F/? decisions.

For each item, mark the narrowed-list options with a different symbol (star, dash, etc.). Items are listed in logical order, alphabetically or numerically. When looking for an option such as "xanthinuria," do not start at the beginning of the list. Looking in the appropriate place saves valuable seconds.

TEST WISENESS

How a question is worded can often influence your response to it. Most clues about "test psychology" are a function of the way in which a question is worded—test constructors cannot rename body parts, drugs, diseases, and so forth. Being aware of the psychology behind the wording can often help you answer the test question.

Using techniques of test psychology to arrive at a correct answer has limited value on standardized exams because those who construct the exams are well aware of the use of these techniques. Nonetheless, being wise to these techniques of test psychology may add another point or two to your score, and they can also enhance your sense of control. Knowing these techniques provides additional strategies to employ should the question temporarily stump you.

The best way to take any exam is to be totally prepared with a strong knowledge base and personal test confidence. The following techniques should be used only if you have exhausted your knowledge base, eliminated all distractors, and cannot come up with the answer even with logical thinking and sound reasoning. Such techniques are **not** a substitute for knowledge, nor are they foolproof.

- **Identify common ideas or themes within the options and between the stem and options.**
  - Circle repeated words in the options.
  - Select the option with the most repeated words or phrases.
  - Circle words repeated in both stem and options.
  - Select the option that contains key words or related words from the stem. This is a stem/option repetition.
- **Beware of words that narrow the focus or are too extreme because they tend to be incorrect.**

Circle such words as *all, always, every, exclusively, never, no, not, none.*

- **Options that are look-alikes are good candidates for exclusion.**
- **Note qualifiers that broaden the focus because they may be correct.**

Circle words such as *generally, probably, most, often, some, usually.*

- **Identify antonyms or two opposing statements as potentially correct options.**

Test constructors may use pairs of opposites, so this tip may lose its effectiveness.

- **Select the most familiar-looking option.**

Always go from what you know. Alternatives with unknown terms may be likely distractors.

- **Select the longest, most inclusive answer.**

This would include "All of the above" as a strong potential response.

- **In numerical items, knock out the high and low alternatives and select one in the middle that seems most plausible.**
- **In negatively stemmed questions, categorize responses; the one that falls out of the category is a likely candidate.**
- **Mark the same alternative consistently throughout the test if you have no best guess and cannot eliminate distractors.**

Before the test, decide which letter (A, B, C, D, E) will be your choice. In this way, if you have given a question your best effort and cannot decide, mark you favorite response and move to questions that cover more comfortable material.

AFTER THE EXAM

- **Between booklets and overnight:**
  - Take a well-deserved break. Eat nutritionally.
  - If you feel the urge to study, study material that is comfortable, from a source with which you are familiar (e.g., personally developed study cards or your annotated review book.)
  - If you discovered a recurring "theme," you might desire to consult that set of information.
  - Do something pleasurable. Relax. Get a good night's rest.
- **After the final booklet:**
  - Recognize that this exam is a measure of what you know on a given day for a given set of information at a given point in time. Keep a reasonable perspective.
  - **Celebrate!**

References

Bushan V, Le T, Amin C: *First aid for the USMLE Step 1,* ed 5, Norwalk, Conn, 1995, Appleton & Lange.

MONEY-BACK GUARANTEE

We are confident that ACE THE BOARDS will prepare you for passing the USMLE. We are so sure of this, that we'll offer you a money back guarantee should you fail the USMLE. To receive your refund, simply mail us a copy of your failed USMLE report, plus the original receipt for this product. Mail these materials to:

Marketing Manager, Medical Textbooks
Mosby-Year Book, Inc.
11830 Westline Industrial Drive
St. Louis, MO 63146

CONTENTS

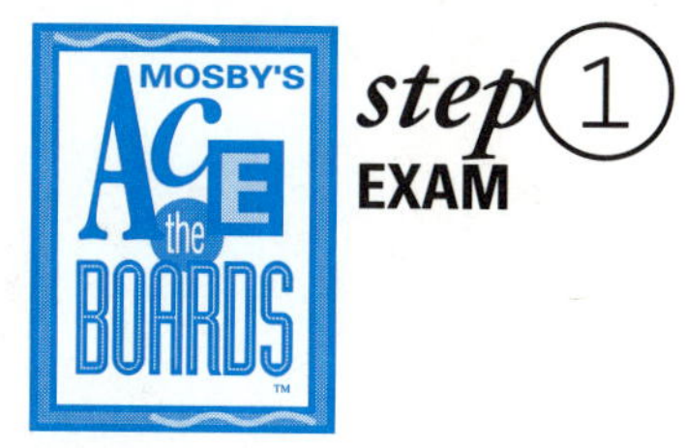

Basic Sciences

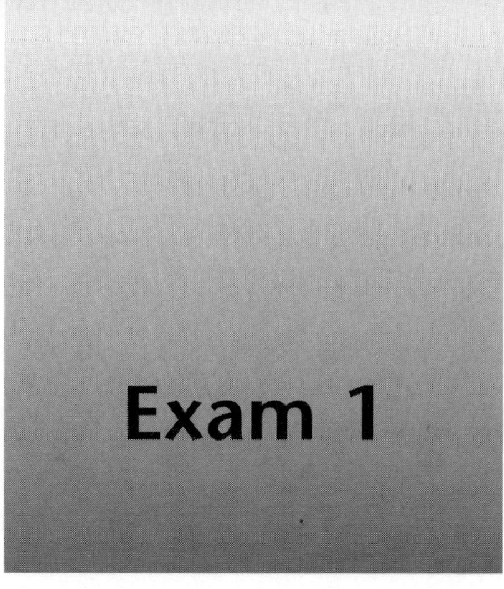

Exam 1

1. C5a is a product of complement activation that has important functions during the acute inflammatory response. Which of the following statements concerning C5a is *not* true?

   a. C5a is a vital component of the final "attack" complex that causes bacteriolysis.
   b. C5a is produced during the activation of complement by the classical pathway.
   c. C5a is produced during the activation of complement by the alternate pathway.
   d. C5a is the major contributor to chemotaxis of neutrophils in acute inflammation.
   e. C5a is not a major inducing agent of endothelial cell adhesion molecules.

2. Which of the following drugs would *not* be used prophylactically in asthmatic patients between attacks?

   a. Epinephrine
   b. Theophylline
   c. Methylprednisolone
   d. Cromolyn sodium
   e. Methotrexate

3. Which of the following causes a competitive block of Uptake I?

   a. Tyramine
   b. Clonidine
   c. Isoproterenol
   d. Cocaine
   e. Oxymetazoline

4. Which of the following statements about phenylalanine metabolism is *correct?*

   a. Phenylpyruvate, phenyllactate, and phenylacetate accumulate in low phenylalanine diets.
   b. Phenylalanine hydroxylase catalyzes the formation of phenylalanine from tyrosine.

   c. The most common form of phenylketonuria (PKU) has a deficiency in the enzyme phenylalanine hydroxylase.
   d. Phenylalanine hydroxylase requires a vitamin B6 (pyridoxal phosphate) cofactor.
   e. PKU is treated by pharmacologic agents that block the synthesis of tyrosine from phenylalanine.

5. Spirochetes are the etiologic agents of all *except* which of the following syndromes?

   a. Tick-borne relapsing fever
   b. Louse-borne relapsing fever
   c. Louse-borne typhus fever
   d. Lyme disease
   e. Syphilis

6. The surgical procedure you are conducting on your patient involves ligation of the infundibulopelvic ligament (suspensory ligament of the ovary) near the pelvic brim. Which of the following structures is most at risk during this ligation?

   a. Sympathetic chain ganglia
   b. Ureter
   c. Obturator nerve
   d. Inferior epigastric vessels
   e. Uterine artery

7. Concerning important adverse effects, which of the following statements is *false?*

   a. Aspirin causes GI disturbances.
   b. Phenacetin is nephrotoxic.
   c. Acetaminophen is hepatotoxic.
   d. Indomethacin causes agranulocytosis.
   e. Ibuprofen is cardiotoxic.

8. The major sensory input layer of the cerebral cortex is which of the following?

   a. Layer II
   b. Layer III

    c. Layer IV
    d. Layer V
    e. Layer VI

9. Figure 1 shows known transmembrane signaling mechanisms.

    1. Intracellular receptors that regulate gene expression
    2. Ligand-regulated transmembrane enzymes (i.e., protein tyrosine kinase)
    3. Ligand-gated channels
    4. G-proteins and second messengers

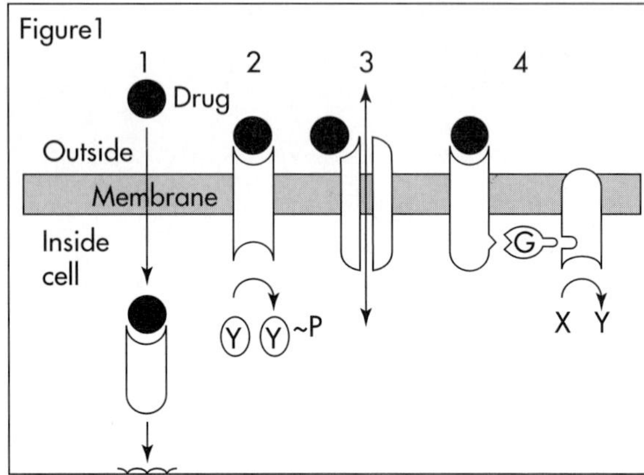

Which of the following agents are *not known* to function at site 4?

    a. Beta-adrenergic agonists
    b. Muscarinic agonists that stimulate phosphoinosite turnover via a G protein
    c. Adrenocorticotropic hormone (ACTH)
    d. Parathyroid hormone (PTH)
    e. Thyroid hormone

10. Patients may show signs of psychosis after receiving large doses of which of the following?

    a. Growth hormone
    b. Deoxycorticosterone
    c. Potassium iodide
    d. Cortisone
    e. Calcitriol

11. If a bacterium is capable of adhering to epithelial cells in the absence of mannose, but not in the presence of mannose, what is the most likely explanation?

    a. Mannose is present in the epithelial receptor for this organism.
    b. Mannose forms a bridge between two fimbrial structures on the bacterial surface to make a new structure, which now can adhere to the epithelial cell.
    c. The bacterium contains mannose on its surface.
    d. Mannose is not present in the epithelial receptor for this organism.
    e. Mannose is not an essential growth factor for this bacterium.

12. The pathogenesis of some bacteria is partially due to the presence of a capsule or slime layer external to the cell wall of the organism. Why does the capsule or slime layer act as a virulence factor?

    a. It often contains components of bacterial endotoxin.
    b. It contains beta-lactamases.
    c. It contains enzymes that degrade host cell membranes.
    d. It is immunogenic.
    e. It is antiphagocytic.

13. Which tissue possesses little, if any, inorganic material per mm^3?

    a. Lens
    b. Dentin
    c. Endochondral bone
    d. Cementum
    e. Enamel

14. Edema can be caused by which of the following?

    a. An increase in plasma protein concentration
    b. A decrease in capillary permeability
    c. A decrease in plasma protein concentration
    d. A decrease in venous pressure

15. What does Takayasu's arteritis involve primarily?

    a. Major branches of the aorta
    b. Medium-sized muscular arteries
    c. Small muscular arteries
    d. Capillaries
    e. Veins

16. Which of the following represents the correct sequence of events in the cyclic AMP-second messenger pathway?

    a. Vasopressin → cell membrane receptor → G protein → adenylyl cyclase → cAMP → protein kinase A → phosphorylated protein → increased water permeability
    b. Cortisol → cell membrane receptor → G protein → adenylyl cyclase → cAMP → protein kinase A → phosphorylated protein → gluconeogenesis
    c. Vasopressin → adenylyl cyclase → G protein → nuclear receptor → cAMP → protein kinase A → phosphorylated protein → water permeability
    d. Vasopressin → cell membrane receptor → phosphodiesterase → adenylyl cyclase → cAMP → diphosphoinositol → phosphorylated protein → water permeability
    e. Oxytocin → cell membrane receptor → protein kinase A → 5′ AMP → adenylyl cyclase → protein kinase A → cAMP → milk ejection

17. Patients with acute pancreatitis sometimes develop hypocalcemia, which can be of sufficient severity to cause concern. What is the mechanism of this hypocalcemia?

    a. Hormonal response to acute pancreatic injury
    b. Bleeding into the retroperitoneal connective tissue
    c. Enzymatic fat necrosis with formation of insoluble soaps
    d. Reflex release of calcitonin
    e. Increased osteoblastic activity in response to circulating enzymes

18. The anterior spinal artery is formed via the union of two branches derived from which of the following?

    a. Lumbar arteries
    b. Posterior intercostal arteries
    c. Vertebral arteries
    d. Posterior inferior cerebellar arteries
    e. Radicular arteries

19. Which of the following statements concerning oxytocin is *not* correct?

    a. It has a half-life of 30 to 40 minutes.
    b. It is optimally administered by intravenous drip.
    c. In high doses, it produces uterine tetany.
    d. It is used to promote milk "let down."
    e. It is used to control post-partum uterine hemorrhage.

20. Rickettsia causes all of the diseases *except* which of the following?

    a. Typhoid fever
    b. Rocky Mountain spotted fever
    c. Ehrlichiosis
    d. Q fever
    e. Bacillary angiomatosis

21. Complete anesthesia of the labia in the female requires that anesthetic be used to block which of the following nerves?

    a. Iliohypogastric and ilioinguinal nerves
    b. Iliohypogastric and pudendal nerves
    c. Ilioinguinal and pudendal nerves
    d. Pudendal nerve only
    e. Pelvic splanchnic nerves

22. If measurements of glomerular function disclosed the following:

    Glomerular capillary hydrostatic pressure (GCp) = 40 mm Hg
    Hydrostatic pressure in Bowman's space (BSp) = 8 mm Hg
    Glomerular capillary oncotic pressure (GCπ) = 23 mm Hg
    Oncotic pressure in Bowman's space (BSπ) = zero

    What would net ultrafiltration pressure equal?

    a. 5 mm Hg
    b. 9 mm Hg
    c. 15 mm Hg
    d. 31 mm Hg
    e. 40 mm Hg

23. Contraction of which of the following muscles produces movement at more than one joint?

    a. Gastrocnemius
    b. Piriformis
    c. Iliacus
    d. Obturator internus
    e. Vastus intermedius

24. The addition of a noncompetitive inhibitor to an enzyme catalyzed reaction leads to which of the following?

    a. Both an increase in the V_{max} and an increase in the Km
    b. A decrease in the observed V_{max}
    c. A decrease in Km and in V_{max}
    d. An increase in Km but no change in V_{max}
    e. Irreversible inhibition

25. How does the resistance of two muscular arteries A and B of equal length compare, if the diameter of A = 6 mm, and the diameter of B = 2 mm?

    a. The resistance of A is 3 times greater than B.
    b. For equal lengths, the resistances must be equal.
    c. The resistance of A is ⅓ that of B.
    d. The resistance of B is ⅑ that of A.
    e. The resistance of A is ¹⁄₈₁ that of B.

26. Which of the following statements is *true* of a spindle primary sensory axon (1A)?

    a. It conveys data about muscle tension.
    b. It conveys data about length and velocity of stretch.
    c. It reports cerebellar commands to muscles.
    d. It synapses with Renshaw cells in the cord.
    e. It terminates upon dorsal column neurons.

27. Which of the following statements concerning fibrocystic change of the female breast is *not* true?

    a. Fibrocystic change (disease) is unusual except in kindreds who have a history of breast malignancy.
    b. Nonproliferative fibrocystic change has no increased risk for the development of carcinoma.
    c. Proliferative fibrocystic change has an increased risk of about 1.5 × for the development of carcinoma.
    d. Atypical proliferation increases the risk for cancer by a factor of about 5.
    e. Proliferative lesions are bilateral and multifocal. Risk of subsequent development of cancer is equal in both breasts.

28. A 26-year-old, slightly overweight, woman and her husband seek your help because she is unable to conceive. Further history suggests her menstrual cycle is irregular and her periods have been scanty to absent. On physical examination she is slightly hirsute and her ovaries are palpable and seem somewhat enlarged. Ultrasound shows her ovaries to be enlarged and to contain numerous cysts of varying size. What is the proposed pathophysiology for her inability to conceive and her abnormal body habitus?

    a. There is a deficit in the link between her hypothalamus and her adenohypophysis.
    b. There is end organ failure of her endometrium to respond to hormonal stimuli.
    c. There is chronic anovulation with LH induced ovarian overproduction of androgens.
    d. This is a case of testicular feminization and no ovaries are present.
    e. This is a case of Turner's syndrome.

29. Muscles used in performing a high jump are dependent primarily on ______ for the immediate source of ATP, while muscles used in a marathon depend primarily on ______. (Fill in the blanks.)

    a. Oxidation of fatty acids; preformed creatine phosphate
    b. Oxidation of fatty acids; anaerobic glycolysis
    c. Glycogenesis; oxidation of amino acids

    d. Preformed ATP and phosphocreatine; aerobic metabolism

    e. Performed ATP; preformed creatine phosphate

30. Which of the following is a characteristic of dietary fructose?

    a. It is metabolized by a separate pathway from the glycolytic pathway.

    b. It enters into glycolysis after conversion to fructose 6-phosphate.

    c. It is converted into UDP-fructose and then epimerized into UDP-glucose.

    d. It is metabolized in the liver by aldolase B, an enzyme that recognizes fructose 1-phosphate.

    e. It must be phosphorylated by phosphofructokinase prior to entering glycolysis.

31. Nonselective cholinergic agonists may increase blood pressure when atropine is simultaneously administered because they stimulate which of the following?

    a. Alpha receptors of blood vessels, directly

    b. The release of nitric oxide

    c. The myocardium, directly

    d. The release of catecholamines from the adrenal medulla

    e. Beta receptors of the blood vessels

32. Human slow virus diseases such as Kuru and Creutzfeldt-Jakob disease are *not* characterized by which of the following?

    a. Presence of protein

    b. Disinfected by formaldehyde

    c. Spongiform encephalopathy

    d. Individuals at risk include surgeons and transplant and brain surgery patients

    e. Filterable, infectious agents

33. The characteristic background brainwave frequency of a normal awake person is which of the following?

    a. Alpha

    b. Beta

    c. Delta

    d. Gamma

    e. Theta

34. Which of the following statements describes the side chain of the amino acid serine?

    a. It contains a hydroxyl group.

    b. It can form disulfide bonds.

    c. It can participate in hydrophobic interactions.

    d. It has a nitrogen-containing ring structure.

    e. It is charged at physiologic pH.

35. Which of the following types of tissue is *not* characterized by a preponderance of type I collagen fibers?

    a. Medulla of lymph node

    b. Aponeurosis

    c. Lamina propria of duodenum

    d. Submucosa of esophagus

    e. Tunica adventitia of muscular artery

36. Which of the following is derived from pro-opiomelanocortin?

    a. C-peptide

    b. Adrenocorticotropic hormone

    c. Glucagon

    d. Parathyroid hormone

    e. Somatostatin

37. The anatomical substrate for the biological clock is which of the following?

    a. Arcuate nucleus

    b. Habenular nucleus

    c. Lateral mammillary nucleus

    d. Nucleus proprius

    e. Suprachiasmatic nucleus

38. The events associated with the activation of T cells following receptor-ligand binding include all *except* which of the following?

    a. Phosphatidylinositol-phospholipase C-gamma 1 catalyzed hydrolysis of phosphatidylinositol 4,5-bisphosphate

    b. Increased levels of cytoplasmic inositol 1,4,5-triphosphate and diacylglycerol

    c. Rapid efflux of cytosolic calcium

    d. Activation of protein kinase C

    e. Activation by calmodulin or kinases other than protein kinase C and phosphatases

39. The cell wall of gram-positive bacteria may contain which of the following components that is absent in gram-negative bacterial cell walls?

    a. Peptidoglycan

    b. Lipoteichoic acid

    c. Lipopolysaccharide

    d. Lipid A

    e. O antigen

40. Which of the following cell types is *not* found in the epithelium of the small intestine?

    a. Enterocytes

    b. Goblet cells

    c. Paneth cells

    d. Ciliated epithelial cells

    e. Stem cells

41. What is the temperature that is achieved in an autoclave set at 15 pounds per square inch, and which is effective in killing both vegetative bacterial cells as well as spores?

    a. 95° C

    b. 102° C

    c. 121° C

    d. 212° F

    e. 225° F

42. Lamina VII of Rexed in the spinal cord contains all *except* which of the following?

    a. Intermediolateral cell column

    b. Nucleus dorsalis of Clark

    c. Sacral parasympathetic nucleus

d. Spinal border cells
e. Substantia gelatinosa

43. A peripheral lesion of the trigeminal nerve might cause which of the following?

    a. Cough
    b. Dysphonia
    c. Dysphagia
    d. Loss of taste on the same side
    e. Loss of corneal reflex on the same side

44. The sensory retina is a complex association of cells and basic tissues. Which of the following cell types is *not* part of the sensory retina?

    a. Multipolar neuron
    b. Epithelial cell
    c. Bipolar neuron
    d. Smooth muscle cell
    e. Melanocyte

45. You have a patient who has painless jaundice and after an exhaustive diagnostic evaluation has been diagnosed as having carcinoma of the pancreas. The patient has asked you what the prognosis is in this disease. What would you tell the patient concerning the 5-year survival rate in this disease?

    a. The 5-year survival rate is 50%.
    b. The 5-year survival rate is 25%.
    c. The 5-year survival rate is 10%.
    d. The 5-year survival rate is 5%.
    e. The 5-year survival rate is <5%.

46. A right-handed elderly patient was brought to the emergency room unable to speak and paralyzed on the right side, except for the foot. The patient was alert, cooperative, and able to understand verbal commands. Six weeks later he had spasticity and hyperreflexia in his right arm. His speech was telegraphic, containing mostly nouns and verbs and no articles. His lesion is consistent with a stroke in which of the following arteries?

    a. Anterior spinal artery
    b. Left anterior cerebral artery
    c. Left middle cerebral artery
    d. Right anterior cerebral artery
    e. Right middle cerebral artery

47. How does oligomycin interfere with synthesis of high-energy compounds?

    a. It blocks the transfer of electrons from cytochrome b to cytochrome c.
    b. It uncouples electron transport from oxidative phosphorylation.
    c. It closes the proton channel through the stalk of ATP synthetase.
    d. It inhibits the adenine nucleotide carrier in the inner mitochondrial membrane.
    e. It inhibits the oxidation of NADH.

48. Which one of the following statements about protein structure is *correct?*

    a. The alpha-helix is stabilized primarily by ionic interactions between the side chains of amino acids.
    b. In order to form a disulfide bond, the two participating amino acids must be next to each other in the primary structure of the protein.
    c. Quaternary structure is stabilized by covalent bonding between the subunits.
    d. Irreversible loss of secondary and tertiary structure always results from the process of denaturation.
    e. The information for the correct folding of a protein is contained in the specific sequence of amino acids along the polypeptide chain.

49. Which of the following is the only depolarizing neuromuscular blocker commonly used clinically today?

    a. Tubocurarine
    b. Tetrodotoxin
    c. Succinylcholine
    d. Methacholine
    e. Bethanecol

50. In the laboratory diagnosis of infection by *Enterobius vermicularis,* the method of choice would include which of the following?

    a. Microscopic examination of a stool sample for parasites
    b. Microscopic examination of a blood smear for parasites
    c. Microscopic examination of centrifuged spinal fluid for parasites
    d. An anal impression smear to look for parasite eggs
    e. Microscopic examination of a skin snip to look for parasites in macrophages

51. Which of the following is *not* found in a representative section of cancellous (spongy) bone?

    a. Osteoblasts
    b. Osteoclasts
    c. Osteocytes
    d. Osteone (Haversian system)
    e. Lacuna

52. Blood from the internal iliac artery or its branches is distributed to all *except* which of the following?

    a. Pelvic viscera
    b. Gluteal region
    c. Labia majora
    d. Iliacus and psoas major muscles
    e. Testes

53. A patient has normal comprehension and fluent spontaneous speech but is unable to repeat spoken phrases. He also has some paraphasias in his spontaneous speech. His lesion is in which of the following?

    a. Arcuate fasciculus
    b. Cingulum
    c. Corpus callosum
    d. Inferior occipitofrontal fasciculus
    e. Uncinate fasciculus

54. Absence (petit mal) seizures are generally characterized by all *except* which of the following?

    a. Duration of 30 seconds or less
    b. Immediate mental clearing after seizure
    c. Normal interictal EEG

    d. Olfactory or visual aura
    e. Onset in childhood (4 to 12 years)

55. Which of the following begins as individual chromosomes become visible? As the chromosomes enlarge, they are seen to consist of two structures known as which of the following?

    a. The cell cycle, centromeres
    b. The synthesis phase, kinetochores
    c. Prophase, chromatids
    d. Interphase, diplotenes
    e. Metaphase, leptotenes

56. What do the characteristics of the Na^+, K^+ ATPase of mammalian cell membranes include?

    a. Extrusion of one Na^+ from the cell in exchange for one K^+
    b. Electrogenic exchange of three Na^+ for two K^+
    c. A requirement for binding of K^+ at an intracellular site
    d. Active transport of Na^+ from the extracellular space into the cell
    e. A requirement for binding of Na^+ at an extracellular site

57. Which of the following causes an increase in the level of phosphorylation of the pyruvate dehydrogenase complex (PDC)?

    a. Coenzyme A
    b. Thiamine pyrophosphate
    c. NADH
    d. Insulin
    e. Lipoic acid

58. A "motor unit" is defined as which of the following?

    a. A set of extrafusal muscle fibers innervated by the same alpha motor neuron
    b. A corticospinal cell and all the alpha motor neurons it innervates
    c. A corticocerebellar neuron and its reticulospinal branches
    d. A large muscle fiber and all the alpha motor neurons contacting it
    e. One gamma motor neuron and all the intrafusal fibers it innervates

59. What is the cause of leukocytoclastic vasculitis thought to be?

    a. IgE dependent immunologic reaction
    b. Complement activation
    c. T lymphocyte cytotoxicity
    d. Autoimmunity
    e. Circulating immune complexes

60. All *except* which of the following statements regarding the ischioanal fossa is correct?

    a. It typically contains an abundance of adipose tissue.
    b. It contains the pudendal canal.
    c. It contains the inferior rectal nerves.
    d. It contains the inferior rectal arteries.
    e. It is in direct communication with the superficial perineal space.

61. Which of the following is *true* of *Vibrio cholerae?*

    a. It commonly causes bacteremia and sepsis.
    b. It is commonly found only in the Nile River Valley.
    c. It has recently become much more prevalent as a diarrheal pathogen world-wide.
    d. It can always be treated effectively with antibiotics.
    e. It is a commensal organism found in the bowel of normal individuals.

62. Which of the following types of proteins does a prokaryotic regulatory gene synthesize?

    a. The promoter
    b. The operator
    c. The repressor
    d. The enhancer
    e. The inducer

63. In both animal models and in human transplantation, acute graft-versus-host disease may be best minimized by which of the following?

    a. Depletion of host bone marrow B lymphocytes
    b. Depletion of host bone marrow T lymphocytes
    c. Depletion of donor bone marrow B lymphocytes
    d. Depletion of donor bone marrow T lymphocytes

64. Which of the following factors increases blood flow from peripheral veins toward the heart?

    a. Dilation of the peripheral veins
    b. Increased activity of the skeletal muscle pump
    c. Decreased respiratory rate
    d. Decreased blood volume
    e. Decreased sympathetic stimulation of the veins

65. Microglia do *not* contribute to which of the following functions?

    a. Phagocytosis of cellular debris at sites of CNS injury
    b. Regeneration of cut peripheral axons
    c. Release of cytokines in response to CNS injury
    d. Scar tissue formation in the CNS
    e. Stimulation of astroglial proliferation

66. All *except* which of the following factors increases the rate of passive, nonfacilitated diffusion of a solute across a cell membrane?

    a. An increase in solute concentration gradient
    b. An increase in lipid solubility of the solute
    c. A decrease in membrane thickness
    d. An increase in surface area of the membrane
    e. An increase in water solubility of the solute

67. Which of the following is *not* considered as having a retroperitoneal location?

    a. Ureter
    b. Suprarenal gland
    c. Celiac ganglion
    d. Spleen
    e. Descending colon

68. What is the laboratory test that most easily differentiates staphylococci from streptococci and enterococci?

    a. Resistance to novobiocin
    b. Sensitivity to bacitracin
    c. Ability to coagulate plasma
    d. Catalase activity
    e. Hemolytic pattern

69. The structure forming the anterior boundary of the carotid triangle is which of the following?

    a. Anterior border of the sternomastoid muscle
    b. Anterior border of the trapezius muscle
    c. Inferior border of the mandible
    d. Posterior belly of the digastric muscle
    e. Superior belly of the omohyoid muscle

70. All *except* which of the following statements regarding the ophthalmic artery is correct?

    a. It arises from the internal carotid artery.
    b. It gives rise to the central artery of the retina.
    c. It lies superiorly to the optic nerve during part of its course in the orbit.
    d. It enters the orbit through the superior orbital fissure.
    e. It supplies the lacrimal gland.

71. What is the mechanism of glucose transport from lumen to cytoplasm in intestinal and renal tubular epithelial cells?

    a. Secondary active cotransport with Na^+
    b. Primary transport via a glucose, ATPase
    c. Facilitated diffusion
    d. Antiport with Na^+
    e. Cotransport with K^+

72. Which of the following statements about allelic exclusion is *true?*

    a. It allows deletion of allelic genes on homologous chromosomes.
    b. It is characteristic of both B and T lymphocyte receptors for antigens.
    c. It occurs in B lymphocytes but not T lymphocytes.
    d. It allows dual specificity since both parental alleles can be expressed.
    e. It allows for production of both kappa and lambda light chains to be produced by a single B lymphocyte.

73. A 24-year-old patient has had a 6 year history of diarrhea and rectal bleeding, which has waxed and waned in severity. For the last month, it has become severe. The patient appears pale and has a low fever. On physical examination the abdomen is focally tender to deep palpation. Flexible sigmoidoscopy shows the mucosa of the large bowel to be widely ulcerated, edematous, and rather inflammed. The process seems to be more severe in the rectum and sigmoid colon, but it does extend to the hepatic flexure. Representative biopsies show the process to be limited to the mucosa. In a few areas of regeneration, the colonic muscoa appears mildly atypical. Laboratory studies show a mild degree of leukocytosis and a moderate microcytic anemia. Which of the following is *not* a complication of this disease?

    a. Uveitis
    b. Ankylosing spondylitis
    c. Sclerosing cholangitis
    d. Toxic megacolon
    e. Spread to jejunem

74. Which mild central nervous system stimulant has slightly less effect on food intake and on blood pressure than d-amphetamine?

    a. Phenytoin
    b. Diazepam
    c. Methylphenidate
    d. Amitriptyline
    e. Dextropropoxyphene

75. The nucleus that gives rise to preganglionic parasympathetic neurons that terminate in the ciliary ganglion, is which of the following?

    a. Inferior salivatory nucleus
    b. Edinger-Westphal nucleus
    c. Nucleus solitarius
    d. Nucleus ambiguus
    e. Superior salivatory nucleus

76. Which of the following is true of methotrexate used in the management of asthma?

    a. It can be given by aerosol.
    b. It is an effective bronchodilator.
    c. It is not effective when given in one dosage each week.
    d. It potentiates the action of beta agonists and theophylline.
    e. It is used for its anti-inflammatory properties.

77. Which of the following is a common immunological finding in Hodgkin's disease?

    a. Acquired agammaglobulinemia
    b. Hypocomplementemia
    c. Increased serum IgM
    d. Absent serum IgA
    e. Anergy to skin test antigens

78. Which of the following is a constant secondary finding in patients afflicted with osteopetrosis?

    a. Increased incidence of cartilaginous tumors
    b. Increased incidence of osteosarcoma
    c. Synthesis of abnormal type I collagen
    d. Severe anemia
    e. Foci of heterotopic bone formation

79. The tectum is part of which of the following?

    a. Diencephalon
    b. Mesencephalon
    c. Myelencephalon
    d. Prosencephalon
    e. Thalamus

80. The nucleus solitarius is involved in all *except* which of the following activities?

    a. Gastrointestinal motility
    b. Maintenance of blood pressure
    c. Respiration
    d. Somatic afferent sensation
    e. Taste

81. Which drug is used for immunosuppressive therapy but not cancer chemotherapy?

 a. Vincristine
 b. Cyclophosphamide
 c. Methotrexate
 d. Cyclosporine
 e. Dacarbazine

82. A patient was diagnosed with gout (chronic tophaceous gout). Serum uric acid levels were high, but urinary excretion of uric acid was not excessive. Treatment with sulfinpyrazone was slowly beginning to exert beneficial effects, but gastrointestinal disturbances were adversely affecting compliance. Treatment with sulfinpyrazone was discontinued for 2 weeks with an exacerbation of symptoms. Treatment with allopurinol was initiated, but the patient soon complained of joint pain and inflammation.

The patient's arthritic symptoms should be treated with which of the following?

 a. Methotrexate
 b. Colchicine
 c. Probenecid
 d. Aspirin
 e. Discontinuation of allopurinol

83. Digoxin differs significantly from digitoxin in which of the following ways?

 a. Therapeutic index
 b. Site of action on the heart
 c. Incidence of nausea and vomiting
 d. Duration of action
 e. Usual route of administration

84. Which of the following statements concerning the introduction of recombinant DNA into bacteria is *false?*

 a. When a bacteriophage is used to introduce DNA into a bacteria, the technique is called transformation.
 b. Plasmid DNA can be taken up by bacteria without being degraded.
 c. Plasmid DNA carries a gene for resistance to specific antibiotics.
 d. Recombinant DNA in bacteriophage vectors substitutes for a portion of the original chromosome.
 e. Insertion of recombinant DNA into plasmids linearizes the DNA.

85. Which of the following is *true* for bilirubin metabolism?

 a. Bilirubin is converted directly to biliverdin.
 b. UDP-glucuronyl transferase activity is needed to increase the water solubility of bilirubin.
 c. Absence of UDP-glucuronyl transferase increases the concentration of direct reacting bilirubin.
 d. The conversion of bilirubin to urobilinogen is catalyzed by enzymes in the mucosa of the small intestine.
 e. Bile acids are derived from the conjugation of bilirubin.

Questions 86 through 88

86. A young epileptic is brought to the ER after an attempt at suicide with drugs at home. On arrival, he is semi-conscious, BP is 110/65. Heart rate 80, rectal temp is 99.5° F (37.5° C). In the ER, he has a brief generalized seizure with rapid recovery. He has intermittent muscle twitches with gross movements of his arms and legs.

From these signs which of the following drugs is *most likely* the one taken in the suicidal attempt?

 a. Morphine
 b. Phenytoin
 c. Diphenhydramine
 d. Chlorpromazine
 e. Not enough information

87. With the additional information that the pupils are dilated and respiratory rate is 25/min, which drug would you now rule out as a toxicant?

 a. Morphine
 b. Phenytoin
 c. Diphenhydramine
 d. Chlorpromazine
 e. Guanethidine

88. At this point you have gavaged the patient and seizures have become continuous. What would you do now?

 a. Wait for laboratory tests for blood levels of drugs
 b. Give nalorphine
 c. Give diazepam intravenously
 d. Give phenytoin intramuscularly
 e. Give physostigmine intramuscularly

89. Which of the following is *not* a component of the enamel organ?

 a. External (outer) enamel epithelium
 b. Dental papilla
 c. Stellate reticulum
 d. Internal (inner) enamel epithelium
 e. Stratum intermedium

90. Figure 2 shows the degree of action versus time for the following three insulin preparations in a fasting patient with

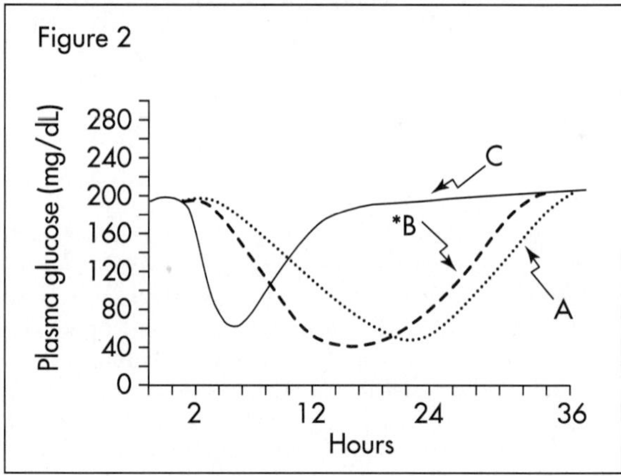

diabetes: isophane insulin (NPH), protamine zinc insulin (PZI), and regular insulin (CZI, insulin injection). Select the hypoglycemic time curve that best describes the actions of isophane (NPH) insulin.

91. Which of the following is most likely to produce convulsions in sensitive patients when administered intravenously in moderately high therapeutic doses?

    a. Quinidine
    b. Hydralazine
    c. Phenytoin
    d. Lidocaine
    e. Bretylium

92. A mixed tumor of salivary gland takes its histologic appearance by what mechanism?

    a. Divergent differentiation of a single cell line of parenchymal cells
    b. A mixture of tumor cells of both mesenchymal and parenchymal origin
    c. Collision of two separately developing, benign tumors
    d. Malignant transformation of the connective tissue elements
    e. Malignant transformation of the parenchymal element

93. Structural proteins in skeletal muscle cells do *not* include which of the following?

    a. Titin
    b. C protein
    c. Spectrin
    d. Myomesin
    e. Alpha-actinin

94. An elderly man had a large stroke involving the right middle cerebral artery. On examination he also has which of the following?

    a. Left gaze palsy and a left hemiparesis
    b. Left gaze palsy and a right hemiparesis
    c. Right gaze palsy and a right hemiparesis
    d. Right gaze palsy and a left hemiparesis
    e. Achromatopsia

95. Which of the following statements about pulmonary vascular resistance is *false?*

    a. Resistance increases as lung volume approaches total lung capacity.
    b. Pulmonary vascular resistance is determined primarily by autonomic nervous activity.
    c. Resistance decreases as cardiac output increases.
    d. Normally, pulmonary vascular resistance is about $\frac{1}{10}$ of systemic resistance
    e. Decreasing alveolar PO_2 below normal increases pulmonary vascular resistance.

96. The thalamic nucleus through which taste information is relayed to the cortex is which of the following?

    a. Anterior nucleus
    b. VA
    c. VPM

    d. VPL
    e. VL

97. Secretomotor fibers (parasympathetic) to the lacrimal gland are *not* located in which of the following?

    a. Pterygopalatine ganglion
    b. Facial nerve
    c. V2 (maxillary division of trigeminal nerve)
    d. V1 (ophthalmic division of trigeminal nerve)
    e. Greater petrosal nerve

98. Which of the following is the most frequent cause of hepatic cirrhosis in the United States?

    a. Viral hepatitis
    b. Biliary disease
    c. Alcoholism
    d. Alpha$_1$-trypsin deficiency
    e. Hemachromatosis

99. Which of the following is the class of lymphocyte that bears CD16, an F_c receptor for IgG, and is important in antibody-dependent cellular cytotoxicity?

    a. B lymphocyte
    b. T helper lymphocyte
    c. T cytotoxic lymphocyte
    d. Natural killer lymphocytes
    e. No lymphocyte bears CD16.

100. The larynx is composed of a complex of basic tissues that function to produce a series of sounds that we interpret as language. Which phrase does *not* describe the histology of the larynx?

    a. Serous and mucous glands in the true vocal chords
    b. Epiglottis is supported mainly by elastic cartilage
    c. Respiratory epithelium lines the lumen adjacent to the false vocal chords
    d. Vocalis ligament composed mainly of elastic fibers
    e. Skeletal muscle is the true vocal chords

101. Which of the following statements correctly describes the cross-bridge cycle in skeletal muscle?

    a. Ca^{2+} binds to myosin $\rightarrow$ myosin activated $\rightarrow$ actin-myosin interaction $\rightarrow$ actin filaments move past myosin $\rightarrow$ Ca^{2+} binds to myosin $\rightarrow$ myosin charged and released from actin
    b. Myosin charged by ATP binding $\rightarrow$ Ca^{2+} activation $\rightarrow$ ADP and PI released from myosin $\rightarrow$ actin-myosin interaction $\rightarrow$ actin filaments move past myosin $\rightarrow$ ATP binds to myosin $\rightarrow$ myosin charged and released from actin
    c. Actin charged by tropomyosin binding $\rightarrow$ Ca^{2+} activation $\rightarrow$ ADP and PI released from actin $\rightarrow$ actin-myosin interaction $\rightarrow$ actin filaments move past myosin $\rightarrow$ ATP binds to myosin $\rightarrow$ actin charged by tropomyosin binding

    d. Myosin charged by ATP hydrolysis → Ca^{2+} inactivation → ADP and PI released from myosin → actin-myosin interaction → actin filaments move past myosin → ATP hydrolyzed → myosin charged and released from actin

    e. Action potential → tropomyosin binds ATP → Ca^{2+} inactivation → ADP and PI released from myosin → actin-myosin interaction → actin filaments move past myosin → ATP binds to tropomyosin

102. Three of the four basic tissues are represented in the cornea. Which cell type listed below is *not* a constituent of one of the these three basic tissues?

    a. Endothelium cell
    b. Fibrocyte (fibroblast)
    c. Epithelial cell
    d. Smooth muscle cell
    e. Nerve cell

103. Preganglionic neurons of both the sympathetic and parasympathetic systems secrete which of the following?

    a. Acetylcholine
    b. Epinephrine
    c. Norepinephrine
    d. Serotonin
    e. Substance P

104. Sexual differentiation of the brain in humans occurs approximately at which of the following stages?

    a. 5 months in utero
    b. Birth
    c. 1 to 2 years of age
    d. 5 to 8 years of age
    e. Puberty

105. What is the opening between the pterygopalatine fossa and the infratemporal fossa termed?

    a. Sphenopalatine foramen
    b. Superior orbital fissure
    c. Ptyergoid canal
    d. Pterygomaxillary fissure
    e. Inferior orbital fissure

106. Which of the following parasitic diseases usually is *not* transmitted by the bite of an arthropod or other insect vector?

    a. *Cutaneous leishmaniasis*
    b. *Falciparum malaria*
    c. *African trypanosomiasis*
    d. *American trypanosomiasis*
    e. *Giardiasis*

107. When absence seizures occur alone, which agent is the antiepileptic drug of choice?

    a. Valproic acid
    b. Ethosuximide
    c. Trimethadione
    d. Thiopental (intravenously)
    e. Carbamazepine

108. Which of the following is an antimetabolite that inhibits dihydrofolate reductase and is used to treat certain leukemias and choriocarcinoma and whose bone marrow depression and gastrointestinal effects can be reduced by co-administering "leucovorin rescue"?

    a. Trimethoprim
    b. Pyrimethamine
    c. Methotrexate
    d. Cytarabine
    e. 5-fluorouracil

109. Which of the following is true of renal compensation for respiratory acidosis?

    a. It is a result of decreased plasma P_{CO_2}.
    b. It includes hyperventilation.
    c. It depends on renal generation of HCO_3^-.
    d. It is nearly complete within minutes of the start of the acidosis.
    e. It results from a decrease in urinary NH_4^+ excretion.

110. Which of these cells possess nuclei that are *not* characterized by abundant heterochromatin?

    a. Fibrocytes in adult tendon
    b. Unilocular adipocytes in the panniculus adiposis
    c. Orthochromatophilic erythroblasts in red bone marrow
    d. Perineuronal oligodendrocytes in gray matter of the spinal cord
    e. Hepatocytes in liver cords

111. One would *not* expect to see which of the following morphologic characteristics in cells that are actively secreting protein for export?

    a. Numerous mitochondria
    b. Abundant rER
    c. A nucleus with abundant euchromatin
    d. A well-developed Golgi complex (apparatus)
    e. A large nucleolus

112. What is the major predisposing cause in the development of acute cholecystitis?

    a. Trauma
    b. Sepsis
    c. Postpartum state
    d. Gallstones
    e. Hepatic steatosis

113. Which of the following tumor-suppresser genes requires deletion of only one allele in order for a tumor to form?

    a. WT-1
    b. Rb
    c. P53
    d. DCC
    e. NF-1

114. What is the coronary sulcus?

    a. A groove between the atria above and ventricles below
    b. A groove between the two atria
    c. A groove between the two ventricles
    d. Located only on the posterior aspect of the heart
    e. Located only on the anterior aspect of the heart

115. Given these data concerning capillary hydrostatic and oncotic pressures:

    Capillary hydrostatic pressure (Pcap) = 23 mm Hg
    Interstitial hydrostatic pressure (Pin) = 2 mm Hg
    Capillary protein oncotic pressure (πcap) = 19 mm Hg
    Interstitial protein oncotic pressure (πin) = 5 mm Hg

    What is a net pressure equal to?

    a. 14 mm Hg favoring filtration
    b. 7 mm Hg favoring filtration
    c. 21 mm Hg favoring reabsorption
    d. 7 mm Hg favoring reabsorption
    e. 0 mm Hg

116. Which of the following statements concerning myesthenia gravis is *not* true?

    a. Patients with myesthenia gravis have a positive tensilon test.
    b. Patients with myesthenia gravis frequently have thymic hyperplasia.
    c. Patients with myesthenia gravis are usually female.
    d. Patients with myesthenia gravis have early involvement of the extraocular muscles.
    e. Patients with myesthenia gravis show demyelination of the corticospinal tract.

117. Thrombosis of the anterior spinal artery at T4 would probably *not* affect which of the following tracts?

    a. Anterior corticospinal tract
    b. Fasciculus gracilis
    c. Lateral corticospinal tract
    d. Posterior spinocerebellar tract
    e. Spinothalamic tract

118. Which of the following is *not* correct with respect to Brunn's epithelial nests (nests of von Brunn)?

    a. Brunn's epithelial nests are premalignant proliferations of urothelial cells.
    b. Brunn's epithelial nests are formed from invaginations of surface urothelium.
    c. Brunn's epithelial nests are examples of epithelial hyperplasia.
    d. Brunn's epithelial nests may be found in any urothelial covered structure.
    e. Cystitis cystica is a Brunn's epithelial nest with a central slit or space.

119. Viruses are transmitted to humans by all *except* which of the following mechanisms?

    a. Fomites
    b. Direct contact with infectious secretions
    c. Zoonotic
    d. Aerosol
    e. Transfection

120. Based on your knowledge of the urinary system, you would expect that the presence of large amounts of protein in the urine (proteinuria) would indicate abnormalities in which of the following?

    a. Distal convoluted tubule
    b. Urethra
    c. Urinary bladder
    d. Renal corpuscle
    e. Collecting duct

121. Which of the following statements is *false*?

    a. Protamine is an antidoate to heparin overdose.
    b. Vitamin K is an antidote to warfarin overdose.
    c. Plasmin selectively attacks thromboemboli.
    d. Heparin is not administered orally or intramuscularly.
    e. Warfarin is a racemic mixture of two enantiomers that have different anticoagulant potencies.

122. What is the role of tropomyosin in muscle contraction?

    a. To form cross-bridges with actin-myosin complex
    b. To pump Ca^{2+} into the sarcoplasmic reticulum
    c. To hydrolyze ATP during the "power stroke"
    d. To cover myosin binding sites on actin molecules when the muscle is at rest
    e. To prevent ATP from binding to actin during cross-bridge formation

123. *Staphylococcus epidermidis* is an important cause of which of the following?

    a. Necrotizing fasciitis
    b. Folliculitis
    c. Postinfectious glomerulonephritis
    d. Urinary tract infections in young, sexually active women
    e. Bacteremia associated with indwelling vascular catheters

124. Which of the following is true of ampicillin?

    a. It is absorbed slowly from intramuscular site.
    b. In its acid stable form, it is lactamase-resistant.
    c. In its penicillinase-resistant form, it is orally effective.
    d. As a broad-spectrum penicillin, it is lactamase-sensitive.
    e. It is penicillinase-resistant and acid labile.

125. Lysosomal storage diseases may be defined as autosomal recessive traits that are characterized by the accumulation of normal substrates in the lysosomes due to the absence of specific acid hydrolases. Which of the following is *not* a lysosomal storage disease?

    a. Alcaptonuria
    b. Tay-Sachs disease
    c. Gaucher's disease
    d. Niemann-Pick lipidoses
    e. Mucopolysaccharidoses

126. As the ventilation/perfusion ratio ($\dot{V}_A/\dot{Q}$) increases, alveolar gas composition (P_{O_2} and P_{CO_2}) changes to more closely resemble the gas composition of which of the following?

    a. Mixed venous blood
    b. Systemic capillary blood
    c. Systemic arterial blood
    d. Inspired air
    e. Pulmonary arterial blood

127. Which of the following inhibits HMG-CoA reductase to lower plasma LDL?

    a. Clofibrate
    b. Cholestyramine
    c. Lovastatin

    d. Nicotinic acid
    e. Enalapril

128. Which of the following statements is *true* of blood flow at the onset of exercise?

    a. Intestinal blood flow increases due to increased sympathetic nerve activity.
    b. Skeletal muscle blood flow increases primarily due to parasympathetic vasodilation.
    c. There is little or no change in brain blood flow.
    d. Contraction of skeletal muscle in the legs impedes venous return to the heart.
    e. Venous return is increased during expiration.

129. Which of the following correctly compares the DNA from "Pollyanna" virus (22 mole percent cytosine) with DNA from medical students (32 mole percent thymine)?

    a. The T_m of medical student DNA will be lower than that of "Pollyanna" virus.
    b. Medical student DNA has more thymine than adenine.
    c. The T_m of medical student DNA will be identical to that of "Pollyanna" virus.
    d. "Pollyanna" virus has more cytosine than guanine.
    e. Medical student DNA has a greater molecular weight than "Pollyanna" virus.

130. A decrease in the ventilation/perfusion ratio ($\dot{V}_A/\dot{Q}$) causes alveolar P_{O_2} to _______ and alveolar P_{CO_2} to _______:

    a. increase, increase.
    b. decrease, increase.
    c. decrease, decrease.
    d. increase, decrease.
    e. increase, not change.

131. Patients with xeroderma pigmentosum are liable to develop malignant and premalignant lesions of the skin such as basal cell carcinoma, squamous cell carcinoma, and malignant melanoma. What mechanism accounts for their unusual susceptibility to these skin tumors?

    a. Acquired loss of P53 tumor-suppressor genes
    b. Activation of the *ras* oncogene
    c. Abnormal melanin synthesis
    d. Unusual sensitivity to infrared light
    e. Defective DNA repair of ultraviolet light damage

132. All *except* which of the following statements regarding the erector spinae muscle is correct?

    a. It is surrounded by thoracolumbar fascia.
    b. The iliocostalis represents its most lateral component.
    c. It is the deepest of the intrinsic back muscles.
    d. It is innervated by ventral rami of spinal nerves.
    e. The spinalis represents its most medial component.

133. How does an action potential in skeletal muscle initiate contraction?

    a. By causing the opening of Ca^{2+} channels in the sarcoplasmic reticulum
    b. By stimulating the Ca^{2+} pump in the sarcoplasmic reticulum
    c. By activating acetylcholinesterase in the presynaptic membrane

    d. By opening Na^+ channels in the transverse tubules
    e. By opening of K^+-specific channels in the sarcolemma

134. As a general principle, the increase in bulk of a tumor is caused primarily by what mechanism?

    a. Tumor necrosis with reactive cellular swelling
    b. Abnormal tumor angiogenesis and interstitial hemorrhage
    c. Imbalance in tumor cell proliferation and tumor cell death
    d. Markedly higher mitotic rate when compared with normal tissues
    e. Excessive connective tissue proliferation in tumors

135. By what rate does the risk increase for people who smoke one pack of cigarettes per day to develop lung cancer, as compared with those who do not smoke?

    a. $1\times$
    b. $2\times$
    c. $5\times$
    d. $10\times$
    e. $>10\times$

136. The chemical substance released by free nerve endings, which causes degranulation of mast cells and blood vessel dilation, is which of the following?

    a. Bradykinin
    b. Histamine
    c. Prostaglandins
    d. Serotonin
    e. Substance P

137. Arteriolar vasoconstriction will result in which of the following?

    a. An increase in capillary hydrostatic pressure
    b. A decrease in capillary hydrostatic pressure
    c. An increase in fluid filtration out of the capillary
    d. An increase in blood flow to the tissue supplied by the arteriole
    e. An increase in lymph flow from the tissue

138. A muscle of the foot attached to the tendon of the flexor digitorum longus is known as which of the following?

    a. Abductor digiti minimi
    b. Adductor hallucis
    c. Flexor hallucis brevis
    d. Flexor digiti minimi brevis
    e. Quadratus plantae

139. Which of the following tracts *do not* terminate in the VL nucleus of the thalamus?

    a. Ansa lenticularis
    b. Dentatothalamic tract
    c. Lenticular fasciculus
    d. Nigrothalamic tract
    e. Subthalamic fasciculus

140. In order for two reactions to be coupled, which of the following is absolutely necessary?

    a. The reactions should have a common transition state.
    b. The reactions have a combined standard free energy that is negative.

c. The rate of the second reaction should be significantly faster than the first reaction.

d. A metabolic intermediate should be common to both reactions.

e. The activation energies of both reactions do not exceed the total free energy change.

141. The fornix originates from neurons in which of the following?

    a. Amygdala
    b. Anterior nucleus of the thalamus
    c. Cingulate gyrus
    d. Hippocampus
    e. Subthalamic nucleus

142. In some persons, sudden and complete internal carotid occlusion results in large strokes, while in others, occlusions are asymptomatic. This is best explained by variations in which of the following?

    a. Autoregulation
    b. Blood pressure
    c. Blood volume
    d. Race
    e. The circle of Willis

143. The increase in heart rate that often occurs while donating blood is most likely a result of which of the following?

    a. The baroreceptor reflex
    b. A decrease in cardiac contractility
    c. The hemorrhage inhibiting secretion of vasopressin
    d. The Frank-Starling law of the heart
    e. Increased parasympathetic stimulation of the sino-atrial nodal cells

144. What is the complementary sequence for a DNA strand having a sequence of pG-C-T-A-G-C-C-C?

    a. pC-G-A-T-C-G-G-G
    b. pC-C-C-G-A-T-C-G
    c. pG-G-G-C-T-A-G-C
    d. pG-C-T-A-G-C-C-C
    e. pG-G-G-C-U-A-G-C

145. For six months, a 39-year-old patient has had midgastric abdominal pain about 1 to 2 hours after eating. Drinking milk or taking an over-the-counter antacid provides temporary relief. The patient has not noticed any change in stool or bowel habits. An upper GI x-ray film series shows an erosion of the duodenal mucosa. A capsule biopsy of the stomach shows a mild degree of atrophic gastritis and numerous faintly staining bacilli clinging to the luminal aspect of the columnar epithelium or embedded in gastric mucus. What is the organism that was found?

    a. *Helicobacter pylori*
    b. *Yersinia enterocolitica*
    c. *Eschericia coli*
    d. *Proteus mirabilis*
    e. *Pseudomonas aeruginosa*

146. Which of the following is *not* associated with the development of diffuse alveolar damage (DAD)?

    a. High inspired concentrations of oxygen for a prolonged period of time
    b. A severe crush injury of the lower extremity with development of hypovolemic shock
    c. Treatment of a metastatic neoplasm with Beomycin
    d. Inhalation of paraquat while working in a field
    e. Development of alveolar proteinosis in a patient with non-Hodgkin's lymphoma.

147. In which of the following joints is movement restricted to the vertical axis of rotation?

    a. Radioulnar
    b. Humeroulnar
    c. Humeroradial
    d. Radiocarpal

148. What is the most common cause of diabetes insipidus?

    a. Tumors
    b. Trauma
    c. Hypophysectomy
    d. Granulomatous disease (tuberculosis, etc.)
    e. Idiopathic

149. In which of the following diseases are exotoxins *not* important?

    a. Brucellosis
    b. Scalded skin syndrome
    c. Whooping cough
    d. Scarlet fever
    e. Diphtheria

150. Where are the cell bodies of all somatosensory receptors below the neck located?

    a. Dorsal root ganglia
    b. Dorsal horn of the spinal cord
    c. Nucleus dorsalis of Clark
    d. Lamina VII of Rexed
    e. Terminal ganglia

151. When a foul odor was noticed by a security officer, a homeless person was found dead in an abandoned office. In examining the scene, the medical examiner noticed that brown paper had been taped to the windows and in the center of the room there was a cast iron hibachi in which ashes of charcoal briquettes were found. A few unburned briquettes were found near the hibachi. Despite a moderate degree of decomposition, the skin of the victim was a fairly bright red. Which of these laboratory examinations might be critical in determining this person's demise?

    a. Toxicologic analysis of the stomach contents for barbiturates
    b. Analysis of the blood for alcohol
    c. Analysis of the blood for carboxyhemaglobin
    d. Analysis of the serum for evidence of HIV
    e. Analysis of the blood for cocaine and its metabolites

152. Prokaroytic organisms such as bacteria have all *except* which of the following structures?

   a. Ribosomes
   b. Mesosomes
   c. Cytoplasmic membrane
   d. Nuclear membrane
   e. Single molecule of double-stranded DNA

153. Consider a gene for a protein that contains 200 amino acids and is composed of two exons and one intron. Which of the following mutations would be the *most likely* to prevent synthesis of a protein?

   a. An insertion mutation in the second exon
   b. A five base deletion from the promoter region of the gene
   c. A nonsense mutation in the intron
   d. A nonsense mutation in the second exon
   e. A base substitution mutation in the first intron

154. Epithelial tissue in the kidney *cannot* be classified as which of the following?

   a. Simple squamous
   b. Transitional
   c. Simple cuboidal with numerous microvilli
   d. Stratified cuboidal with numerous stereocilia
   e. Simple columnar

155. Which of the following describes an effector for an allosteric enzyme?

   a. A coenzyme that is required for the activity of the enzyme
   b. A ligand, other than the substrate, that binds to the active site
   c. A ligand, other than the substrate, that binds to the enzyme but not to the active site
   d. A competitive inhibitor
   e. A noncompetitive inhibitor

156. Fibers of the ventral ramus of C1 travel with the hypoglossal nerve for a short distance before innervating which of the following muscles?

   a. Thyrohyoid
   b. Sternohyoid
   c. Sternothyroid
   d. Omohyoid
   e. Cricothyroid

157. Secretion of atrial natriuretic peptide (ANP) occurs in response to which of the following?

   a. Activation of arterial baroreceptors
   b. Increased activity of cardiac parasympathetic nerves
   c. Increases in plasma osmolality
   d. Increases in plasma [angiotensin II]
   e. Stretch of the atria

158. Which of the following is not a complication of levodopa?

   a. Constipation
   b. Dystonia
   c. Nightmares
   d. Chorea
   e. Psychosis

159. Which of the following is *true* during RNA synthesis by DNA-dependent RNA polymerase?

   a. Inorganic phosphate is cleaved from the precursor nucleotides.
   b. Only one of the DNA strands in a chromosome can serve as a template.
   c. Nucleotides are added to the 5′ end of the growing chain.
   d. There appear to be specific sites on DNA for initiating and terminating RNA synthesis.
   e. The polymerase exhibits an active proofreading function.

160. A semisynthetic penicillin that has a broader spectrum of antibacterial activity than penicillin G but which is *not* resistant to penicillinase is which of the following?

   a. Methicillin
   b. Amoxicillin
   c. Nafcillin
   d. Benzathine penicillin
   e. Oxacillin

161. Swallowing can be initiated by water touching all *except* which of the following?

   a. Anterior two thirds of the tongue
   b. Arytenoid cartilages
   c. Epiglottis
   d. Posterior pharyngeal wall
   e. Tonsillar pillars

162. Of the following, which is *not* mediated by apoptosis?

   a. Endometrial cellular breakdown during the menstrual cycle
   b. Destruction of immune cells by the administration of hydrocortisone
   c. Atrophy of the prostate following castration
   d. Organogenesis in a fetus
   e. Myocardial necrosis following thrombosis of a coronary artery

163. Endotoxin (lipopolysaccharide) is *not* capable of eliciting which of the following responses?

   a. Activation of the complement cascade by the traditional pathway
   b. Activation of the complement cascade by the alternate pathway
   c. Activation of the tumor necrosis factor
   d. Fever production
   e. Activation of interleukin-1 and prostaglandins

164. Which of the following statements is *true* of fatty acid synthetase?

   a. It produces oleic acid when a reductase skips an NADPH-requiring step.
   b. It can produce odd-chain fatty acids.
   c. It produces mainly palmitate.
   d. It is found in the mitochondrial matrix.
   e. It is found in the adipose tissue but not in the liver.

165. The periodontal ligament attaches to which of the following?

    a. Cementum to alveolar bone
    b. Enamel to cementum
    c. Enamel to alveolar bone
    d. Dentin to enamel
    e. Dentin to alveolar bone

166. Which of the following is an example of the effect of Starling's law of the heart on cardiac output?

    a. An increase in stroke volume occurring just after lying down
    b. An increase in stroke volume with no change in end-diastolic ventricular volume
    c. A decrease in cardiac output occurring in response to sympathetically mediated constriction of the veins
    d. The decrease in systolic blood pressure that occurs with decreased compliance of the aorta
    e. The increase in cardiac output with parasympathetic stimulation of the sinoatrial node

167. A patient was placed on a second generation antidepressant agent and after a while developed symptoms that looked to be tarvive dyskinesia. This effect would have been most likely associated with which of the following agents?

    a. Fluoxetine
    b. Tranylcypromine
    c. Amoxapine
    d. Trazodone
    e. Bupropion

168. Which of the following bacteria are *not* free-living?

    a. *Haemophilus influenzae*
    b. *Coxiella burnetii*
    c. *Gardnerella vaginalis*
    d. *Bacteroides fragilis*
    e. *Clostridium perfringens*

169. Which of the following is *not* true concerning Grave's disease?

    a. Grave's disease is primarily caused by hypersecretion of TSH by the pituitary.
    b. Grave's disease is an autoimmune disease.
    c. Exophthalmus in Grave's disease is caused by an increase in mass of the extraocular muscles within the orbit.
    d. Grave's disease is 7 to 10× more common in women than in men.
    e. Grave's disease has a higher level of concordance in monozygotic than dizygotic twins.

170. Which agent is considered the drug of choice for treatment of partial seizures and also effective in the treatment of trigemine neuralgia?

    a. Primidone
    b. Ethosuximide
    c. Carbamazepine
    d. Valproic acid
    e. Phenytoin

171. Which of the following antibodies recognizes the antigen combining site of the heavy chain and light chain of an immunoglobulin molecule?

    a. Anti-allotypic antibodies
    b. Anti-alloreactive antibodies
    c. Anti-idiotypic antibodies
    d. Anti-isotypic antibodies
    e. Anti-xenotypic antibodies

172. A serious blood disorder, granulocytopenia, is mainly associated with which one of the following antipsychotic drugs?

    a. Thiothixene
    b. Thioridazine
    c. Clozapine
    d. Haloperidol
    e. Trifluoperazine

173. Compared to skeletal muscle, smooth muscle has which of the following properties?

    a. Has more extensive sarcoplasmic reticulum
    b. Is dependent on a myosin-Ca^{2+}-calmodulin complex for contraction.
    c. Contains a large amount of troponin
    d. Exhibits very rapid cross-bridge cycling
    e. Responds only to direct neural stimulation

174. Atrial natriuretic hormone is secreted by which of the following?

    a. Endothelial cells in the endocardium
    b. Simple columnar epithelial cells in the myocardium
    c. Neuron cell bodies in the endocardium
    d. Cardiac muscle cells (myocardial fibers)
    e. Smooth muscle cells in the myocardium

175. Semen is a complex fluid that is composed of secretory products from all *except* which of the following?

    a. Prostate gland
    b. Bartholin's glands
    c. Seminal vesicles
    d. Testes
    e. Bulbourethral (Cowper's) glands

176. Which of the following is true according to the Starling's law of the heart (Frank-Starling mechanism)?

    a. Stroke volume decreases with sympathetic stimulation of the heart.
    b. Cardiac output is inversely related to sarcomere length of cardiac muscle cells.
    c. Stroke volume is proportional to end-diastolic ventricular volume.
    d. Stroke volume decreases if pulse pressure increases.
    e. Stroke volume increases when venous return decreases.

177. Which of the following best describes the Hering-Breuer reflex?

    a. Stimulation of stretch receptors in the bronchi sends a signal via myelinated fibers in the vagus, resulting in inhibition of inspiration.
    b. Irritant receptors in the bronchial smooth muscle acting via unmyelinated sympathetic afferents induce a cough reflex.

   c. J receptors in the bronchial mucosa respond to changes in alveolar air by inducing slow, deep respirations.
   d. Pain causes hyperventilation.
   e. Intercostal muscle spindles sense elongation and reflexively influence respiratory rate.

178. Stimulation of beta-adrenergic receptors causes all *except* which of the following?

   a. Bronchodilation
   b. Calorigenesis
   c. Cardiac slowing
   d. Intestinal relaxation
   e. Vasodilation

179. ACE inhibitors have *all except* which of the following potential adverse reactions?

   a. Syncope
   b. Hypokalemia
   c. Cough
   d. Neutropenia
   e. Angioedema

180. Which of the following is the most common form of X-linked muscular dystrophy?

   a. Duchenne's muscular dystrophy
   b. Fasioscapulohumeral muscular dystrophy
   c. Becker's muscular dystrophy
   d. Oculopharnygeal muscular dystrophy
   e. Limb-girdle dystrophy

181. Which of the following glands *do not* possess either intercalated or striated ducts?

   a. Pancreas
   b. Liver
   c. Parotid
   d. Sublingual
   e. Submandibular

EXTENDED MATCHING QUESTIONS

Directions for Questions 182 through 200: Each set of questions has several lettered options, followed by several numbered items. For each numbered item, select ONE lettered option that is most closely associated with it. Each lettered option may be used once, more than once, or not a all.

Questions 182 through 188

   a. Parietal cell (oxyntic cells)
   b. D cells
   c. G cells
   d. Chief cells
   e. Mucous cells

For each description, select the gastric cell most closely associated with it.

182. Secretes pepsinogen

183. Secretes gastrin

184. Stimulated by histamine

185. Gastric H^+ secretion

186. Source of "alkaline tide"

187. Secretes somatostatin

188. Stimulated by gastrin

Questions 189 through 191

   a. Chaperones
   b. Lymphotoxin
   c. ICAM-1
   d. Phosphotyrosine kinases
   e. Suppressor T lymphocytes
   f. E-selectins
   g. Tumor necrosis factor-alpha

For each description select the most appropriate item from the list above. Each lettered option may be used once, more than once, or not at all.

189. The principal mediator of the host response to gram-negative bacteria synthesized primarily in macrophages, and to some extent in T cells

190. Accessory protein that regulates the delivery and binding of peptides to class II MHC molecules

191. Intercellular adhesion molecule that mediates the initial attachment of neutrophils to vascular endothelial cells on venules of peripheral tissues

Questions 192 through 193

   a. Release of endotoxin
   b. Release of exotoxins
   c. Intracellular replication
   d. Host immune attack on infected cells
   e. Cellular transformation
   f. Promotion of secondary infection

Choose the best response from the list for the method of injury involved in the specific infections.

192. Hepatitis B viral infection of the liver.

193. *Corynebacterium diphtheria* infection.

Questions 194 through 196

   a. Paracrine effect
   b. Gamma-interferon
   c. Alpha-interferon
   d. Tumor necrosis factor-alpha
   e. Interleukin-1 (IL-1)
   f. Interleukin-2 (IL-2)
   g. Tumor necrosis factor-beta (lymphotoxin)

For each description, select the cytokine most closely associated with it.

194. Produced by stimulated T lymphocytes or natural killer cells this cytokine is capable of activating macrophages.

195.   Produced by activated CD4$^+$ T cells this cytokine induces proliferation of activated T cells, B cells, and natural killer cells.

196.   This cytokine is produced by lymphocytes and is responsible for target cell destruction.

Questions 197 through 200

    a. Abducens nucleus
    b. Caudal central nucleus
    c. Dentate nucleus
    d. Dorsal lamellae of inferior olive
    e. Dorsal motor nucleus of X
    f. Fastigial nucleus
    g. Hypoglossal nucleus
    h. Inferior salivatory nucleus
    i. Interpositus nucleus
    j. Medial parabrachial nucleus
    k. Nucleus ambiguus
    l. Oculomotor nucleus
    m. Red nucleus
    n. Superior olive

For each question, choose the nucleus most closely associated with it.

197.   Which GSE motor nucleus receives only crossed supranuclear innervation?

198.   Which pontine nucleus gives rise to GSE axons that can be involved in an alternating hemiplegia?

199.   Which nucleus receives axonal projections from the interpositus nucleus?

200.   Which nucleus innervates muscles of the larynx and pharynx derived from gill arch IV?

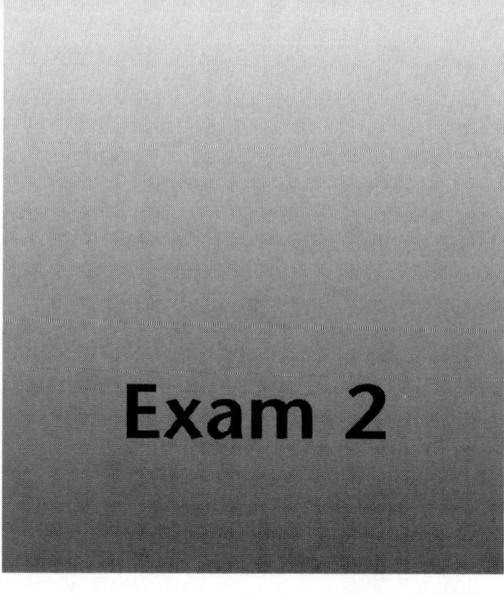

1. Which of the following statements is *true* of restriction endonucleases?

   a. They digest DNA duplex molecules from the 3′-OH ends.
   b. They have a specificity for single-stranded DNA.
   c. They are produced exclusively by bacterial viruses.
   d. They digest double-stranded DNA molecules at random sites.
   e. They can recognize palindromes.

2. A patient was admitted to the coronary care unit after complaining of chest pain. An ECG revealed atrial fibrillation with a ventricular rate of 180. Since the patient was developing pulmonary edema, meperidine was administered by the resident in attendance. The patient's heart rate then exceeded 200, triggering ventricular fibrillation.

   What property of meperidine was most likely implicated here?

   a. Peripheral vasoconstriction
   b. Catecholamine release from the adrenals
   c. Strong antimuscarinic activity
   d. Increased anxiety
   e. Chronic accumulation of normeperidine

3. Which of the following statements is *true* of the dorsalis pedis artery?

   a. Its pulse is palpable immediately anterior to the lateral malleolus.
   b. It is a continuation of the anterior tibial artery.
   c. It arises within the popliteal fossa.
   d. It gives rise to the lateral plantar artery.
   e. It is related to the tendon of the tibialis posterior muscle.

4. Which of the following statements regarding neutrophils is *not* correct?

   a. They are highly motile.
   b. They are members of the mononuclear phagocyte system (MPS) or the reticuloendothelial system (RES).
   c. Their primary function is to ingest and destroy invading microorganisms.
   d. They play a central role in early stages of acute inflammatory response.
   e. They are major constituents of pus.

5. A 6-year-old male has a history of recurrent bacterial infections, particularly of the skin and respiratory tract. A fraternal female twin has developed normally. A maternal uncle died of pneumonia at age 2. An x-ray examination of the patient's head and neck shows hyperlucency of the pharyngeal area. Laboratory studies show nearly absent IgG and no circulating B lymphocytes. What would a histologic examination of his lymph nodes be expected to show?

   a. Multiple granulomas
   b. Lack of germinal centers
   c. Selective hyperplasia of the mantle zone
   d. Diffuse increase in plasma cells
   e. Histologically normal lymph node

6. Which of the following statements about the TCA cycle is *correct?*

   a. Four molecules of NADH are produced per acetyl CoA oxidized to CO_2.
   b. The rate-limiting step is catalyzed by pyruvate carboxylase.
   c. The formation of citrate from acetyl CoA and oxaloacetate is irreversible.

    d. Carbon dioxide is formed at the steps catalyzed by malate dehydrogenase and by succinate dehydrogenase.

    e. The TCA cycle provides over 90% of the ATP requirement for erythrocytes.

7. According to the chemiosmotic hypothesis, what is the driving force for ATP synthesis by oxidative phosphorylation?

    a. A gradient of sodium ions between the matrix and cytosol

    b. An intermediate containing a high-energy bond that is coupled to ATP synthesis

    c. Electron transport from the cytoplasm to the matrix

    d. A hydrogen ion (proton) gradient between the matrix and intermembrane space

    e. Protons are transferred into the mitochondria during electron transport, establishing a pH gradient.

8. All *except* which of the following statements regarding the sphincter urethrae muscle is correct?

    a. It surrounds the shortest part of male urethra.

    b. It is located within deep perineal space.

    c. It is innervated by parasympathetic fibers.

    d. It lies between superior and inferior fascia of the UG diaphragm.

    e. It may be denervated by transecting branches of the pudendal nerves.

9. All *except* which of the following statements regarding the submental triangle is correct?

    a. It is bordered in part by the hyoid bone.

    b. Its floor is formed by the hyoglossus muscle.

    c. Its apex is the symphysis menti.

    d. It is bordered in part by the anterior bellies of the digastric muscles.

    e. It contains lymph nodes that receive lymph from the tip of the tongue.

10. A decrease in hematocrit occurring after a hemorrhage is primarily due to which of the following?

    a. Uptake of erythrocytes by the spleen

    b. Decreased plasma protein concentration

    c. A shift of interstitial fluid into the blood

    d. A decrease in blood volume and venous return

    e. Increased plasma Na^+ concentration due to loss of blood

11. Infection with *Helicobacter pylori* has *not* been associated with the development of which of the following?

    a. Gastric ulcers

    b. Gastric cancer

    c. Epiglottitis

    d. Duodenal ulcers

    e. Gastritis

12. Which of the following is *not* true of shigellosis?

    a. Outbreaks are common in day-care centers, prisons, and homes for the mentally retarded.

    b. The infectious dose is very high, 10^6 to 10^7 bacteria.

    c. *Shigella sonnei* is the most common cause of shigellosis in the industrial world.

    d. The natural habitat is limited to primates.

    e. Children aged 6 months to 10 years have the highest attack rate.

13. Which of the following is *not* a typical result of hepatic failure?

    a. Coagulopathy

    b. Hyperalbuminemia

    c. Hepatorenal syndrome

    d. Testicular atrophy

    e. Hyperbilirubinemia

14. How do muscles generate increasing force?

    a. By decreasing the fatigue resistance of its motor units

    b. By decreasing the oxidative phosphorylation of its muscle fibers

    c. By increasing the conduction velocity of its motor axons

    d. By increasing the number of active motor units

    e. By increasing the number of muscle spindles activated

15. Where is vasopressin (antidiuretic hormone) synthesized?

    a. Dorsomedial nucleus

    b. Nucleus basalis of Meynert

    c. Supraoptic nucleus

    d. Subfornical organ

    e. Ventromedial nucleus of the hypothalamus

16. Of the hepatitis viruses, which of the following does *not* have RNA genomes?

    a. Hepatitis A

    b. Hepatitis B

    c. Hepatitis C

    d. Hepatitis D

    e. Hepatitis E

17. All *except* which of the following passes through the greater sciatic foramen?

    a. Pudendal nerve

    b. Piriformis muscle

    c. Coccygeus muscle

    d. Sciatic nerve

    e. Inferior gluteal artery

18. Which of the following is *true* of the signal peptide found at the amino end of proteins?

    a. It contains a high proportion of hydrophilic amino acids.

    b. It is cleaved off prior to the translocation of the protein across the cell membrane.

    c. It is cleaved off by a protease inside the endoplasmic reticulum.

    d. It is added on to the polypeptide chain as a post-translational modification.

    e. It is used to anchor the protein to the membrane.

19. A straddle injury causing rupture of the proximal portion of the spongy urethra results in the subcutaneous extravasation of urine. Urine will pass subcutaneously into all *except* which of the following?

    a. Anteriorly into the scrotum
    b. Anteriorly into the penis
    c. Anterior abdominal wall
    d. Posteriorly into ischioanal fossa
    e. Superficial perineal space

20. Which of the following is one factor that results in an increase in muscle blood flow during exercise?

    a. Increased parasympathetic activity to the muscle
    b. Increased plasma angiotensin II concentration
    c. Increased P_{CO_2} in muscle interstitial fluid
    d. Flow autoregulation
    e. Decreased lymph flow

21. You are performing a surgical procedure in your female patient to correct urinary stress incontinence. The procedure calls for the placement of sutures in the pectineal ligament. Which of the following is most at risk when placing these sutures?

    a. Obturator nerve
    b. Internal pudendal artery
    c. Obturator artery
    d. Ureter
    e. Pudendal nerve

22. According to Erik Erikson's psycosocial stages of the life cycle, an individual navigates the tasks necessary to develop a sense of adequacy and an ability to perform productive work during a phase termed "industry versus inferiority." Which age range represents the typical timeframe for this stage?

    a. Birth to 1 year
    b. 1 to 3 years
    c. 3 to 5 years
    d. 6 to 11 years
    e. 11 years through adolescence

23. What is the driving force for uptake of oxygen by metabolizing tissues?

    a. The percent saturation of hemoglobin
    b. The difference between PA_{O_2} and PA_{CO_2}
    c. The difference between mean capillary P_{O_2} and mitochondrial P_{O_2}
    d. Arterial P_{O_2} minus venous P_{O_2}
    e. The total amount of O_2 carried by the arterial blood

24. Which of the following is *not* true of capillaries of the blood-brain-barrier (BBB)?

    a. These capillaries allow anesthetics with high-lipid solubility to enter the brain rapidly.
    b. These capillaries keep serum albumin from entering the brain.
    c. These capillaries are fenestrated and allow large molecules to pass freely into the brain.
    d. These capillaries are surrounded by astrocyte foot processes.
    e. These capillaries have many mitochondria in their endothelium when compared with muscle capillaries.

25. What is one role for the second messenger pathways in mediating the effects of hormones on cells?

    a. Amplification of the humoral signal at each level in the pathway
    b. Activation of membrane receptors in response to binding of hormones to cyclic AMP
    c. Induction of intracellular effects by hydrolysis of phosphodiesterase
    d. Direct inhibition of mitochondrial oxidative phosphorylation
    e. Induction of nonspecific intracellular effects of the hormone

26. Symptoms of a IX nerve lesion include all *except* which of the following?

    a. Deviation of the uvula to the side of the intact nerve
    b. Increased gastrointestinal motility
    c. Loss of taste on posterior third of the tongue
    d. Loss of the gag reflex
    e. Loss of sensation in the palatine tonsillar area

27. Which of the following is *not* a feature of *Bordetella pertussis?*

    a. Possesses a filamentous hemagglutinin believed to be important in attachment of the organism to ciliated cells
    b. Produces exotoxins
    c. Is a gram-negative coccobacillus
    d. Causes disease by invading tissues
    e. Causes a highly contagious disease

28. What is the most common endocrinopathy associated with pituitary adenoma?

    a. Hypersecretion of growth hormone
    b. Hypersecretion of ACTH
    c. Hypersecretion of FSH and LH
    d. Hypersecretion of prolactin
    e. Hypersecretion of TSH

29. Which of the following statements best describes oxytocin?

    a. Oxytocin is slowly metabolized by the liver and has a plasma half-life of several hours.
    b. Oxytocin is useful for the stimulation of milk production.
    c. Oxytocin is useful for therapeutic abortions during the first trimester because it produces well-coordinated contractions.
    d. Oxytocin is a polypeptide that is inactivated when given orally.
    e. Contraction effects are blocked by atropine.

30. In describing the most common psychological stages a dying patient experiences, Elisabeth Kübler-Ross included all *except* which of the following?

    a. Denial
    b. Anger
    c. Bargaining
    d. Acceptance
    e. Actualization

31. Parallel fibers in the cerebellum secrete which of the following?

    a. Acetylcholine
    b. Aspartate
    c. GABA
    d. Glutamate
    e. Taurine

32. Which of the following is not applicable to glyceryl trinitrate?

    a. Tolerance occurs with frequent, repeated administration.
    b. Total coronary blood flow is usually not increased.
    c. It may cause reflex tachycardia.
    d. It is most quickly absorbed through the oral mucosa.
    e. It causes methemoglobinemia.

33. Why would oxidation of an odd-numbered chain fatty acid be expected to yield less ATP per carbon than that of an even-numbered chain fatty acid?

    a. Propionyl-CoA cannot be metabolized.
    b. Methylmalonyl-CoA is not completely oxidized to carbon dioxide and water.
    c. Oxidation of propionyl-CoA requires energy input from ATP at a carboxylation step.
    d. Intermediates of propionyl-CoA metabolism inhibit the pyruvate dehydrogenase complex.
    e. Propionyl-CoA enters the TCA cycle at a point after Acetyl CoA.

34. Which of the following is *not* true about *Mycobacterium tuberculosis?*

    a. It may cause localized pulmonary infections or dissemination to other body sites such as the kidneys, meninges, skin, and CNS.
    b. The natural reservoir for *Mycobacterium tuberculosis* is humans.
    c. The host's humoral immune response to *Mycobacterium tuberculosis* causes clinical disease.
    d. The lipid-rich cell wall makes *Mycobacterium tuberculosis* resistant to disinfectants.
    e. *Mycobacterium tuberculosis* can evade phagocytic destruction by inhibiting phagosome-lysosome fusion.

35. The tract that is the sole source of climbing fiber input to the cerebellum is which of the following?

    a. Anterior spinocerebellar tract
    b. Cuneocerebellar tract
    c. Olivocerebellar tract
    d. Posterior spinocerebellar tract
    e. Trigeminocerebellar tract

36. The AIDS virus infects and kills cells that have T4 (also called CD4) receptors on their plasma membranes. Which of the following cells can be infected by the AIDS virus?

    a. Helper T lymphocytes
    b. All B cells
    c. Mast cells
    d. Eosinophils
    e. Neutrophilic myelocytes

37. Immune function abnormalities that result from HIV-1 infection do *not* include which of the following?

    a. Decreased cytotoxic T cell activity against virus-infected cells
    b. Increased release of tumor necrosis factor (TNF) and other cytokines
    c. Increased interleukin-1 (IL-1) production by monocytes
    d. Decreased microbicidal activity
    e. Decreased antigen-specific humoral responses

38. Bacteria may display resistance to certain antibiotics for all *except* which of the following reasons?

    a. Failure of the antibiotic to penetrate through the outer membrane
    b. The presence of proteolytic enzymes in the periplasmic space that degrade the antibiotic
    c. Failure to bind to the target site
    d. Hydrolysis of the antibiotic by beta-lactamases
    e. Point mutations in genes

39. Depth of anesthesia inhalation is closely proportional to which of the following?

    a. Partial pressure of the agent in the brain
    b. Concentration of the agent in intracellular fluid
    c. Partial pressure of the agent in the alveoli
    d. Concentration of the agent in the blood
    e. Concentration of the agent in the alveoli

40. Which of the following is *true* of cross-resistance in reference to drug resistance?

    a. It is transferred to other microorganisms.
    b. It is transferred between patients.
    c. It is one agent induced by another.
    d. It is transferred from bacteria to eukaryotes.
    e. It is transferred from plasmid to chromosome.

41. Which of the following statements about hemoglobin and myoglobin is *true?*

    a. The common genetic disorders of hemoglobin involve mutations affecting the heme binding site.
    b. The greater oxygen affinity of fetal hemoglobin makes possible the transfer of oxygen from the maternal circulation adult hemoglobin to the fetal circulation.
    c. The myoglobin oxygen saturation curve has a sigmoidal shape.
    d. The hemoglobin oxygen saturation curve has a hyperbolic shape.
    e. The heme groups are different for hemoglobin and myoglobin.

42. After attempting to donate blood, a 23-year-old patient who is a chronic intravenous drug abuser is diagnosed as having an HIV infection. At what point will this patient most likely begin to show rapid progression in the development of symptoms of AIDS?

    a. When the $CD8^+$ lymphocyte and $CD4^+$ lymphocyte populations are approximately equal in numbers
    b. When the $CD4^+$ lymphocyte population is greater than 500 cells per microliter of blood
    c. When the $CD4^+$ lymphocyte population is between 200 and 500 cells per microliter of blood

d. When the CD4$^+$ lymphocyte population is 200 or fewer cells per microliter of blood
e. When there is an absolute circulating monocytosis

43. Which of the following statements is *true* of paradoxical cold?

 a. It is an adaptation response to prolonged cold exposure.
 b. It results when there is injury to the hypothalamic heat conservation center.
 c. It is an example of labeled line coding.
 d. It results when thermal nociceptors are stimulated.
 e. It is part of the thermoregulatory process.

44. Which of the following factors do *not* influence autoregulation?

 a. Blood P_{CO_2}
 b. Blood pH
 c. Local transluminal activity
 d. Stimulation of the organum vasculosum
 e. Tissue and blood P_{O_2}

45. Myasthenia gravis results from which of the following?

 a. Decreased tryptophan hydroxylase activity in the central nervous system
 b. Increased tyrosine hydroxylase activity in the central nervous system
 c. Increased monoamine oxidase activity in the peripheral nervous system
 d. Loss of dopamine in the substantia nigra
 e. Loss of acetylcholine receptors due to an autoimmune process

46. All *except* which of the following cells is a component of the mononuclear phagocyte system (MPS).

 a. Langerhan's cell
 b. Histiocyte
 c. Type II pneumocyte
 d. Mesangeal cell
 e. Osteoclast

47. The cruciate anastomosis in the upper thigh is formed by the anastomosis of branches from all *except* which of the following arteries?

 a. Inferior gluteal
 b. Superior gluteal
 c. Lateral circumflex femoral
 d. Medial circumflex femoral
 e. First perforating branch of profunda femoris

48. What are the two major factors that determine the pulse pressure?

 a. Mean arterial pressure and blood volume
 b. Heart rate and arteriolar resistance
 c. Ventricular contractility and the length of systole
 d. Stroke volume and arterial compliance
 e. End-systolic ventricular volume and heart rate

49. The postsynpatic receptor in skeletal muscle functions as which of the following?

 a. Voltage gated Ca^{2+} channel
 b. Na^+, K^+ ATPase
 c. Chemically gated Na^+, K^+ channel
 d. Voltage gated K^+ channel
 e. Fast Na^+ channel

50. What structure (layer or cell) is present in thin skin and *not* present in thick skin?

 a. Duct of common sweat gland
 b. Reticular layer of the dermis
 c. Dermal papillae
 d. Sebaceous gland
 e. Langerhan's cell

51. In metabolic acidosis, buffering of excess H^+ includes all *except* which of the following mechanisms?

 a. Buffering by intracellular proteins and organic phosphates
 b. Reaction of H^+ with extracellular NH_4^+
 c. Reaction of H^+ with carbonates of bone mineral
 d. Reaction of H^+ with extracellular fluid HCO_3^-
 e. Buffering of H^+ by plasma proteins

52. The lytic unit of the classical complement pathway is formed in which of the following ways?

 a. C5 convertase splits C5 into C5a and C5b. C5a binds to the cell membrane with the subsequent addition of C6, C7, C8, and C9.
 b. C5 convertase splits C5 into C5a and C5b. C6 binds to the cell membrane with the subsequent addition of C7, C8, and C9.
 c. C5 convertase splits C5 into C5a and C5b. C5b binds to the cell membrane with the subsequent addition of C6, C7, C8, and C9.
 d. C5 convertase splits C5 into C5a and C5b. C5a and C5b both bind independently to the cell membrane with the subsequent addition of C6, C7, C8, and C9.
 e. C5 convertase catalyzes the binding of C4b3b2a to the cell membrane with subsequent addition of C6, C7, C8, and C9.

53. Which of the following does *not* represent a way to increase the power of a research study?

 a. Increase the effect size
 b. Increase the sample size
 c. Use one-tailed tests
 d. Decrease the alpha
 e. Maintain equal sample sizes

54. A 27-year-old woman has a Pap test as part of her annual physical examination. The cytopathologist reports that the Pap smear shows low-grade intraepithelial neoplasia. Which of the following is *not* true concerning that diagnosis?

 a. Fifty percent of cases will regress to normal.
 b. Ten percent of cases may progress to high-grade cervical intraepithelial neoplasia.
 c. Progression to carcinoma in situ would take more than 10 years.

    d. The atypical cell contains HPV type 6 DNA incorporated into their genome.
    e. The patient should be examined culposcopically.

55. All *except* which of the following statements about pathogenic strains of *Staphylococcus aureus* are true?

    a. They are rarely hemolytic on sheep blood agar.
    b. They may produce beta-lactamases that inactivate some penicillins.
    c. Capsules and other cell wall components inhibit phagocytosis.
    d. They produce coagulase.
    e. They are the most frequent cause of pyogenic infections such as boils and abscesses.

56. A right-handed female visited her doctor with a chief complaint of severe headache, nausea, frequent falling, and gradual hearing loss in her left ear. Physical examination confirmed the hearing loss and an ataxia, which caused her to fall to the left. She had some weakness of her left facial muscles. The lesion that could account for this is which of the following?

    a. A stroke of the left vertebral artery
    b. A stroke of the right posterior inferior cerebellar artery
    c. A stroke of the right anterior inferior cerebellar artery
    d. A cerebello-pontine angle tumor on the left
    e. A pinealoma

57. Which of the following is *not* a clinical manifestation of polyarteitis nodosa?

    a. Fever
    b. Weight loss
    c. Glomerulonephritis
    d. Hypertension
    e. Abdominal pain

58. The intestinal absorption of lipids involves all *except* which of the following?

    a. Solubilizing of fatty acids and monoglycerides by formation of micelles with bile salts
    b. Active transport of triglycerides across the luminal membrane of enterocytes
    c. Passive diffusion of lipids across the luminal membrane of enterocytes
    d. Reconstitution of triglycerides from monoglycerides and fatty acids within the enterocyte
    e. Incorporation into chylomicrons and very-low-density lipoproteins within enterocytes

59. Which statement about neural regulation of gastrointestinal function is *true?*

    a. The only neurotransmitters involved in regulation of GI function are acetylcholine and norepinephrine.
    b. Parasympathetic stimulation of the enteric nervous system enhances activity of most GI functions.
    c. Increased sympathetic activity increases the rate at which food boluses move through the intestine.
    d. The enteric nervous system acts independently of the autonomic nerves.
    e. In the GI tract, unlike blood vessels, the primary sympathetic neurotransmitter is vasoactive intestinal polypeptide (VIP).

60. Which of the following tumors is a malignant tumor of skeletal muscle origin?

    a. Spindle cell carcinoma
    b. Rhabdomyosarcoma
    c. Rhabdomyoma
    d. Leiomeioma
    e. Leiomyosarcoma

61. Which of the following statements regarding the vas (ductus) deferens is *not* correct?

    a. It lies lateral to inferior epigastric vessels at the deep inguinal ring.
    b. It dilates to form an ampulla near the bladder.
    c. It joins the duct of the seminal vesicle to form the ejaculatory duct.
    d. It is homologous to the round ligaments of the uterus.
    e. Contraction of its muscular walls is under autonomic control.

62. Which of the following is a cause of acute adrenal insufficiency associated with meningococcal septisemia?

    a. Withdrawal of exogenous corticosteroid therapy
    b. Waterhouse-Friderichsen syndrome
    c. Isolate ACTH deficiency
    d. Tuberculosis
    e. Oat cell carcinoma of the lung

63. In addition to producing bone marrow depression, which of the following produces neurotoxicity and is a cell-cycle-dependent agent?

    a. Busulfan
    b. 5-fluorouracil
    c. Vincristine
    d. Actinomycin D
    e. Etoposide (VP-16)

64. According to the "gate control theory," pain sensation transmitted via C-fibers can be reduced by concurrent activation of which of the following?

    a. Adjacent substance P-releasing C-fibers
    b. Glutamate-releasing A-delta fibers
    c. High-threshold polymodal nociceptors
    d. Mechanoreceptor fibers
    e. Spinoreticular tract

65. Which of the following statements about penicillin is incorrect?

    a. It is the least toxic of the antimicrobial antibiotics.
    b. It may produce anaphylactic reactions in sensitive patients.
    c. It is bactericidal.
    d. Its action on gram-positive organisms is potentiated by tetracycline.
    e. It is secreted by the renal tubules.

66. The cell of origin in virtually all carcinomas of the pancreas is which of the following?

    a. The ascinar cells
    b. The islet beta cells
    c. The islet alpha cells
    d. The interstitial fibroblasts
    e. The ductular epithelium

67. A sample of cerebrospinal fluid (CFS) is routinely obtained by a needle inserted into the subarachnoid space between the spinous processes of which of the following vertebrae?

    a. T11 and T12
    b. T12 and L1
    c. L1 and L2
    d. L2 and L3
    e. L4 and L5

68. Which of the following is *not* located in the superficial perineal space of the male?

    a. Ischiocavernosus muscle
    b. Bulb of the penis
    c. Superficial transversus perinei muscle
    d. Bulbourethral glands
    e. Crura of the penis

69. A patient becomes easily annoyed during an office visit, perceiving a physician's comments as judgmental. Later, the physician discovers that the patient's reaction resulted from excessive criticism from a father, who had many traits similar to the physician. The patient's response is an example of which of the following?

    a. Projection
    b. Transference
    c. Regression
    d. Reflection
    e. Tangentiality

70. Where is the major site of renin synthesis?

    a. Granular cells of the intralobular arteriole
    b. Granular cells of the afferent arteriole
    c. The nucleus tractus solitarius
    d. The paraventricular nucleus
    e. The posterior pituitary gland

71. All *except* which of the following may characterize sickle cell anemia?

    a. The disease can be diagnosed in fetal DNA by restriction enzyme digestion.
    b. Sickling occurs when there is a high concentration of the oxygenated form of hemoglobin S.
    c. Hb S has an unchanged electrophoretic mobility relative to normal hemoglobin.
    d. Hb S is altered by the deletion of a single amino acid in the beta chain.
    e. The solubility of oxygenated Hb S is abnormally low.

72. The placental barrier separates maternal blood from fetal blood. The respiratory barrier separates blood from air in much the same way as the placental barrier separates maternal blood from fetal blood. In the latter half of the first trimester, the placental barrier is composed of all *except* which of the following?

    a. Endothelium of fetal capillaries
    b. Decidua basalis
    c. Mesenchyme in fetal villi
    d. Basal lamina of fetal capillaries
    e. Syncytiotrophoblast

73. Compliance is defined as which of the following?

    a. Change in volume per unit change in pressure
    b. Pressure/resistance
    c. Flow $\times$ resistance
    d. Stroke volume/end-diastolic ventricular volume
    e. CO $\times$ MAP

74. Which of the following disorders may *not* be associated with a subcortical dementia?

    a. AIDS
    b. Alzheimer's disease
    c. Huntington's disease
    d. Parkinson's disease
    e. Wilson's disease

75. A 50-year-old male patient (70 kg) is given oral atenolol (50 mg once a day) to treat hypertension. Atenolol has the following characteristics:

    Volume of distribution = 1 L/kg
    Oral bioavailability (F) = 0.60
    Half-life   = 6 hr

    What is the concentration of atenolol at a steady state in this patient?

    a. 50 nanograms/ml
    b. 150 nanograms/ml
    c. 50 micrograms/ml
    d. 150 micrograms/ml
    e. 1 milligram/ml

76. Which of the following ganglia does *not* receive preganglionic sympathetic or parasympathetic input?

    a. Ciliary ganglion
    b. Otic ganglion
    c. Pterygopalatine ganglion
    d. Submandibular ganglion
    e. Vestibular ganglion

77. Which of the following morphological changes is associated with **lethal** cellular injury?

    a. Cytoplasmic vacuolation
    b. Nuclear pyknosis
    c. Fatty change
    d. Dense amorphous densities in the mitochondria
    e. Karyorrhexis

78. Which of the following is mimicked by the antibiotic puromycin?

    a. Peptidyl-tRNA
    b. Aminoacyl-tRNA
    c. Peptidyl transferase
    d. Translation release factors
    e. Formylmethionyl-tRNA

79. Which of the following is not an indication for chloramphenicol?

    a. Carrier state of typhoid
    b. *H. influenzae* meningitis
    c. Meningococcal meningitis in penicillin allergic patients
    d. Brain abscess
    e. Symptomatic *Salmonella* infection, e.g., typhoid fever

80. Which of the following syndromes occurs in 20% to 40% of patients chronically treated with phenothiazines and is a late-occurring syndrome of abnormal choreoathetoid movements?

    a. Parkinson's disease
    b. Tardive dyskinesia
    c. Acute dystonic reactions
    d. Akathisia
    e. Perioral tremor

81. Which tract is part of the descending autonomic output from the hypothalamus to the brain stem and spinal cord?

    a. Dorsal longitudinal fasciculus
    b. Fornix
    c. Medial lemniscus
    d. Medial longitudinal fasciculus
    e. Tectospinal tract

82. Which of the following best describes erythromycin estolate?

    a. Has a range of activity restricted to gram-negative infections
    b. Exhibits a penicillin cross-sensitivity of 50%
    c. Must be given with caution to patients in renal failure because of its rapid renal excretion
    d. Interferes with bacterial cell wall synthesis
    e. Is the drug of choice in Legionnaires' disease

83. Which of the following statements regarding rifampin is *false?*

    a. Adverse reactions to rifampin include an orangish-pink coloration of body fluids, such as tears.
    b. Rifampin is poorly absorbed orally and should be given intramuscularly.
    c. Rifampin decreases the effectiveness of oral contraceptives.
    d. Para-aminosalicylic acid delays absorption of rifampin.
    e. Rifampin is primarily excreted in the biliary and urinary tracts.

84. Which of the following statements concerning *Vibrio cholerae* infection is *false?*

    a. Cholera causes severe, watery diarrhea, which may be life threatening.
    b. *V. cholerae* releases a potent exotoxin which causes an increase in cellular cAMP.
    c. *V. cholerae* binds to gut epithelial cells and releases its exotoxin after it enters the cell.
    d. The diarrhea fluid produced by *V. cholerae* infection is unusual because it contains few acute inflammatory cells.
    e. *V. cholerae* infection may be successfully treated by oral replacement of the massive fluid loss from the gut.

85. A patient with a III nerve lesion may exhibit all *except* which of the following?

    a. External strabismus
    b. Loss of accommodation
    c. Mydriasis
    d. Nystagmus
    e. Ptosis

86. Axons of the spiral ganglion carrying auditory information synapse first in which of the following?

    a. Dorsal and ventral cochlear nuclei
    b. Inferior colliculus
    c. Medial geniculate
    d. Superior colliculus
    e. Superior temporal gyrus

87. What is the major, direct determinant of the resting membrane potential of most cells?

    a. An electroneutral Na^+, K^+ ATPase
    b. An electrogenic Na^+, K^+ ATPase
    c. The diffusion potential for K^+
    d. The diffusion potential for Na^+
    e. Na^+, glucose cotransport

88. The lateral vestibulospinal tract can be found in which of the following?

    a. Basilar pons
    b. Lateral funiculus of the spinal cord
    c. Tectum of the mesencephalon
    d. Tegmentum of the mesencephalon
    e. Ventral funiculus of the spinal cord

89. Which of the following components of *Klebsiella pneumoniae* is most closely associated with its pathogenesis?

    a. Urease
    b. Capsule
    c. Fimbriae
    d. Hemolysin
    e. Flagella

90. GALT does *not* include which of the following?

    a. Palatine tonsils
    b. Lymphoid nodules in the tracheal mucosa
    c. Peyer's patches
    d. Lymphoid nodules in the mucosa of the esophagus
    e. Lymphoid nodules in the mucosa of the appendix

91. Zollinger-Ellison syndrome is caused by gastrin-secreting tumors. What is the most effective drug for treating this disease?

    a. Sucralfate
    b. Famotidine
    c. Misoprostol
    d. Omeprazole
    e. 5-aminosalicylic acid

92. Which of the following is *not* a physiological effect of angiotensin II?

    a. Vasoconstriction of systemic arterioles
    b. Stimulation of drinking
    c. Stimulation of aldosterone secretion
    d. Stimulation of K^+ reabsorption
    e. Stimulation of proximal tubular Na^+ reabsorption

93. What is the renal autoregulatory response to an increase in arterial blood pressure?

    a. A proportional increase in glomerular filtration rate (GFR) and renal blood flow (RBF)
    b. Little or no change in either GFR or RBF
    c. A proportional increase in GFR, but no change in RBF
    d. A proportional increase in RBF, but no change in GFR
    e. Vasodilation of the afferent arteriole

94. Which of the following are the most common dose-related adverse effects associated with the use of valproic acid?

    a. Cardiovascular related
    b. Renal related
    c. Gastrointestinal related
    d. Visual disturbances
    e. Mental confusion

95. Ciprofloxacin acts in which of the following ways?

    a. Interference with cell wall synthesis
    b. Competitive antagonism of folic acid synthesis
    c. Alteration of function of plasma membrane
    d. Inhibition of DNA synthesis (DNA topoisomerase-II)
    e. Inhibition of protein synthesis

96. What is the mechanism of action for calmodulin?

    a. Activates adenylate cyclase when complexed with alpha-subunit of Gs-protein
    b. Binds to receptors on endoplasmic reticulum causing release of calcium into the cytoplasm
    c. Binds calcium to become an activator of several cellular enzymes
    d. Acts to increase the activity of membrane bound protein kinase C
    e. Activates protein kinase A to become a regulator of enzymes by phosphorylation

97. When neurons in the CNS die, the dead cells are removed by macrophages via the process of phagocytosis. The damaged area is then repaired by proliferation of which of the following?

    a. Astrocytes
    b. Microglia
    c. Oligodendroglia
    d. Ependymal cells
    e. Meningeal neutrophils

98. Which of the following connect the right and left occipital lobes?

    a. Anterior commissure
    b. Arcuate (U) fibers
    c. Corpus callosum
    d. Cingulum
    e. Posterior commissure

99. All *except* which of the following statements regarding the piriformis muscle is correct?

    a. Its tendon attaches to the greater trochanter of the femur.
    b. It functions as a lateral (external) rotator of the thigh.
    c. It has attachments to the pelvic surface of the sacrum.
    d. It is innervated by branches of the sacral plexus.
    e. In the gluteal region, it lies inferior to the tendon of the obturator internus muscle.

100. Hemorrhagic fever is *not* commonly associated with which of the following viruses?

    a. Hantaan
    b. Ebola
    c. Lassa fever
    d. Hepatitis A
    e. Marburg

101. Which of the following ligaments is commonly called the "spring ligament"?

    a. Long plantar
    b. Plantar calcaneocuboid
    c. Deltoid
    d. Plantar calcaneonavicular
    e. Calcaneofibular

102. During a laboratory experiment a rat is trained to press a bar to avoid receiving a painful electric shock. Based on the principles of operant conditioning the electric shock is known as which of the following?

    a. Conditioned stimulus
    b. Conditioned response
    c. Punishment
    d. Positive reinforcer
    e. Negative reinforcer

103. Which of the following statements is *not* true regarding medical students and physicians?

    a. Suicide rates in male physicians are 4 times higher than in the general male population.
    b. Suicide rates in female physicians are 4 times higher than in the general female population.
    c. As many as one out of five medical students seek psychiatric services during their education.
    d. Medical students seeking psychiatric services typically have adjustment, depression, and marital conflict issues.
    e. As many as one out of three practicing physicians seek outpatient psychiatric services yearly.

104. Which of the following statements is *true* of viruses that have negative sense RNA genomes?

    a. They have early genes that encode DNA-binding proteins and enzymes.
    b. They contain an RNA polymerase.
    c. They require a DNA intermediate to replicate.
    d. They do not undergo recombination.
    e. They are all inhibited by amantadine.

105. Which of the following is *not true* for supersecondary structure motifs?

    a. They can bind metal ions such as zinc.
    b. They are composed only of arrangements of alpha helices.
    c. The stability of motif structure forms domains within the protein molecule.
    d. This is not another term for tertiary structure.
    e. The same motif can appear in different proteins with similar function.

106. All *except* which of the following statements is true?

    a. Dietary control is needed for type II (non-insulin-dependent) diabetes.
    b. The subcutaneous injection of insulin may cause lipodystrophies.
    c. Insulin requirements are often increased by infection.
    d. Regular exercise reduces insulin requirement.
    e. The site of insulin injection should be kept constant to ensure uniform onset and duration of action.

107. Which of the following is *not* true about CSF formation?

    a. CSF formation is decreased when there is local arteriolar vasoconstriction.
    b. CSF formation is decreased when the patient is hypotensive.
    c. Hyperventilation causes decreased CSF formation.
    d. The ventricles make approximately 2000 ml/day.
    e. Vasodilation increases CSF formation.

108. An amphitrichously flagellated bacterium would have which of the following?

    a. Flagella surrounding the entire cell
    b. No flagella
    c. One flagellum at one end of the cell
    d. Two or more flagella at one or both ends
    e. One or more flagella at each end

109. In the following partial sequence of a messenger RNA, what effect on the protein product is most likely after a mutation in the DNA changes codon 91 to UAG? (Nonsense codons are UGA, UAA, UAG.)

88	89	90	91	92	93	94
GTC	GAC	CAG	AAG	GGC	UAA	CCG

    a. There will be no alteration since only the wobble position was affected.
    b. It will be completely inactivated due to a frameshift mutation.
    c. The mutation in the DNA will be repaired, restoring the original codon.
    d. There will be a mild effect due to substitution with a similar amino acid.
    e. It will be shortened by only two amino acids.

110. Which of the following is *not* an X-linked recessive disorder?

    a. Hemophilia A
    b. Hemophilia B
    c. Duchenne-Becker muscular dystrophy
    d. Adult polycystic kidney disease
    e. Chronic granulomatous disease

111. The facial nerve innervates all of the following muscles *except* which of the following?

    a. Stylohyoid
    b. Tensor tympani
    c. Stapedius
    d. Buccinator
    e. Posterior belly of digastric

112. Which of the following may induce anginal attacks and ECG changes characteristic of myocardial ischemia?

    a. Methyldopa
    b. Hydralazine
    c. Guanethidine
    d. Hydrochlorothiazide
    e. Reserpine

113. The conversion of 11-cis retinal to all-trans retinal is caused by which of the following?

    a. Absorption of a photon by a rhodopsin molecule
    b. Inactivation of transducin
    c. Inactivation of phosphodiesterase
    d. Hyperpolarization of the photoreceptor
    e. Closing of sodium channels in the photoreceptor plasma membrane

114. Stable-cell wall-less bacteria that may arise either spontaneously or through induction by antibiotics, are known as which of the following?

    a. Protoplasts
    b. Mycoplasmas
    c. L-forms
    d. Spheroplasts
    e. Prions

115. In determining the utility of a diagnostic measure, if A = True Positives, B = False Positives, C = False Negatives and D = True Negatives, then what does A/A + C represent?

    a. Sensitivity
    b. Validity
    c. Reliability
    d. Specificity
    e. Variability

116. When the brachial plexus is injured in the axilla from the improper use of a crutch, producing a condition often called "crutch palsy," which of the following nerves is most typically injured?

    a. Thoracodorsal nerve
    b. Long thoracic nerve
    c. Suprascapular nerve
    d. Radial nerve
    e. Ulnar nerve

117. Ultraviolet damage of DNA in skin is associated with which of the following?

    a. DNA ligase detects damaged areas.
    b. Pyrimidine dimers are formed.
    c. Both strands are cleaved by an endonuclease.
    d. Thymine is converted to adenine.
    e. DNA fragments.

118. Lymphocytes or their stem cells move back and forth between the blood vascular system and the lymphatic tissue compartment by passing through the walls of all *except* which of the following?

    a. Sinusoids in red bone marrow
    b. Central arterioles/arteries in the spleen
    c. Capillary loops in the thymus
    d. Venous sinusoids in the spleen
    e. Postcapillary venules in lymph nodes

119. Four general classes of hypersensitivity reaction are given below. Match the type of reaction to the clinical scenario.

    A 32-year-old patient with lupus erythematosis develops progressive renal failure. On renal biopsy, there is marked damage and destruction of the glomeruli.

    a. Type I hypersensitivity reaction
    b. Type II hypersensitivity reaction
    c. Type III hypersensitivity reaction
    d. Type IV hypersensitivity reaction

120. Which of the following statements about sulfonamides is *true?*

    a. They prevent the synthesis of dihydrofolate reductase.
    b. They are effective against only those bacteria that synthesize their own folate.
    c. They are used with trimethoprim, but they are not synergistic.
    d. They are especially useful against *Pseudomonas aeruginosa.*
    e. They are the drugs of choice for meningococcal carrier state because no resistant strains have ever been reported.

121. What is the effect of an increase in plasma acidity (decrease in pH) on oxygen carriage by hemoglobin?

    a. Decreases the percent saturation at any level of P_{O_2}
    b. Increases the percent saturation at any level of P_{O_2}
    c. Increases the affinity of hemoglobin for carbon monoxide
    d. Decreases the amount of oxygen released to exercising tissues at any level of P_{O_2}
    e. Shifts the hemoglobin-oxygen dissociation curve to the left

122. Which pair of nerves below is intimately related to a portion of the humerus and can be injured by fractures of the humerus?

    a. Axillary and musculocutaneous
    b. Axillary and median
    c. Axillary and radial
    d. Ulnar and musculocutaneous
    e. Median and radial

123. A physician receives a consultation request to evaluate a patient to determine whether the patient is demented or delirious. In conducting the evaluation the physician should remember which of the following true statements?

    a. Dementia's onset is gradual, whereas, delirium has a sudden onset.
    b. Demented patients show more difficulty maintaining alertness.
    c. In dementia, fluctuations in cognitive functioning over the course of a day are more likely.
    d. Demented patients cannot have comorbid symptoms of a depressive disorder.
    e. Dementia cannot be the result of a general medical condition.

124. Which of the following is most useful in treating paralytic ileus without obstruction?

    a. Neostigmine
    b. Succinylcholine
    c. Acetylcholine
    d. DFP (diisopropylfluorophosphate)
    e. Ephedrine

125. Which of the following corticosteroids has long-lasting actions and has minimum sodium-retaining liability?

    a. Prednisone
    b. Cortisone
    c. Dexamethasone
    d. Fludrocortisone
    e. Desoxycorticosterone

126. The section of the brain stem between the superior and inferior colliculi leads to which of the following:

    a. Ataxia
    b. Ballism
    c. Decerebrate rigidity
    d. Epilepsy
    e. Insomnia

127. Which one of the following statements about high-energy compounds is *true?*

   a. ATP can be synthesized from ADP by phosphate transfer from phosphoenolpyruvate.

   b. Phosphocreatine can substitute for ATP as a high-energy compound in muscle tissues.

   c. Reactions that are energetically unfavorable must hydrolyze ATP to ADP and inorganic phosphate to be spontaneous.

   d. Hydrolysis of ATP to AMP and pyrophosphate is used in some synthetic reactions, because of the extra energy released from that bond.

   e. ATP is synthesized exclusively in the mitochondrion, while GTP is synthesized exclusively in the cytoplasm.

128. The ras oncogene is the most commonly mutated oncogene found in human solid malignancies. What is the function of the *ras* oncogene?

   a. Prevents apoptosis

   b. Activates multiple kinases

   c. Receives growth factor

   d. Activates DNA transcription

   e. Produces growth factor

129. What structure is most at risk during surgical removal of the right suprarenal gland?

   a. Portal vein

   b. Abdominal aorta

   c. Right renal artery

   d. Inferior vena cava

   e. Hepatic portal vein

130. A patient with Korsakoff's syndrome will often create fictitious events to compensate for unrecoverable memories. This phenomena is known as which of the following?

   a. Perseveration

   b. Confabulation

   c. Flight of ideas

   d. Malingering

   e. Neologisms

131. Fertilization usually occurs in which of the following?

   a. Uterus

   b. Ampulla of oviduct

   c. Vagina

   d. Cervix

   e. Intramural portion of the oviduct

132. What effect does the increase of mean arterial pressure (MAP) have on the frequency of firing of baroreceptor action potentials?

   a. It decreases.

   b. It changes very little over the normal pressure range.

   c. It increases.

   d. It increases to a peak at normal MAP, then decreases.

   e. It decreases to a minimal value at normal MAP, then increases.

133. Stem cells are easily injured and killed when adult cancer patients receive radiation and chemotherapy. Stem cells are *not* present in which of the following?

   a. Bone marrow

   b. Nerve fascicles

   c. Gastric pits/glands

   d. Hair follicles

   e. Crypts of Lieberkühn

134. Suppression of the immune response may be accomplished by preventing lymphocyte activation. Mechanisms by which this may occur do *not* include which of the following?

   a. Feedback-inhibition by antibodies

   b. Immunologic tolerance

   c. Feedback inhibition by cytokines

   d. Regulation of networks of idiotypes and anti-idiotypes

   e. Constant stimulation of antigen levels

135. Which of the following is *not* consistent with a leukemoid reaction?

   a. Toxic granulation of neutrophils

   b. Döhle inclusion bodies in neutrophils

   c. High neutrophil leukocyte alkaline phosphatase

   d. Majority of circulating neutrophils are myelocytes

   e. Presence of circulating promyelocytes

136. At what blood alcohol level is lethal coma a likely result?

   a. 50 mg/dl

   b. 100 mg/dl

   c. 150 mg/dl

   d. 200 mg/dl

   e. 300 mg/dl

137. What is the morphologic finding in the kidneys of patients who die with severe liver disease and hepatorenal syndrome?

   a. Diffuse glomerulopathy with mesangial widening

   b. Necrotizing glomerulonephritis

   c. Proximal tubular necrosis

   d. Severe medullary interstitial nephritis

   e. No intrinsic morphologic change

138. Which of the following is *not* a true statement concerning crytorchidism of the testis?

   a. This is an interesting developmental anomaly but is of little concern.

   b. Untreated, the testis will be sterile.

   c. Untreated there is a distinct increase in the incidence of embryonal cell carcinoma.

   d. Untreated there is an increase in the incidence of seminoma.

   e. Orchiopexy should be performed before the second birthday.

139. Bone can be classified according to histologic appearance, gross morphology, and/or embryologic origin. Which of the following is *not* used to classify bone?

    a. Intramembranous ossification
    b. Periosteum
    c. Woven bone
    d. Compact bone
    e. Lamellar bone

140. Anatomic evidence of cholestasis is the presence of bile pigment in the hepatocytes and bile canaliculi. Which of the following would *not* be an expected laboratory finding in cholestasis?

    a. Increase in conjugated bilirubin
    b. Increase in blood cholesterol
    c. Increase in circulating bile acids
    d. Increase in serum alkaline phosphatase
    e. Increase in serum creatine kinase

141. Red blood cells are suspended in a solution that contains 300 millimoles/liter of urea as the only solute. Urea has no electrical charge, and the cell membranes are highly permeable to urea. In this urea solution, what will the red blood cells do?

    a. Remain stable since the osmolality is 300 mOsm/liter, about equal to normal plasma
    b. Swell and lyse as urea diffuses into the cell along its concentration gradient
    c. Shrink, because the osmolality of the solution is double normal plasma osmolality
    d. Initially shrink as urea diffuses into the cell, and then regain their normal volume
    e. Initially swell as urea diffuses into the cell, and then regain their normal volume

142. Which of the following is *not* associated with the development of chronic pancreatitis?

    a. Alcoholism
    b. Biliary tract disease
    c. Hypercalcemia
    d. Hyperlipidemia
    e. Mumps virus infection

143. When obtaining interview data from a psychotic patient, the interviewer should *not* abide by which of the following statements?

    a. Challenge the patient's delusions through confrontation
    b. Interview family members to gain a second source of data
    c. Keep the interview structured and directive
    d. Proceed in a manner that maintains formality
    e. Focus on coping skills and activities of daily living

144. Which of the following factors sets the upper limit on whole body oxygen consumption during exercise?

    a. Pulmonary uptake of oxygen
    b. Caloric intake
    c. Cardiac output
    d. Sensitivity of the baroreceptors
    e. Stroke volume

145. Which of the following is *true* of the velocity of an enzyme-catalyzed reaction?

    a. It is always dependent on substrate concentration.
    b. It is half maximal at the Km.
    c. It will continue to rise with increasing temperature.
    d. It will be independent of the pH.
    e. It is slower at first then increases with time.

146. Which of the following statements concerning Huntington's disease is *not* true?

    a. Huntington's syndrome is caused by a gene on chromosome 4 (4p16.3).
    b. Patients with only one HD allele have a milder form of the disease.
    c. Grossly, the brain shows symmetric atrophy of the caudate nuclei.
    d. Microscopically, the small neurons of the caudate and putamen are especially depleted.
    e. Symptoms usually begin about age 40.

147. What causes lactose intolerance?

    a. Absence of pancreatic amylase
    b. Osmotic diarrhea due to accumulation of sucrose in the bowel
    c. Deficiency of dissacharidases in the brush border membrane of enterocytes
    d. Constipation due to excessive lactose in the bowel
    e. Deficiency of dissacharidases secreted from the pancreas

148. The microtubule is a widely dispersed, nonmembranous organelle that functions in subcellular movement. Microtubule functions do *not* include which of the following?

    a. Cell migration
    b. Intracellular transport of secretory granules
    c. Movement of chromosomes during mitosis
    d. Maintenance of asymmetric shapes (e.g., platelets)
    e. Movement of the plasma membrane (as in cytokinesis and endocytosis)

149. An injured axillary artery is surgically ligated between the thyrocervical trunk and subscapular artery. Subsequent collateral circulation is likely to result in a reversal of blood flow in which of the following?

    a. Circumflex scapular artery
    b. Transverse cervical artery
    c. Posterior intercostal arteries
    d. Suprascapular artery
    e. Profunda brachii artery

150. The symptoms associated with narcolepsy include all *except* which of the following?

    a. Cataplexy
    b. Daytime drowsiness
    c. Enuresis
    d. Hypnagogic hallucinations
    e. Sleep paralysis

151. The chemoreceptive trigger zone (CTZ) for vomiting is which of the following?

    a. Area postrema
    b. Hypothalamus
    c. Organum vasculosum
    d. Pineal gland
    e. Subfornical organ

152. Usual manifestations of severe atropine poisoning do *not* include which of the following?

    a. Hyperthermia
    b. Profuse sweating
    c. Mydriasis
    d. Tachycardia
    e. Hallucinations

153. Rods and cones are both photoreceptors. However, they differ from one another structurally and functionally. Which of the following characteristics does *not* describe a rod?

    a. Possesses rhodopsin
    b. Present exclusively in the fovea centralis
    c. Disks of outer segments are replaced on a regular basis.
    d. Most numerous cell type in the layer of rods and cones
    e. Functions during periods of low-light intensity (for example, at dusk).

154. All *except* which of these statements is a characteristic of a typical cell in the proximal convoluted tubule (PCT)?

    a. Numerous vesicles in the apical cytoplasm
    b. Eosinophilic cytoplasm
    c. Extensive rER
    d. Basal striations created by a large number of basal mitochondria oriented longitudinally with respect to numerous infoldings of the basal cell membrane
    e. Numerous microvilli

155. Repeated stimulation of which receptor leads to a lower threshold and sensitization?

    a. Cold receptors
    b. Golgi tendon organs
    c. Meissner's corpuscles
    d. Pacinian corpuscles
    e. Polymodal nociceptors

156. The many islets of Langerhans are collectively considered to be a diffuse organ that works to regulate blood glucose levels. Secretory products of the islets of Langerhans do *not* include which of the following?

    a. Insulin
    b. Secretin
    c. Vasoactive intestinal peptide (VIP)
    d. Glucagon
    e. Somatostatin

157. Transitional epithelium is a unique tissue associated with only one organ system. Which of the following statements regarding transitional epithelium is *not* true?

    a. It contains cells that protect the underlying tissue from abrasion.
    b. It lines the urinary bladder.
    c. It contains cells that prevent movement of water from the underlying tissues into urine.
    d. It lines the renal pelvis.
    e. It possesses binucleate cells in its most superficial layer.

158. In mutation-derived changes in the hemagglutinins, H1 and H2, which of the following viruses are responsible for "antigenic shifts"?

    a. Adenoviruses
    b. Influenza virus A
    c. Respiratory syncytial virus
    d. Poliovirus
    e. Rhinoviruses

159. Which of the following agents is administered intravenously for treatment of cyanide poisoning?

    a. Glyceryl trinitrate
    b. Amyl nitrite
    c. Papaverine
    d. Sodium nitrite
    e. Erythrityl tetranitrate

160. *Haemophilus influenzae* is *not* commonly associated with which of the following syndromes in children?

    a. Osteomyelitis
    b. Cellulitis
    c. Otitis media
    d. Meningitis
    e. Epiglottitis

161. An 18-year-old woman comes to the emergency room at a local hospital complaining of general malaise, fever, and cough. The symptoms have persisted for about 7 days. A chest x-ray examination shows patchy areas. Gram staining of sputum reveals no bacteria, and the physician orders a test for "cold agglutinins." The titer is ≥ 256. The bacterium that is the most likely cause of this woman's infection is which of the following?

    a. *Streptococcus pneumoniae*
    b. *Klebsiella pneumoniae*
    c. *Chlamydia pneumoniae*
    d. *Mycoplasma pneumoniae*
    e. *Chlamydia psittaci*

162. Which of the following antihypertensive drugs would concurrently inhibit reflex tachycardia?

    a. Metoprolol
    b. Minoxidil
    c. Spironolactone
    d. Sodium nitroprusside
    e. Enalapril

163. Which of the following is *not* true of *Bordetella pertussis* toxin?

    a. It is responsible for many systemic effects of the disease caused by *Bordetella pertussis.*
    b. It is composed of several subunits.
    c. It is an important component of newly developed vaccines against whooping cough.
    d. Its toxic enzymatic activity is associated with ATP hydrolysis.
    e. It aids in the adherence of *Bordetella pertussis* to respiratory epithelial cells.

164. When considering the anesthetics, hepatotoxicity is most often associated with which agent?

    a. Methoxyflurane
    b. Halothane
    c. Diazepam
    d. Nitrous oxide
    e. Thiopental

165. A normal adult is placed on a balanced diet lacking only tyrosine. Which statement describes this person's nitrogen metabolism?

    a. The person would be in negative nitrogen balance.
    b. There would be a transient period of negative nitrogen balance, followed by nitrogen equilibrium.
    c. The rate of synthesis of phenylalanine would decrease
    d. The person would be in nitrogen equilibrium.
    e. Urea excretion would increase above that in the prediet period.

166. Which of the following statements concerning Meckel's diverticulum is *not* true?

    a. Meckel's diverticulum may cause appendicitis-like symptoms.
    b. Meckel's diverticulum may contain ectopic foci of gastric mucosa.
    c. Meckel's diverticulum may contain ectopic foci of pancreatic tissue.
    d. Meckel's diverticulum is a pseudodiverticulum lacking one or more layers.
    e. Meckel's diverticulum arises from persistence of the vitelline duct.

167. Of the following statements concerning venous thrombosis and pulmonary embolism, which is *not* true?

    a. Most pulmonary emboli arise in the lower extremities.
    b. Deep vein thrombosis is associated with venous stasis.
    c. Most pulmonary emboli result in pulmonary infarction.
    d. Deep vein thrombosis is associated with oral contraceptives.
    e. Large pulmonary emboli may be quickly fatal.

168. Which of the following is a sexually transmitted disease, which left untreated, may result in genital elephantiasis and rectal stricture?

    a. Gonorrhea
    b. Syphilis
    c. Chancroid
    d. Mycoplasma
    e. Lymphogranuloma venereum

169. Which of the following viruses is *not* transmitted to humans by the bite of an arthropod vector?

    a. Dengue
    b. St. Louis encephalitis
    c. Hantaan virus
    d. Eastern equine encephalitis
    e. Powassan

170. All *except* which of the following tracts enters the cerebellum through the inferior cerebellar peduncle?

    a. Cuneocerebellar tract
    b. Olivocerebellar tract
    c. Pontocerebellar tract
    d. Posterior spinocerebellar tract
    e. Reticulocerebellar tract

171. All *except* which of the following are characteristics of carrier-mediated transport (facilitated diffusion)?

    a. Transport of hydrophilic molecules at rates higher than expected based on their lipid solubility
    b. Direct dependence on hydrolysis of ATP for transport
    c. Transport saturates at high substrate concentration
    d. Only specific substances bind to specific carriers
    e. Competitive inhibition of transport may occur with similar substrates

172. A patient has a tumor that is releasing large amounts of parathyroid hormone (PTH). Which of the following findings would you expect?

    a. Erosion of bone due to loss of both organic and inorganic calcium
    b. Formation of $24,25\text{-}(OH)_2$ cholecalciferol from $25\text{-}(OH)$ calciferol is inhibited.
    c. Formation of $1,25\text{-}(OH)$ cholecalciferol from $25\text{-}(OH)$ cholecalciferol is inhibited.
    d. Formation of cholecalciferol from 7-dehydrocholesterol is inhibited.
    e. Calcium uptake by the intestinal mucosa is inhibited.

173. Which of the following sensations do C fibers transmit?

    a. Discriminative touch
    b. Flutter
    c. Limb proprioception
    d. Slow, burning pain
    e. Vibration

174. The first branches of the middle cerebral artery are prone to stroke because of their small size. However, they innervate the posterior limb of the internal capsule and can induce both sensory and motor deficits. What are these called?

    a. Central (rolandic) branches
    b. Callosomarginal arteries
    c. Lenticulostriate arteries
    d. Pericallosal arteries
    e. Recurrent artery (of Heubner)

175. When a kidney is transplanted, the sympathetic nerve supply to the kidney is interrupted for a prolonged period. During this period, infusion of a given dose of norepinephrine causes a greater renal vasoconstriction than when the same dose is given if the renal nerves are intact. What is the characteristic of the adrenergic receptors that is responsible for this increased responsiveness termed?

    a. Specificity
    b. Ligand gating
    c. Supersensitivity
    d. Down regulation
    e. Saturation

176. The predominant glial cell found in white matter is which of the following?

    a. Ependymal cell
    b. Fibrous astrocyte
    c. Interfascicular oligodendroglia
    d. Perineuronal oligodendroglia
    e. Tanycyte

Questions 177 and 178 refer to the figure.

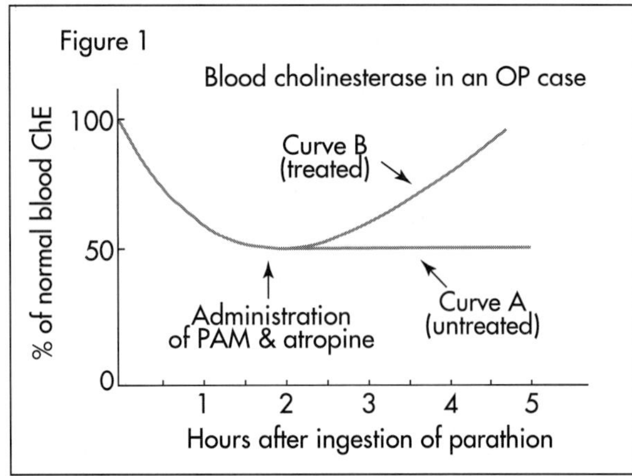

177. The marked inhibition of the cholinesterase activity in this patient is the indirect result of which of the following?

    a. Inhibition of the synthesis of acetylcholinesterase
    b. Increased secretion of the cholinesterase inhibitor
    c. Inactivation of the cholinesterase following the binding of paraoxon to the enzyme
    d. The conversion of paraoxon to parathion
    e. Increased catabolism of the cholinesterase

178. Reactivation of the blood cholinesterase after drug therapy (curve B) is due to which of the following?

    a. Increased synthesis of cholinesterase in the liver
    b. Increased complex by neostigmine therapy
    c. Pralidoxime therapy
    d. Decreased catabolism of the cholinesterase inhibitor
    e. Blocking of cholinergic effects by atropine

179. Which of the following symptoms is *not* characteristic of arsenic poisoning?

    a. Nausea, anorexia, and diarrhea
    b. Dermatitis of the skin
    c. Thinning of the skin of the palms and soles
    d. Capillary damage
    e. Personality changes

180. Of the following organisms that cause diarrhea, which causes enterocolitis that does not produce fecal leukocytosis?

    a. *Salmonella typhi*
    b. *Shigella* sp.
    c. *Yersinia enterocolitica*
    d. Enterohemorrhagic *E. coli*
    e. *Vibrio cholerae*

EXTENDED MATCHING QUESTIONS

Directions for Questions 181 through 200: Each set of questions has several lettered options, followed by several numbered items. For each numbered item, select ONE lettered option that is most closely associated with it. Each lettered option may be used once, more than once, or not at all.

Questions 181 through 185

    a. *Clostridium difficile*
    b. *Clostridium tetani*
    c. *Clostridium perfringens*
    d. *Clostridium botulinum*
    e. *Fusobacterium nucleatum*
    f. *Actinomyces israelii*
    g. *Bacteroides fragilis*
    h. *Peptostreptococcus*

Match each organism with the disease it causes.

181. Infection by this bacterium is characterized by multiple abscesses connected by sinus tracts and by the production of sulfur granules.

182. This bacterium produces a lecithinase and is a cause of food poisoning.

183. This bacterium is associated with pseudomembranous colitis and is an important nosocomial pathogen.

184. This gram-positive bacillus produces a neurotoxin which blocks the release of acetylcholine.

185. This bacterium produces a neurotoxin that blocks release of neurotransmitters of inhibitory synapses.

Questions 186 and 187

- **a.** Paranoid personality disorder
- **b.** Antisocial personality disorder
- **c.** Histrionic personality disorder
- **d.** Avoidant personality disorder
- **e.** Obsessive-compulsive personality disorder

For each of the following patient scenarios select the most appropriate diagnosis based on the data available.

186. During an interview, a patient appears to be interacting with a physician in a seductive, dramatic manner. The patient's past history suggests that the individual has had difficulty maintaining close relationships.

187. A patient reports having occupational difficulties. Upon questioning, the patient admits that a preoccupation with rules, orderliness, and neatness has caused an inability to perform tasks in a timely manner.

Questions 188 and 189

- **a.** Seminoma
- **b.** Embryonal carcinoma
- **c.** Yolk sac tumor
- **d.** Choriocarcinoma
- **e.** Teratoma
- **f.** Sertoli cell tumor
- **g.** Leydig cell tumor

Match each tumor with its description.

188. This tumor is a tumor of male children that is largely composed of a reticular (net like) pattern of undifferentiated medium- to large-sized cells with multiple microcysts and papillary projections. Multiple Schiller-Duval bodies are present. The tumor and the patient's serum are both positive for the presence of alpha-1-fetoprotein.

189. This is the most common germ cell tumor found in males.

Questions 190 and 191

- **a.** Tarasoff I
- **b.** Tarasoff II
- **c.** Wyatt v. Stickney
- **d.** M'Naghten Rule
- **e.** Durham Rule

For each of the following patient-related legal decisions, select the court ruling that addressed the issue.

190. Duty to warn

191. Right to appropriate treatment

Questions 192 and 193

- **a.** Mumps virus
- **b.** Parainfluenza virus 1
- **c.** Respiratory syncytial virus
- **d.** Measles virus
- **e.** Influenza virus A
- **f.** Parainfluenza virus 3
- **g.** Arenaviruses
- **h.** Coronaviruses
- **i.** HIV-1

Match each virus with its description.

192. After rhinoviruses this virus is the next most prevalent cause of the common cold.

193. The polyprotein gp160 of this virus is cleaved into the glycoproteins, gp 41 and gp120.

Questions 194 through 197

- **a.** Alpha-amylase
- **b.** Trypsin
- **c.** Elastase
- **d.** Chymotrypsin
- **e.** Carboxypeptidase

For each of the numbered options related to digestive enzymes, select the lettered item most closely associated with it.

194. An exopeptidase

195. Secreted in saliva

196. Cleaves amino acids from the carboxyl end of a peptide

197. Cleaves peptide linkages containing a carboxyl group from arginine or lysine

Questions 198 through 200

- **a.** Ischemic phase of endometrium
- **b.** Luteinizing hormone peak
- **c.** Proliferation of endometrium
- **d.** Menstruation
- **e.** Increasing plasma progesterone

For each of the lettered options listing factors related to the menstrual cycle, select the numbered item with which it is most closely associated.

198. Late follicular phase of cycle

199. Increasing plasma estradiol

200. Secretory phase of endometrium

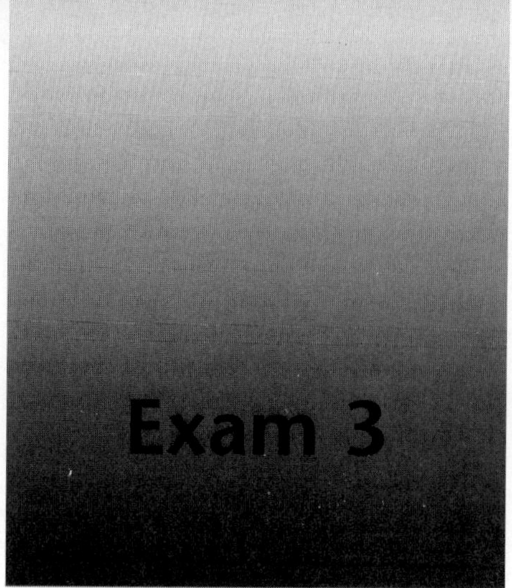

Exam 3

1. Within a few minutes after intravenous injection of insulin, all *except* which of the following changes occur in plasma?

   a. Glucose concentration decreases
   b. Amino acid concentrations increase
   c. Free fatty acid concentrations decrease
   d. Concentration of ketone bodies decreases
   e. K^+ concentration decreases

2. Injury to the superior gluteal nerve, either by direct trauma or disease, will usually result in paralysis of which of the following?

   a. Gluteus maximus muscle
   b. Gluteus medius muscle
   c. Obturator internus muscle
   d. Piriformis muscle
   e. Quadratus femoris muscle

3. A 37-year-old woman had a small lump in the upper out quadrant of her right breast, which did not change character during her menstrual cycle. Mammography showed suspicious calcification, but the lesion measured only about 1 cm in diameter. The lesion was biopsied, and the result was a diagnosis of infiltrating ductal adenocarcinoma. The patient opted for treatment with a lumpectomy and adjuvant radiation to the site. No additional tumor was found at the original biopsy site, and a sampling of axillary lymph nodes was negative for tumor. What is the likelihood of a 5-year cure in this patient?

   a. 100%
   b. 90%
   c. 80%
   d. 70%
   e. 60% or less

4. Which is the correct equation for calculating alveolar ventilation? $V_A =$

   a. $(V_{ECO2} + P_{ACO2})/K$
   b. $P_{I02} - P_{ACO2} [F_{I02} + 1]$
   c. $(P_{ICO2} \times V_{ECO2})/K$
   d. $(V_{ECO2} \times K)/P_{ACO2}$
   e. $(P_{ICO2} - P_{ECO2})/V_{ECO2})$

5. Which of the following agents are antimusarinic agents and used in drug-induced (antipsychotic) Parkinsonism?

   a. Carbidopa
   b. Bromocriptine
   c. Amantadine
   d. L-DOPA
   e. Trihexyphenidyl

6. Brainwave activity includes all *except* which of the following types?

   a. Alpha
   b. Beta
   c. Gamma
   d. Delta
   e. Theta

7. Which of the following conditions is *not* commonly associated with coxsackie virus infections?

   a. Aseptic meningitis
   b. Herpangina
   c. Pleurodynia
   d. Vesicular lesions
   e. Renal failure

8. Most cases of which of the following mycotic diseases in the United States occur in a small geographic area of the southwest?

   a. North American blastomycosis
   b. Histoplasmosis
   c. Coccidioidomycosis
   d. Candidiasis
   e. Cryptococcosis

9. Given that total lung capacity (TLC) = 6 liters, vital capacity (VC) = 4.8 liters, functional residual capacity (FRC) = 2.4 liters, and tidal volume (VT) = 0.5 liters, what would the calculation be for expiratory reserve volume (ERC) and inspiratory reserve volume (IRV)?

   a. ERV = 3.1 L, IRV = 1.2 L
   b. ERV = 1.9 L, IRV = 1.2 L
   c. ERV = 1.7 L, IRV = 0.7 L
   d. ERV = 1.2 L, IRV = 3.1 L
   e. ERV = 1.2 L, IRV = 1.7 L

10. Which hormone is *not* involved in the morphologic and physiologic changes that occur in the endometrium and ovary during the menstrual cycle?

    a. Estrogen
    b. Inhibin
    c. Progesterone
    d. Luteinizing hormone
    e. Follicle-stimulating hormone

11. Transport of glucose from plasma to a muscle cell may be increased by all *except* which of the following?

    a. An increase in the glucose concentration gradient from plasma to interstitial fluid
    b. A decrease in the rate of metabolism of glucose by the cell
    c. An increase in blood flow to the muscle
    d. An increase in the number of open capillaries in the muscle
    e. An increase in the number of fused vesicle channels in the capillary endothelium

12. How is secretion of ADH from the posterior pituitary increased?

    a. An increase in blood pressure
    b. A decrease in blood volume
    c. A decrease in plasma osmolality
    d. An increase in extracellular fluid volume
    e. A decrease in plasma K^+ concentration

13. Stimulation of the myenteric plexus results in all *except* which of the following?

    a. Increased tone of the intestinal wall
    b. Increased strength of the rhythmical contractions
    c. Increased rate of rhythmic contractions
    d. Decreased velocity of peristaltic waves
    e. Inhibited contraction of the pyloric sphincter

14. Which of the following statements is *not* true?

    a. Chloramphenicol inhibits the metabolism of tolbutamide.
    b. Disulfiram (Antabuse) inhibits the metabolism of ethanol.
    c. Isoniazid inhibits the metabolism of coumarin.
    d. Phenytoin inhibits the metabolism of digitoxin.
    e. Cimetidine inhibits the metabolism of diazepam.

15. *Mycoplasma pneumoniae* infection in humans usually is acquired by which of the following?

    a. The bite of an arthropod vector
    b. Inhalation of aerosolized droplets
    c. Aspiration of contaminated food
    d. Inoculation through a break in the skin
    e. Immunocompromising an individual by drug therapy

16. The abducens nucleus belongs to which of the following classifications?

    a. It is a general somatic efferent nucleus.
    b. It is a general visceral afferent nucleus.
    c. It is a special somatic afferent nucleus.
    d. It is a special visceral efferent nucleus.
    e. It is a general visceral efferent nucleus.

17. What does closure of the atrioventricular valves cause, and when does it occur?

    a. The second heart sound, during atrial contraction
    b. The first heart sound, at the start of the isovolumetric ventricular contraction
    c. The second heart sound, at the start of the isovolumetric ventricular relaxation
    d. The first heart sound, at the beginning of diastole
    e. The first heart sound, near the end of ventricular ejection

18. In addition to *Pseudomonas aeruginosa,* which of the following bacteria is frequently associated with cystic fibrosis?

    a. *Pseudomonas cepacia*
    b. *Pseudomonas maltophilia*
    c. *Pseudomonas pseudomallei*
    d. *Moraxella catarrhalis*
    e. *Acinetobacter calcoacetius*

19. A neurologist notes that his patient has loss of fine tactile discrimination, conscious proprioception, and vibration sense on the left side below T12. Pain and temperature sensation were absent below T12 on the right side. A spastic paresis, hyperreflexia, and increased muscle tone were present on the left along with a Babinski sign below L1. This patient probably has which of the following?

    a. Anterior spinal artery infarct
    b. Left hemisection of the spinal cord at T12
    c. Left posterior inferior cerebellar artery infarct
    d. Right posterior spinal artery infarct
    e. Right vertebral artery infarct

20. What is the most serious sequela of developing Barrett's esophagus in long-standing esphageal reflux?

    a. Esophageal stricture
    b. Esophageal varices
    c. Mallory-Weiss syndrome
    d. Hematemesis
    e. Adenocarcinoma

21. Viruses that do *not* affect the central nervous system include which of the following?

    a. Herpes simplex
    b. Enterovirus
    c. Rotavirus
    d. Rabies
    e. Measles

22. Darling's disease is caused by a dimorphic fungus in which the yeast phase is found almost exclusively in macrophages. What is another name for this disease?

    a. Coccidioidomycosis
    b. Histoplasmosis
    c. Cryptococcosis
    d. Mucormycosis
    e. Aspergillosis

23. What is the primary mechanism regulating secretion of bile salt synthesis?

    a. Decreased parasympathetic stimulation
    b. Increased sympathetic stimulation
    c. Secretion of cholecystokinin
    d. Release of motilin from the gastric mucosa
    e. Negative feedback from hepatic portal venous bile salt concentration

24. A patient with a long history of diabetes mellitus and peripheral neuropathies might *not* show which of the following?

    a. Babinski's sign
    b. Decreased deep tendon reflexes
    c. Decreased muscle tone
    d. Fasciculations
    e. Muscle atrophy

25. Which of the following statements referring to Type II, or maturity onset diabetes, is correct?

    a. A high correlation exists between the occurrence of this condition and obesity.
    b. Plasma insulin levels are often low or absent.
    c. Rapid breakdown of fats produces pronounced ketoacidosis.
    d. The prevalence of cataracts is due to glycosylation of cellular proteins in the eye.
    e. In a poorly-controlled diabetic, there is a pronounced decrease in blood levels of hemoglobin A_{1c}.

26. Which of the following structures accompanies the posterior interventricular artery within the posterior interventricular groove?

    a. Great cardiac vein
    b. Middle cardiac vein

    c. Small cardiac vein
    d. Anterior cardiac veins
    e. Coronary sinus

27. What does increased sympathetic nervous activity do?

    a. It increases the duration of systole.
    b. It induces relaxation in the arterioles in most organs.
    c. It increases the slope of the SA nodal pacemaker potential.
    d. It decreases ventricular contractility.
    e. It hyperpolarizes the membrane of sinoatrial nodal pacemaker.

28. A 72-year-old female patient was seen for a routine yearly physical examination. The patient's history revealed that the patient had not been eating a balanced diet and rarely had eaten red meat. The patient complained of chronic fatigue and upon physical examination had a somewhat yellowish hue to her skin. The CBC came back with a hematocrit of 18 and an MCV of 104. The chemistry screening examination was largely unremarkable, except for an LDH of 1852. What diagnosis is most fitting in this scenario?

    a. Iron deficiency anemia
    b. Anemia of chronic disease
    c. Red cell aplasia
    d. Myelophthistic anemia
    e. Pernicious anemia

29. Which of the following statements is *not* true of *Shigella?*

    a. It is usually associated with fecal-oral transmission.
    b. It has no lower animal reservoirs.
    c. It can invade the intestinal mucosa.
    d. It often causes a watery diarrhea without blood or mucus.
    e. It often causes bacteremia.

30. Which of the following is *not* secreted by enteroendocrine cells?

    a. Somatostatin
    b. Gastrin
    c. Intrinsic factor
    d. Secretin
    e. Cholecystokinin

31. In an obstructive lung disorder such as emphysema, all are reduced *except* which of the following?

    a. Total lung capacity
    b. Forced vital capacity (FVC)
    c. Time forced expiratory volume (FEV_1)
    d. Percent of forced vital capacity exhaled in 1 second ($FEV_1/FVC\%$)
    e. Forced midexpiratory flow ($FEF_{25\text{-}75}$)

32. How would the overall metabolic effect of insulin best be described?

    a. Increasing plasma glucose concentration in response to hypoglycemia
    b. Stimulating oxidation of lipids, glycogen, and protein
    c. Acting primarily to stimulate oxidation of glucose only
    d. Promoting storage of glycogen, fat, and protein
    e. Primarily lipolysis in liver and muscle

33. All *except* which of the following statements regarding the bulbourethral (Cowper's) glands is correct?

    a. Their ducts open into the membranous urethra.
    b. They are located within the deep perineal space.
    c. They are embedded within the fibers of the sphincter urethrae muscle.
    d. They are homologous with the greater vestibular (Bartholin's) glands in the female.
    e. Their ducts pierce the perineal membrane.

34. Systemic administration of an alpha$_1$ agonist such as phenylephrine would be expected to produce which of the following?

    a. Mydriasis, dry mouth, urinary retention, hypotension
    b. Increase in mean blood pressure, decrease in heart rate and mydriasis
    c. Relaxation of the uterus, decrease in gastrointestinal tone, increase in blood flow to skeletal muscle
    d. Tachycardia
    e. Increase in gastrointestinal tone, increase in heart rate, increase in blood flow to the kidneys

35. Which of the following inhibits glucagon secretion?

    a. Insulin
    b. Hypoglycemia
    c. Arginine
    d. Acetylcholine
    e. Catecholamines

36. Which of the following conditions does not predispose a patient to the development of bacterial endocarditis?

    a. Previous myocardial infarction
    b. Mitral valve prolapse
    c. Congenital heart disease
    d. Rheumatic valvulitis
    e. Intravenous drug use

37. Stability of the glenohumeral (shoulder) joint depends primarily on which of the following?

    a. Glenoid labrum
    b. Deltoid muscle
    c. Shape of the articular surfaces
    d. Tendons of the "rotator cuff" muscles
    e. Short head of the biceps brachii

38. What is one effect on the kidney of an increase in plasma parathyroid hormone (PTH) concentration?

    a. It decreases the formation of 1,25 dihydroxyvitamin D3.
    b. It stimulates proximal tubular reabsorption of phosphate.
    c. It stimulates Ca^{2+} secretion by the distal tubule.
    d. It increases renal tubular reabsorption of Ca^{2+}.
    e. It stimulates phosphate secretion by the loop of Henle.

39. The tract that connects the hippocampus to the septal area (nuclei) is which of the following?

    a. Arcuate fasciculus
    b. Dorsal longitudinal fasciculus
    c. Fasciculus retroflexus
    d. Fornix
    e. Stria medullaris thalami

40. With what is granulomatous inflammation typically associated?

    a. Increased production of IgM
    b. Increased production of IgG
    c. Deficiency of complement
    d. T-cell mediated immunity
    e. Abscess formation

41. Which of the following statements concerning antiparasitic chemotherapy is *false?*

    a. Mebendazole is a broad spectrum anthelmintic and is the drug of choice for infections due to ascaris, enterobius (pinworm), or hookworms (necator and ancylostoma).
    b. Praziquantel is the drug of choice for the treatment of tapeworm infections.
    c. Pyrantel pamoate is used for the treatment of pinworm (enterobiasis).
    d. Metronidazole is used for the treatment of schistosomiasis.
    e. Metronidazole is effective in the treatment of trichomonas and giardia infections.

42. Which of the following statements is *not* true of Alzheimer's disease?

    a. There is generalized cortical neuronal loss.
    b. Neuronal loss is prominent in the nucleus basalis of Meynert.
    c. Brain acetylcholine is higher than in healthy brains.
    d. Neurofibrillary tangles are prominent.
    e. Granulovacuolar degeneration occurs.

43. The metabolites of arachidonic acid are very important in mediating inflammation. Of the following arachidonic acid metabolites, which does *not* act to produce vasodilatation?

    a. PGL_2
    b. PDG_2
    c. PGF_{2a}
    d. TXA_2
    e. LTB_4

44. Which of the following is *least* likely to affect the V_{max} of an enzyme?

    a. A change in pH
    b. A change in temperature
    c. Addition of a noncompetitive inhibitor
    d. Addition of a competitive inhibitor
    e. Increased ionic strength

45. Axons originating in the cornea synapse on which of the following nuclei?

    a. Chief sensory nucleus of nerve V
    b. Facial nucleus
    c. Mesencephalic nucleus of nerve V
    d. Nucleus solitarius
    e. Spinal nucleus of nerve V

46. Carbon dioxide is carried in the blood in three forms: dissolved CO_2, carbamino compounds, and HCO_3^-. Normally, what percent of the total CO_2 is carried in each form?

    a. 20% HCO_3^-, 65% carbamino compounds, 15% dissolved CO_2
    b. 40% HCO_3^-, 40% carbamino compounds, 10% dissolved CO_2
    c. 50% HCO_3^-, 10% carbamino compounds, 40% dissolved CO_2
    d. 75% HCO_3^-, 5% carbamino compounds, 20% dissolved CO_2
    e. 90% HCO_3^-, 5% carbamino compounds, 5% dissolved CO_2

47. Spike potentials (action potentials) in intestinal smooth muscle have all *except* which of the following characteristics?

    a. They are caused by opening of slow Ca^{2+} channels.
    b. Ca^{2+} entering during the action potential reacts with calmodulin to activate myosin.
    c. They occur when slow potentials are hyperpolarized (more negative).
    d. They are slower then action potentials in large myelinated nerve fibers.
    e. Unlike slow waves, they initiate contraction of smooth muscle.

48. Most axons arising from the nucleus gracilis will terminate in which of the following?

    a. Contralateral VA nucleus
    b. Contralateral VPL nucleus
    c. Ipsilateral postcentral gyrus
    d. Ipsilateral VPM nucleus
    e. Ipsilateral VL nucleus

49. The tendon of which of the following muscles attaches at the most inferior facet of the greater tubercle of humerus?

    a. Supraspinatus
    b. Infraspinatus
    c. Subscapularis
    d. Teres major
    e. Teres minor

50. Which of the following is not associated with the development of Cushing's syndrome?

    a. Adrenal cortical adenoma
    b. Corticotrope hyperplasia of the adenohypophysis
    c. Diffuse adrenal hyperplasia
    d. Exogenous corticosteroids
    e. Chromophobe adenoma of the hypophysis

51. A middle-aged man is taking high, anti-inflammatory doses of aspirin to control his rheumatoid arthritis. To alleviate occasional stomach pain, he takes ranitidine or Rolaids. His impacted wisdom tooth is causing him more and more pain so he decided to have his wisdom tooth pulled. The surgery is accompanied by excessive bleeding, which surprises the patient because he had no previous bleeding disorders.

What is the likely cause of the patient's excessive bleeding?

    a. Activation of the fibrinolytic system by raniditine.
    b. Late onset (adult form) hemophilia
    c. Inhibition of thromboxane synthesis by aspirin
    d. Raniditine-induced thrombocytopenia
    e. Antacid-induced deficiency of vitamin K

52. Which of the following drugs is given in an inactive form and not activated until it reaches the liver?

    a. Doxorubicin
    b. Bleomycin
    c. Cyclophosphamide
    d. L-asparaginase
    e. Methotrexate

53. All *except* which of the following drugs will inhibit the release of ACTH from the pituitary?

    a. Cortisone
    b. Reserpine
    c. Morphine
    d. Methyrapone
    e. Chlorpromazine

Questions 54 and 55 refer to the following figure.

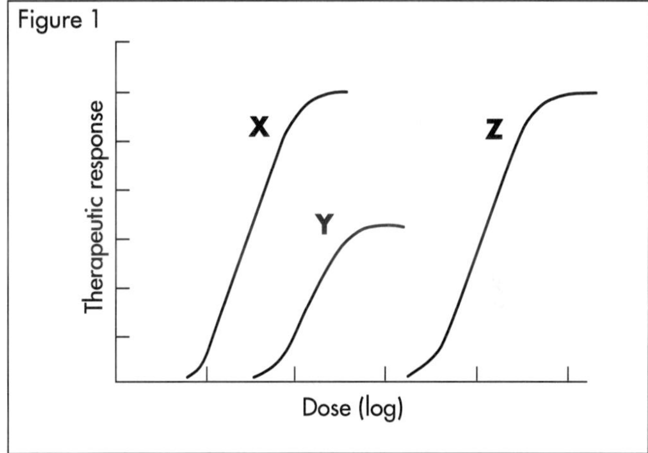

54. Which drug in Figure 1 has the greatest potency?

    a. X
    b. Y
    c. Z
    d. X and Z are similar.

55. Which drug has the greatest efficacy in Figure 1?

    a. X
    b. Z
    c. Y
    d. X and Z are similar.

56. Which of the following statements is true with regard to prokaryotic DNA replication?

    a. Polymerization is continuous on both the leading and the lagging strands of the helix.
    b. The process is unidirectional from the origin of replication.

    c. DNA-directed RNA polymerase is required.
    d. Nucleotides are added at the 5′ end of new strands.
    e. Proofreading by DNA ligase reduces mutations.

57. Thalamic pain is an example of which of the following?

    a. Pain resulting from excitation of A delta fibers
    b. Pain unrelated to nociceptor activation
    c. Referred pain
    d. Subliminal pain
    e. Visceral pain

58. Lyme disease can be assumed to be the clinical disease in question if which one of the following criteria is *not* met?

    a. Isolation of *Borrelia burgdorferi* from the patient
    b. Demonstration of diagnostic levels of IgG or IgM antibodies
    c. Transient exposure to the tick vector in an endemic area
    d. Significant increase in antibody titer between acute and convalescent serum samples to *Borrelia burgdorferi.*
    e. Erythema migrans $\geq$ 5 cm in diameter as a result of a bite

59. In which of the following diseases is toxemia *not* an important component?

    a. Diphtheria
    b. Whooping cough
    c. Syphilis
    d. Scarlet fever
    e. Plague

60. Which of the following statements concerning the Arnold-Chiari malformation of the brain is *true?*

    a. This malformation is associated with an enlarged posterior fossa.
    b. The cerebellar vermis is absent.
    c. A midline ependymal-lined cyst is present, replacing the cerebellar vermis.
    d. There is usually associated hydrocephalus and lumbar meningomyelocele.
    e. A cervical syrinx is usually present.

61. Which of the following is *not* a useful criterion for distinguishing leiomyosarcoma from leiomyoma?

    a. Extensive necrosis
    b. Cellular atypia
    c. > 10 mitotic figures per high power field
    d. Irregular extension into the surrounding myometrium
    e. Subserosal location

62. Stimulation of the posterior hypothalamus does *not* lead to which of the following?

    a. An increased basal metabolic rate
    b. A search for clothing
    c. Shivering
    d. Sweating
    e. Vasoconstriction

63. Which of the following blocks alpha$_1$ receptors?

    a. Metoprolol
    b. Clonidine
    c. Butoxamine
    d. Labetalol
    e. Pindolol

64. The coagulase and fibrinolysin of *Yersinia pestis* play a key role in the pathogenesis of infection by coagulating blood in which of the following?

    a. Human and dissolving the clot in the flea
    b. Rat and dissolving the clot in the flea
    c. Rat and dissolving the clot in the human
    d. Flea and dissolving the clot in the human
    e. Human and dissolving the clot in the rat

65. Which is the major force contributing to stabilization of the native (tertiary) structure of a protein?

    a. Electrostatic bonding
    b. Hydrogen bonding
    c. Hydrophobic bonding
    d. Disulfide bonds
    e. Peptide bonds

66. As the secretion of saliva is stimulated, what changes occur in saliva as compared to its composition in the resting state?

    a. Increasing acidity to aid in digestion of protein
    b. Decreasing osmolality
    c. Increasing of HCO_3^-
    d. Decreasing amylase concentration
    e. Increasing K^+ concentration

67. Which structure is *not* lined with stratified squamous epithelium (keratinized, nonkeratinized, or parakeratinized)?

    a. External auditory meatus
    b. Corneal epithelium
    c. Dorsal surface of the tongue
    d. Lip
    e. Anterior surface of the lens

68. BAL is not an effective antidote for which of the following pesticides?

    a. Sodium fluoride
    b. Corrosive sublimate (mercuric chloride)
    c. Arsenic trioxide
    d. Paris green (copper-aceto-arsenite)
    e. Tartar emetic (antimony potassium tartrate)

69. During a ventricular muscle cell action potential, the initial, rapid depolarization is primarily due to which of the following?

    a. Increase in K^+ permeability
    b. Increase in Cl^- permeability
    c. Increase in Na^+ permeability
    d. Decrease in Na^+ permeability
    e. Decrease in Ca^{2+} permeability

70. Looking at the cut surface of a midsagittal section of the brain, which of the following is *not* seen?

    a. Anterior commissure
    b. Corpus callosum
    c. Fornix
    d. Globus pallidus
    e. Lamina terminalis

71. Histologically, what is the major prognostic feature in a malignant melanoma?

    a. The width of the radial growth phase
    b. The number of mitotic figures per high power field
    c. The depth of invasion (Breslow thickness)
    d. The presence of a lymphocytic infiltrate at the tumor base
    e. Evidence of tumor regression

72. Which of the following is *true* for eukaryotic gene expression?

    a. Enhancers only work when they are close to the promoter.
    b. The promoters of actively regulated genes often lack the TATA box.
    c. CG islands near housekeeping genes are heavily methylated.
    d. Enhancers may be located downstream from the genes that they regulate.
    e. Enhancers act by inhibiting termination of transcription in eukaryotic genes.

73. The fibers of the corona radiata converge to form a compact band known as which of the following?

    a. Anterior commissure
    b. Corpus callosum
    c. External medullary lamina
    d. Fornix
    e. Internal capsule

74. Which organ(s) normally has (have) the *least* resistance to blood flow?

    a. Brain
    b. Heart
    c. Lungs
    d. Liver
    e. Kidneys

75. Of the following, which is *not* mediated primarily by alpha-adrenergic receptors?

    a. Cutaneous vasoconstriction
    b. Increased sweating
    c. Coronary vasodilation
    d. Contraction of the radial muscle of the iris
    e. Increased cardiac glycogenolysis

76. Which of the following produces the most significant stimulation of fatty acid release from adipose tissue?

    a. Isoproterenol
    b. Methoxamine
    c. Dopamine
    d. Phenylephrine
    e. Oxymetazoline

77. Mesosomes of bacteria are thought to function as which of the following?

    a. Attachment sites for flagella
    b. An intermediary in endospore formation
    c. Receptors for chemotactic stimuli
    d. An attachment site for the replicating bacterial chromosome
    e. Attachment sites for fimbriae

78. During the swing phase of walking, the most important muscle stabilizing the hip is which of the following?

    a. Gluteus maximus
    b. Semitendinosus
    c. Gluteus medius
    d. Long head of the biceps femoris
    e. Obturator externus

79. As the ventilation/perfusion ratio $\dot{V}_A/\dot{Q}$ increases, alveolar gas composition (P_{O_2} and P_{CO_2}) changes to more closely resemble the gas composition of which of the following?

    a. Mixed venous blood
    b. Systemic capillary blood
    c. Systemic arterial blood
    d. Inspired air
    e. Pulmonary arterial blood

80. Individuals who are at high risk for drug-induced hemolytic anemia are deficient in which of the following?

    a. Pseudocholinesterase
    b. Cytochrome P-450 2B1
    c. N-acetyltransferase
    d. Alcohol dehydrogenase
    e. Glucose-6-phosphate dehydrogenase

81. Labetalol should *not* be used to treat which of the following?

    a. Hypertensive patients with cardiac failure
    b. Patients with second degree heart block
    c. Hypertensive patients with peripheral vascular disease
    d. Hypertensive patients with chronic obstructive pulmonary disease (COPD)
    e. The young, physically active hypertensive patient

82. Groups of epithelial cells are held together by intracellular contacts. All *except* which of the following is an intracellular contact observed between adjacent epithelial cells?

    a. Zonula occludens
    b. Macula occludens
    c. Desmosomes
    d. Tight junctions
    e. Macula adherens

83. Which sequence listed below represents diuretic effectiveness?

	Loop diuretics	Potassium-sparing diuretics	Thiazide diuretics
a.	+++	++	+
b.	+++	+	++
c.	++	+	+++
d.	++	+++	+
e.	+	++	+++

    +++ Most effective
    ++ Somewhat effective
    + Least effective

84. Which of the following parasites is able to evade the normal immune response by localizing itself in vacuoles within macrophages?

    a. *Ascaris lumbricoides*
    b. *Schistosoma mansoni*
    c. *Trypanosoma brucei*
    d. *Leishmania donovani*
    e. *Toxoplamsa gondii*

85. The parathyroid glands produce parathyroid hormone (PTH), which functions to increase the blood-calcium level via a feedback system. With this in mind, which of the following is *not* a function of PTH?

    a. Enhances bone resorption
    b. Reduces excretion of calcium by the kidneys
    c. Stimulates absorption of calcium by bones
    d. Stimulates osteoclast activity
    e. Stimulates absorption of calcium by the small intestine

86. Which of the following is *not* a component of the respiratory epithelium?

    a. Brush cell
    b. Basal cell
    c. Goblet cell
    d. Ciliated cell
    e. Sustentacular cell

87. Cancer of the prostate is very common. Since early malignant tumor growth does not impinge on the urethra, symptoms of prostate cancer are often masked until the tumor is inoperable. Based on this information, which region in the prostate is most likely to be affected by prostate cancer?

    a. Main prostatic gland
    b. Submucosal gland
    c. Mucosal gland
    d. Epithelium of prostatic urethra
    e. Epithelium of prostatic utricle

88. The reservoir of the plague *bacillus* is in rats, but the organism is usually transmitted by which of the following?

    a. Fleas
    b. Mites
    c. Ticks
    d. Mosquitoes
    e. Lice

89. Which of the following statements regarding the dens is *not* correct?

    a. It occupies a position within the vertebral foramen of the atlas.
    b. It articulates with the posterior arch of the atlas.
    c. Developmentally, it represents the body of the first cervical vertebra.
    d. It is also known as the odontoid process.
    e. It is attached to the occipital bone by a ligament.

90. The pudendal (Alcosk's) canal is a fascial compartment located on the lateral wall of the ischioanal fossa. In this location it lies along the inferior border of which of the following muscles?

    a. Coccygeus
    b. Obturator internus
    c. Pubococcygeus
    d. Iliococcygeus
    e. Piriformis

91. A patient with a tumor involving the cerebellum may exhibit all *except* which of the following?

    a. Dysarthria
    b. Dysdiadochokinesis
    c. Dysmetria
    d. Nystagmus
    e. Resting tremor

92. How is dapsone used?

    a. Used to treat tuberculosis
    b. Used systemically to treat leishmaniasis
    c. Used systemically to treat deep, mycotic infections
    d. Orally effective agent used to treat superficial, mycotic infections
    e. Used to treat leprosy

93. Tinea infections are likely to involve which of the following microorganisms?

    a. *Cryptococcus neoformans*
    b. *Trichosporon beigelii*
    c. *Trichophyton schoenleinii*
    d. *Sporothrix schenckeii*
    e. *Candida albicans*

94. A 50-year-old male (70 kg) is given oral atenolol (50 mg once a day) to treat hypertension. Atenolol has the following characteristics:

    Volume of distribution = 1 L/kg
    Oral bioavailability (F) = 0.60
    Half-life = 6 hr

    The total body clearance of atenolol in this patient is about which of the following?

    a. 50 ml/min
    b. 100 ml/min
    c. 135 ml/min
    d. 250 ml/min
    e. 600 ml/min

95. A patient has been treated for schizophrenia and has developed severe tardive dyskinesia. This patient is placed on a different medication for his schizophrenia but has to have frequent blood tests. The doctor is very insistent that these tests be taken.

    What drug was likely prescribed for this patient?

    a. Carbamazapine
    b. Clozapine

c. Meperidine
d. Maprotiline
e. Trazodone

96. All *except* which of the following statements regarding the phrenic nerves is correct?

   a. They supply a portion of the parietal pleura.
   b. They are in contact with parietal pleura.
   c. They contain motor as well as sensory nerve fibers.
   d. A portion of them lie within the superior mediastinum.
   e. They arise from spinal cord segments C5-C7.

97. Which one of the following statements about purine and pyrimidine biosynthesis is *correct?*

   a. Thymidine 5'-phosphate is formed in a reaction involving the direct participation of PRPP and thymidine.
   b. Only the *de novo* synthesis of pyrimidines is inhibited by methotrexate.
   c. The ring structures of purines and pyrimidines are built first and then are attached to PRPP.
   d. The committed step in pyrimidine biosynthesis is catalyzed by orotate decarboxylase.
   e. AMP and GMP regulate each other's rate of synthesis.

98. Which of the following does *not* relate to Hantavirus infection or transmission?

   a. Aerosol transmission
   b. Rodent reservoir
   c. Hemorrhagic fever
   d. Nephritis
   e. Mosquito vector

99. What causes reflex bradycardia?

   a. Isoproterenol
   b. Terbutaline
   c. Phentolamine
   d. Clonidine
   e. Methoxamine

100. A patient with a tumor invading only the optic chiasm could have which of the following?

   a. Bitemporal hemianopsia
   b. Contralateral hemianopsia
   c. Scotomas
   d. Total blindness
   e. Upper contralateral quadrantic anopsia

101. A painful lesion is associated with disease caused by which of the following organisms?

   a. *Brucella abortus*
   b. *Borrelia burgdorferi*
   c. *Mycobacterium leprae*
   d. *Haemophilus ducreyi*
   e. *Treponema pallidum*

102. Compared to healthy individuals, lung compliance in a person with obstructive lung disease is __________ , and compliance in restrictive lung disease is __________ .

   a. Decreased, decreased
   b. Decreased, increased

c. Increased, decreased
d. Increased, not changed
e. Not changed, increased

103. Which of the following statements about digoxin and digitoxin is *not* true?

   a. Digitoxin is eliminated primarily by metabolic transformation in the liver.
   b. Digitoxin is more completely absorbed from the gastrointestinal tract than digoxin.
   c. Total body equilibrium following daily administration is reached more rapidly with digitoxin than with digoxin.
   d. The margin of safety is narrow for both glycosides.
   e. Digitoxin binds to plasma proteins more than digoxin.

104. The nucleus ambiguus supplies axons found in all *except* which of the following cranial nerves?

   a. Glossopharyngeal nerve
   b. Hypoglossal nerve
   c. Spinoaccessory nerve
   d. Vagus nerve

105. In chronic obstructive lung disease, what is the primary drive maintaining ventilation?

   a. Changes in PaO_2 sensed by peripheral chemoreceptors
   b. Increased PCO_2 sensed by the aortic body
   c. Increased plasma HCO_3^- concentration increasing CSF H^+
   d. Changes in arterial pH sensed by peripheral chemoreceptors
   e. Changes in PO_2 sensed by medullary chemoreceptors

106. In acute inflammation, what is the vascular structure most commonly involved in the movement of neutrophils into the extravascular space?

   a. Regional artery
   b. Precapillary arteriole
   c. Capillary
   d. Postcapillary venule
   e. Regional vein

107. All *except* which of the following statements regarding the prostatic urethra is correct?

   a. It may be obstructed as a result of benign prostatic hypertrophy.
   b. It is the most dilatable portion of the urethra.
   c. The urethral crest is located along its anterior wall.
   d. The ejaculatory ducts open onto the colliculus seminalis.
   e. The prostatic ductules open into prostatic sinuses.

108. B-lymphocytes do *not* predominate in which of the following?

   a. The PALS of the spleen
   b. Palatine tonsils
   c. Peyer's patches
   d. Spleen follicles
   e. The outer cortex of the lymph node

109. What is the isoelectric point of a protein?

  a. The pH at which each carboxyl group is protonated and each amino group is unprotonated
  b. When the pH is equal to the pK
  c. The pH at which all groups are unprotonated
  d. The pH at which the net charge on the molecule is 0
  e. The pH at which all groups have a positive charge

110. Histologically, what does Paget's disease of the bone show?

  a. Lack of bony remodeling with a woven appearance
  b. Heightened osteoclastic activity with significant enlargement of the Haversian canals
  c. A mosaic pattern of lamellar bone with a jigsaw puzzle appearance
  d. Overgrowth of inadequately mineralized cartilage

111. Which of the following nerves is at risk during surgical removal of the axillary tail of the breast?

  a. Thoracodorsal
  b. Upper subscapular
  c. Lower subscapular
  d. Long thoracic
  e. Phrenic

112. How does an RNA primer formed during replication differ from other RNA?

  a. It is always hybridized with DNA.
  b. It is formed by helicase.
  c. It is synthesized by DNA polymerase.
  d. It always contains a $3'$-triphosphate group.
  e. It contains thymidine in place of uracil.

113. Which of the following statements concerning pernicious anemia is *false*?

  a. A loading dose of 1000 μg cyanocobalamin is futile because most of the drug will be excreted.
  b. In the absence of a neurologic disorder, the anemia should be treated with folic acid.
  c. The therapeutic goal is to support hemoglobin and red cell synthesis and replete liver stores of vitamin B_{12}.
  d. Treatment with cyanocobalamin or hydroxocobalamin will continue for life.
  e. The drug of choice is cyanocobalamin because hydroxocobalamin can give rise to allergic reactions.

114. Patients treated with parenteral aminoglycoside antibiotics (e.g., Amikacin, Garamycin, Kanamycin) should be monitored closely for which of the following?

  a. Hearing loss
  b. Insomnia
  c. Resting tremor
  d. Seizures
  e. Tardive dyskinesias

115. Excess secretion of antidiuretic hormone often leads to hyponatremia (low plasma Na^+ concentration). What is likely to happen in a patient with hyponatremia?

  a. Plasma osmolality is increased.
  b. The osmolality of the plasma is decreased, but the osmolality of the interstital fluid is normal.
  c. Total body water is decreased.
  d. The osmolality of the extracellular and intracellular fluids are decreased.
  e. The osmolality of the extracellular and intracellular fluids are increased.

116. Hepatitis D virus (Delta agent) is *not* characterized by which of the following properties?

  a. It is a single-stranded, circular, RNA genome.
  b. It is a defective satellite virus.
  c. It can replicate only in hepatitis C-infected cells.
  d. It is spread in blood, semen, and vaginal fluids.
  e. It is responsible for about 40% of fulminant hepatitis infections.

117. A patient with a lower motor neuron (LMN) lesion of the XII nerve might have all *except* which of the following symptoms?

  a. Atrophy of the tongue muscles
  b. Deviation of the tongue to the side opposite the damaged nerve
  c. Fasciculations of the tongue muscles
  d. Furrowing of the tongue

118. Which of the following is correct regarding the transverse ligament of the atlas?

  a. It connects the atlas with the occipital bone.
  b. It permits nodding of the head, as when indicating approval.
  c. It holds dens in contact with the anterior arch of the atlas.
  d. It connects the atlas with the axis.
  e. It is covered anteriorly by the tectorial membrane.

119. Insulin-induced hypoglycemia may cause all *except* which of the following signs?

  a. Dizziness
  b. Tachycardia
  c. Weakness
  d. Hot dry skin
  e. Confusion

120. Lower animals are important reservoirs for all *except* which of the following?

  a. *Vibrio parahemolyticus*
  b. *Francisella tularensis*
  c. *Salmonella enteritidis*
  d. *Clostridium botulinum*
  e. *Yersinia pestis*

121. Which of the following cells would *not* be found in the buffy coat?

  a. Plasma cells
  b. Lymphocytes
  c. Neutrophils
  d. Monocytes
  e. Eosinophils

122. Which of the following does *not* possess lymphoid nodules?

  a. Peyer's patches
  b. Spleen
  c. Thymus

    d. Lymph nodes
    e. Palatine tonsil

123. The juxtaglomerular (JG) apparatus does *not* include which of the following?

    a. Macula densa cells
    b. Juxtaglomerular cells
    c. Modified smooth muscle cells
    d. Extraglomerular mesangeal cells
    e. Podocyte

124. The extracellular matrix of hyaline cartilage does *not* possess which of the following molecules?

    a. Hyaluronic acid
    b. Keratin sulfate
    c. Chondroitin sulfate
    d. Cytokeratin
    e. Type II collagen

125. Which of the following syndromes is seen with the use of antipsychotic drugs and would most likely respond well to an antimuscarinic agent like benztropine?

    a. Parkinson's disease
    b. Tardive dyskinesia
    c. Acute dystonic reactions
    d. Akathisia
    e. Perioral tremor

126. Which of the following nerves is responsible for innervating the muscles of the extensor compartment of the arm (brachium)?

    a. Axillary
    b. Radial
    c. Musculocutaneous
    d. Median
    e. Ulnar

127. Why is gestational choriocarcinoma unique among human malignant tumors?

    a. It typically has a karyotype of 47,XXY.
    b. It typically has a karyotype of 47,XXX.
    c. It results from parthenogenetic reproduction of an ovum.
    d. It is a tumor allograft from a fetus to the mother.
    e. It results from the dual fertilization of an ovum by two sperm.

128. The anterior spinal artery is usually formed from branches of which of the following?

    a. Anterior inferior cerebellar arteries
    b. Basilar artery
    c. Internal carotid arteries
    d. Posterior inferior cerebellar arteries
    e. Vertebral arteries

129. Which of the following reversibly inhibits utilization of para-aminobenzoic acid in dihydrofolate synthesis?

    a. Sulfadiazine
    b. Tetracycline
    c. Amphotericin B
    d. Methotrexate
    e. Amantadine

130. The lateral hypothalamus is the center for which of the following?

    a. Feeding
    b. Micturition
    c. Satiety
    d. Sexual pleasure
    e. Thirst

131. Which of the effects listed below are likely to occur during antihypertensive treatment with clonidine?

	Renin secretion	Sympathetic nerve activity	Vascular resistance	Blood pressure
a.	increase	decrease	increase	decrease
b.	increase	decrease	decrease	increase
c.	decrease	increase	decrease	increase
d.	decrease	increase	increase	decrease
e.	decrease	decrease	decrease	decrease

132. In adenocarcinoma of the stomach, what is the best predictor of clinical outcome?

    a. The histologic type
    b. The region of the stomach involved
    c. The presence or absence of atrophic gastritis
    d. Achlorhydria
    e. The depth of invasion

133. Which of the following is an intermediate precursor in the synthesis of norepinephrine and dopamine?

    a. 5-HIAA
    b. Choline
    c. Epinephrine
    d. GABA
    e. L-DOPA

134. Which of the following is *not* a characteristic of *Mycoplasma?*

    a. Requires sterols for growth
    b. Lacks a typical bacterial cell wall
    c. Is susceptible to tetracycline
    d. Is susceptible to penicillin
    e. Replicates by binary fission

135. Periodontal disease is caused by the accumulation of calcified food and bacterial debris in which of the following?

    a. Crypts of palatine tonsils
    b. Narrow, moat-like channels that surround circumvallate papillae
    c. Gingival sulci
    d. Dental pulp
    e. Between adjacent filiform papillae

136. The final components of the immunoglobulin heavy chain variable region are assembled at which of the following levels?

    a. DNA level
    b. RNA level
    c. Protein level
    d. DNA and RNA level
    e. RNA and protein levels

137. Beta-endorphin is derived from the prohormone peptide known as which of the following?

    a. Proenkephalin
    b. Prodynorphin
    c. Prolactin
    d. Proopiomelanocortin
    e. Pancreatic polypeptide

138. In gram-negative sepsis (endotoxin shock) bacteria that undergo lysis release lipopolysaccharide from their cell wall. This binds to lipopolysaccharide, which binds protein in the plasma. This complex then binds to receptors on the cell membrane of macrophages. The macrophages are stimulated to release a cytokine, which causes injury to the endothelium and loss of fluid from the vascular to the extravascular space. Which macrophage-produced cytokine is most responsible for the development of endothelial injury?

    a. C5a
    b. C3b
    c. IL-8
    d. Nitric oxide
    e. TNFa

139. The thinnest portion of the blood-air barrier consists of all *except* which of the following?

    a. Cytoplasm of type I pneumocytes
    b. Cytoplasm of alveolar macrophages
    c. Cytoplasm of endothelial cells
    d. Basal lamina of type I pneumocytes
    e. Basal lamina of endothelial cells

140. Second order sensory cell bodies can be found in all *except* which of the following?

    a. Chief sensory nucleus of nerve V
    b. Nucleus cuneatus
    c. Nucleus solitarius
    d. Mesencephalic nucleus of nerve V
    e. Spinal nucleus of nerve V

141. A victim of a drive-by shooting is brought to the medical examiner's office. During the course of the autopsy, it was noted that there was a gunshot wound of the head, which penetrated the skull on both sides. In examining the wound, the pathologist saw that on the right side the defect in the outer table of the skull was wider than that of the inner table. What can be said of the location of the assailant with respect to the victim?

    a. The assailant was to the right of the victim.
    b. The assailant was to the left of the victim.
    c. The assailant was in front of the victim.
    d. The assailant was behind the victim.
    e. The information is inadequate to determine location.

142. A 27-year-old male is diagnosed with Hodgkin's disease. At the time of diagnosis, the patient has no symptoms other than slight lymphadenopathy of his right cervical lymph nodes. A CT scan, bone marrow examination, liver biopsy, and splenectomy all fail to show the presence of Hodgkin's disease, except in the right cervical lymph nodes. Histologically, an involved cervical node was diagnosed as Hodgkin's disease, mixed cellularity. At what stage would this patient be classified using the Ann Arbor Staging System?

    a. Stage I-A
    b. Stage I-B
    c. Stage II-A
    d. Stage II-B
    e. Stage III-A

143. Which of the following is *not* a characteristic finding in Crohn's disease?

    a. Any portion of the GI tract may be involved, from the mouth to the anus.
    b. Surgery at an early stage, when only a single site is involved, often produces a permanent cure.
    c. The most frequent complications are fistula formation and intestinal obstruction.
    d. The inflammation in Crohn's disease is typically transmural and skips from place to place.
    e. Submucosal granulomas are often a prominent part of the inflammatory pattern.

144. At one-half neutralization of a glutamic acid side chain carboxyl by a strong base, which of the following is *true*?

    a. The pK of the carboxyl is changed.
    b. The side chain is in its best buffering range.
    c. The side chain has lost its buffering capacity.
    d. The pH equals 7.0.
    e. The pH is more than the pK.

145. What is the primary mechanism whereby central chemoreceptors respond to changes in arterial P_{CO_2}?

    a. Exchange of HCO_3^- in cerebrospinal fluid (CSF) for Cl^- in blood $\rightarrow$ increased CSF $[H^+]$ $\rightarrow$ stimulate chemoreceptor neurons $\rightarrow$ increased ventilation
    b. Increased Pa_{CO_2} $\rightarrow$ increased CSF P_{CO_2} $\rightarrow$ hydration to carbonic acid $\rightarrow$ dissociation to H^+ and HCO_3^- $\rightarrow$ H^+ stimulates chemoreceptor neurons $\rightarrow$ increased ventilation
    c. Diffusion of H^+ into CSF $\rightarrow$ decreased CSF pH $\rightarrow$ stimulate hypothalamic chemoreceptors $\rightarrow$ decreased ventilation
    d. Increased Pa_{CO_2} $\rightarrow$ decreased CSF P_{O_2} $\rightarrow$ stimulate medullary chemoreceptors $\rightarrow$ decreased ventilation
    e. Decreased Pa_{CO_2} $\rightarrow$ decreased CSF P_{CO_2} $\rightarrow$ decreased CSF pH $\rightarrow$ stimulate medullary chemoreceptors $\rightarrow$ increased ventilation

146. All *except* which of the following are characteristics of eukaryotic chromosome structure?

    a. The repeating unit of chromatin structure is the nucleosome.
    b. Histones are small basic proteins that are components of all nucleosomes.
    c. The nucleosome unit contains about 200 base pairs of DNA.
    d. RNA is an integral component of the nucleosome core.
    e. Some short DNA sequences may be repeated as many as one million times.

147. A 74-year-old patient with a 12-year history of calcific aortic stenosis died of an unrelated cause, and at autopsy was found to have a heart that weighed 780 g (normal < 360 g). What is the mechanism that caused this increase in myocardial weight?

    a. Hypertrophy
    b. Hyperplasia
    c. Metaplasia
    d. Atrophy
    e. Fatty change

148. In acute lymphoblastic leukemia there are two major factors effecting the prognosis. The initial blood leukocyte count at the time of diagnosis is one, what is the other major factor?

    a. The age at onset of the disease
    b. B-cell subtype
    c. T-cell subtype
    d. Null cell subtype
    e. Presence of lymphadenopathy

149. A 62-year-old male patient has a routine physical examination in which urinalysis reveals painless hematuria. The patient is referred to a urologist who performs a cystoscopy. Within the bladder is a frond-like growth, which was biopsied. Histologically there is a delicate frond-like exophytic lesion with a delicate fibrovascular core covered by a layer of normal appearing urothelium. The lesion is limited to the mucosa and shows no suggestion of invasion. What may be said of this lesion?

    a. This lesion is a benign transitional cell papilloma.
    b. This lesion represents transitional cell carcinoma in situ.
    c. This lesion rarely recurs once resected.
    d. One half of patients with this lesion develop invasive carcinoma.
    e. This lesion is a low-grade, transitional cell carcinoma.

150. A genetic deficiency of liver phosphorylase produces a less severe hypoglycemia than when glucose-6-phosphatase is deficient. This is explained by which of the following statements?

    a. Glycolysis cannot occur if phosphorylase is deficient.
    b. Glucagon activates phosphorylase but not glucose-6-phosphatase.
    c. The liver can still regulate blood glucose with a phosphorylase deficiency, but not with a glucose-6-phosphatase deficiency.
    d. Liver phosphorylase is allosterically inhibited by glucose-6-phosphate.
    e. Glucose that is formed from fatty acids can maintain blood glucose within the normal range.

151. Which of the following is *not* an effect of glucocorticoids?

    a. Inhibition of gastric acid secretion
    b. Stimulation of hepatic gluconeogenesis
    c. Inhibition of ACTH secretion and synthesis
    d. Inhibition of bone formation
    e. Decrease in the mass of the thymus

152. Which of the following cells do *not* secrete the antibacterial enzyme lysozyme?

    a. Chief cells in the fundic stomach
    b. Serous cells in the parotid gland
    c. Serous cells in the lacrimal gland
    d. Serous cells in the submandibular gland
    e. Paneth cells in the jejunum

153. Motility of the following bacteria occurs by means of axial filaments with the exception of which of the following?

    a. *Leptospira interrogans*
    b. *Vibrio cholerae*
    c. *Borrelia burgdorferi*
    d. *Treponema carateum*
    e. *Treponema pallidum*

154. Trophic hormones of the adenohypophysis do *not* include which of the following?

    a. Somatotropin
    b. Thyrotropin
    c. Melatonin
    d. Luteinizing hormone
    e. Prolactin

155. Which of the following is a specialized area of epithelium with a rich vascular supply in the lateral wall of the cochlear duct? Some of its cells contain Na-K-ATPase and other enzymes that are involved in ion and fluid regulation.

    a. Stria choroidalis
    b. Vestibular membrane
    c. Endolymphatic sac
    d. Stria vascularis
    e. Pia vascularis

156. Inspection of the left ventricle reveals all *except* which of the following?

    a. Papillary muscles
    b. Trabeculae carneae
    c. Chordae tendineae
    d. Conus arteriosus
    e. Openings of venae cordis minimae

157. The polymerase chain reaction can detect extremely small amounts of specific DNA sequences. This analytical tool requires which one of the following?

    a. Primer sequences added to the target DNA in equimolar quantities
    b. Addition of DNA polymerase after each heating cycle
    c. A sequence of heating and cooling cycles
    d. The entire sequence of the DNA to be detected must be known
    e. Helicase and primase acting as a primosome

158. A dense lymphocytic perivascular infiltrate within the inflammed synovium is one of the histologic findings in rheumatoid arthritis. The lymphocytes in this infiltrate are primarily which of the following?

    a. B cells
    b. Null cells
    c. CD-4 (helper) T cells

    d. CD-8 positive (supressor) cells
    e. Natural killer cells

159. From the following data, calculate Tm glucose (the maximal transport rate).

    Plasma [glucose] = 100 mg/100 ml
    Urine [glucose] = 2 mg/ml
    Glomerular filtration rate = 120 ml/min
    Urine flow = 0.5 ml/min

    a. 119 ml/min
    b. 1.19 mg/min
    c. 119 mg/min
    d. 0; glucose is completely reabsorbed
    e. 50 mg/min

160. The gyrus that is immediately rostral to the central sulcus and dorsal to the lateral fissure is known as which of the following?

    a. Angular gyrus
    b. Postcentral gyrus
    c. Precentral gyrus
    d. Superior temporal gyrus
    e. Supramarginal gyrus

161. All *except* which of the following statements regarding the pretracheal fascia is correct?

    a. It is located superficial to the infrahyoid muscles.
    b. It is continuous laterally with the fascia of the carotid sheath.
    c. It encloses the thyroid gland.
    d. It encloses the esophagus.
    e. It encloses the trachea.

162. In which of the following tapeworm infections does the coracidium leave the egg to be ingested by crustaceans when it develops into a larval stage, is eaten then by fish, and eventually ingested by humans?

    a. *Taenia solium*
    b. *Taenia saginata*
    c. *Hymenolepsis nana*
    d. *Echinococcus granulosus*
    e. *Diphyllobothrium latum*

163. The only cranial nerve to emerge from the dorsal aspect of the brainstem innervates which of the following?

    a. Medial rectus
    b. Superior oblique
    c. Lateral rectus
    d. Inferior oblique
    e. Levator palpebrae superioris

164. The cells located in the PPRF and MPRF that initiate and fire during a saccade, produce the pulse, and then become silent after the saccade are which of the following?

    a. Burst cells
    b. Burst-tonic cells
    c. Oculomotor neurons
    d. Pause cells
    e. Tonic cells

165. The best predictor that HIV-1 infection is progressing toward AIDS is which of the following?

    a. Stable titers of circulating anti-p24 IgM antibodies
    b. Kaposi's sarcoma
    c. Detecting the appearance of reverse transcriptase in the patient's serum
    d. Falling levels of circulating CD4-positive T cells
    e. Occurrence of *Pneumocystis carinii* pneumonia

166. Which of the following is a conspicuous histologic feature of medullary carcinoma of the thyroid?

    a. Papillary growth pattern
    b. Well-developed follicular structure
    c. Presence of lymphoid follicles
    d. Stromal deposition of amyloid
    e. Undifferentiated and anaplastic tumor cells

167. Which agent would be most effective in reversing respiratory depression caused by morphine?

    a. Fentanyl
    b. Sulfentanyl (intravenously)
    c. Dextromethorphan
    d. Naltrexone
    e. Pentazocine

168. Which of the following is *true* of the facilitated transport of glucose?

    a. It can occur up a concentration gradient.
    b. It does not use a specific carrier system.
    c. It is powered by coupling to an energy source.
    d. It will show saturation kinetics.
    e. It occurs on GLUT-1, which is abundant in all tissues.

169. Roughly 70% of the islet (of Langerhans) cells are B cells that function to synthesize insulin, the most abundant secretory product of the endocrine pancreas. Insulin does *not* promote which of the following?

    a. Uptake of glucose from blood
    b. Storage of glucose
    c. Phosphorylation of glucose
    d. Release of glucose into blood
    e. Synthesis of glycogen from glucose

170. Changes in renal function that tend to conserve blood volume include which of the following?

    a. A decrease in renal filtration fraction
    b. Suppression of ADH secretion
    c. Increased renin secretion
    d. Increased glomerular filtration rate
    e. Increased renal medullary blood flow

171. Which of the following applies to H-1 antihistaminics?

    a. Blocks release of histamine from mast cells
    b. Inhibits decarboxylation of histidine
    c. Promotes methylation of histamine
    d. Blocks increased capillary permeability produced by histamine
    e. Inhibits stimulation of gastric acid secretion by histamine

172. A patient with a left internuclear ophthalmoplegia would have which of the following?

   a. A lesion of the right MLF
   b. Interruption of fibers from the right abducens nucleus to the left oculomotor nucleus
   c. Adduction of the left eye on attempted gaze to the right
   d. Failure to abduct the right eye on attempted gaze to the right
   e. Abduction of the left eye on attempted gaze to the right

173. What causes essential (primary) hypertension?

   a. Renal disease
   b. Hyperaldosteronism
   c. Oral contraceptives
   d. Increased intracranial pressure
   e. Idiopathic

174. Which of the following is *true* for the pentose phosphate pathway?

   a. It is absent in red blood cells.
   b. It is regulated by the enzyme glucose-6-phosphate dehydrogenase.
   c. It channels all glucose carbons into the production of ribose.
   d. It can provide the cell with the NADH needed in the synthesis of fatty acids.
   e. One of its functions is to maintain cellular glutathione in the oxidized state.

175. Taste buds associated with fungiform papillae do *not* detect which of the following tastes?

   a. Acid
   b. Sweet
   c. Salty
   d. Bitter
   e. Sour

176. Ischemic heart disease is responsible for approximately what percentage of cardiac deaths in the United States and the industrialized world?

   a. 50%
   b. 60%
   c. 70%
   d. 80%
   e. 90%

177. A 58-year-old patient was fly-fishing with his son when, on making a cast, his right ulna snapped. Other than a history of smoking two packs of cigarettes a day for 40 years and a mild degree of emphysema, he had no pertinent history. He was taken to a local hospital where an x-ray film showed destruction of the ulna in the region of the fracture. Additional films showed a few sharp, punched-out lesions of the skull and ribs measuring about 1 cm in diameter. A screening chemistry examination showed a total protein of 8 g/dl but was otherwise normal. Serum electrophoresis showed a tall spike between the beta and gamma globulin region.

What histologic finding would you expect in this patient's bone marrow?

   a. Infiltration of the marrow by large, clear cells with round nuclei and prominent nucleoli consistent with origin in a renal cell carcinoma
   b. Infiltration of the bone marrow by small, dark cells with irregular nuclei that mold around each other consistent with origin from a small cell carcinoma of lung
   c. Infiltration of the bone marrow by a poorly differentiated squamous cell carcinoma consistent with origin in the lung
   d. Involvement of the bone marrow by chronic lymphocytic leukemia, B-cell type
   e. Normal marrow elements with a plasma cell count of approximately 25% and occasional bizarre forms. The plasma cells were usually present as nodules.

178. Which of the following is considered as belonging to the intermediate group of extrinsic back muscles?

   a. Trapezius
   b. Latissimus dorsi
   c. Serratus posterior
   d. Rhomboid minor
   e. Levator scapulae

179. Which of the following statements is *true* of glycogen synthase?

   a. It catalyzes the synthesis of alpha-1,6 glycosidic linkages.
   b. It catalyzes a freely reversible reaction between UPD-glucose and glycogen.
   c. It is more active when phosphorylated as glycogen synthase b.
   d. It adds glucose 1-phosphate to growing glycogen chain.
   e. It requires a primer with a nonreducing end to initiate a new glycogen molecule.

180. Glaucoma may be precipitated by treatment with which of the following?

   a. Epinephrine
   b. Propranolol
   c. Atropine
   d. Hydrochlorothiazide
   e. Captopril

181. Axons from the dentate nucleus terminate in which of the following?

   a. Globus pallidus
   b. Subthalamic nucleus
   c. VL nucleus
   d. VPM nucleus
   e. VPL nucleus

182. Transmission of an action potential across the neuromuscular junction of skeletal muscle fibers involves which of the following?

   a. Binding of acetylcholine released from Schwann cells to alpha-adrenergic receptors on the muscle cell
   b. Binding of Ca^{2+} to the sarcoplasmic reticulum allowing the action potential to enter T-tubules

   c. Binding of norepinephrine to postsynaptic beta-adrenergic receptors on muscle cells

   d. Binding of acetylcholine released from synaptic vesicles to nicotinic postsynaptic receptors

   e. Sequestration of Ca^{2+} in the sarcoplasmic reticulum when the action potential reaches the T-tubules

EXTENDED MATCHING QUESTIONS

Directions for Questions 183 through 200: Each set of questions has several lettered options, followed by several numbered items. For each numbered item, select ONE lettered option that is most closely associated with it. Each lettered option may be used once, more than once, or not at all.

Questions 183 and 184

   a. Introns
   b. Exons
   c. Signal (leader) peptides
   d. Allogeneic mice
   e. Syngeneic mice
   f. Xenogeneic mice

For each description, select the most appropriate item from the list above.

183.   Mice that are homozygous at every genetic locus and genetically identical to every other mouse in that strain

184.   The removal of transcribed structures from the primary nuclear RNA transcript in the formation of immunoglobulin mRNA is known as RNA splicing.

Questions 185 and 186

   a. Mixed hypertriglyceridemia
   b. Endogenous hypertriglyceridemia
   c. Type III hyperlipoproteinemia
   d. Familial hypercholesterolemia
   e. Familial hypertriglyceridemia

For each finding, select the lipoprotein disorder from the list that is most likely to be associated with it.

185.   Elevated chylomicrons and VLDL, low LDL and HDL

186.   Elevated LDL

Questions 187 and 188

   a. Capillary hemangioma
   b. Glomus tumor
   c. Cavernous hemangioma
   d. Granuloma pyogenicum
   e. Nevus flammeus
   f. Spider telangiectasis
   g. Hemangioendothelioma
   h. Angiosarcoma
   i. Hemangiopericytoma
   j. Kaposi's sarcoma

For each description, select the tumor most closely associated with it.

187.   A malignant tumor found in the liver and associated with exposure to arsenic, Thorotrast or polyvinyl chloride

188.   A painful tumor of the skin frequently found in the distal portion of the digits beneath the fingernails

Questions 189 through 191

   a. Herpes simplex virus I
   b. Herpes simplex virus II
   c. Varicella-zoster virus
   d. Epstein-Barr virus
   e. Cytomegalovirus
   f. Herpesvirus simiae-B virus
   g. HIV-1

For each description, select the virus most closely associated with it.

189.   Systemic spread of this virus through viremia to the skin causes lesions in successive crops in young children and is associated with "shingles" in adults.

190.   This virus is seroepidemiologically associated with human cervical cancer.

191.   Diagnosis of infection by this virus is usually documented by the demonstration of atypical lymphocytes. IgM heterophile antibody to the Paul-Bunnell antigen on sheep and bovine erythrocytes, and by positive serologic findings.

Questions 192 through 196

   a. Insulin
   b. Glucagon
   c. Growth hormone
   d. Cortisol
   e. Testosterone

For each description, match the hormone most closely associated with it.

192.   Increased uptake of K^+ by liver and muscle

193.   Decreased glucose uptake by muscle

194.   Increased facilitated transport of glucose in adipocytes and muscle

195.   Amino acid sequence similar to secretin, vasoactive inhibitory peptide, and gastric inhibitory peptide

196.   Acts only on liver and pancreatic beta cells

Questions 197 and 198

  a. Anterior commissure
  b. Anterior white commissure
  c. Arcuate fasciculus
  d. Claustrum
  e. Corpus callosum
  f. External capsule
  g. External medullary lamina
  h. Extreme capsule
  i. Genu of internal capsule
  j. Hippocampal commissure
  k. Inferior longitudinal fasciculus
  l. Internal medullary lamina
  m. Posterior commissure
  n. Posterior limb of internal capsule
  o. U fibers
  p. Uncinate fasciculus

Match each description with the structure most closely associated with it.

197. This structure separates the dorsal thalamus into a medial and lateral group of nuclei.

198. Damage to this structure can cause a supranuclear facial palsy.

Questions 199 and 200

  a. Carbamoyl phosphate synthetase II
  b. Ornithine transcarbamoylase
  c. Serine hydroxymethyltransferase
  d. Asparagine synthetase
  e. Kinureninase

For each of the descriptions described below, choose the most appropriate enzyme.

199. A genetic deficiency likely to cause hyperammonemia

200. A pyridoxine requiring enzyme that can convert a dietary amino acid to niacin

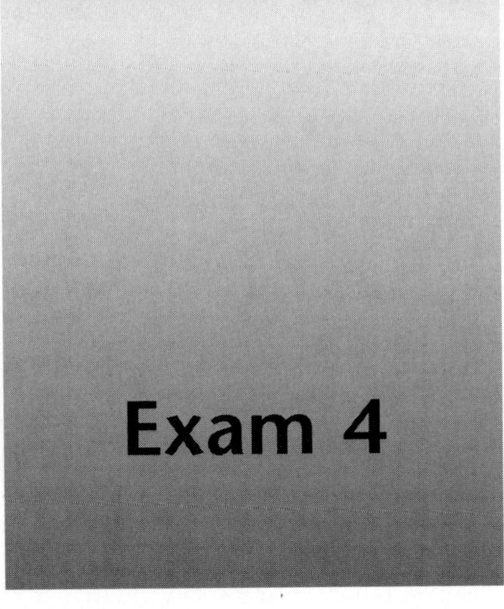

1. During a stressful situation, the symphathetic nervous system would increase all except which of the following?

   a. Arterial pressure
   b. Blood glucose concentration
   c. Glycolysis in muscle
   d. Muscle strength
   e. Salivary secretion

2. Serotonin is the major neurotransmitter of which of the following?

   a. Cerebellar Purkinje cells
   b. Locus ceruleus
   c. Raphe nuclei
   d. Substantia nigra pars compacta
   e. Cerebellar granule cells

3. The most common site of a "rotator-cuff" is which of the following?

   a. Near the insertion of the supraspinatus tendon onto the greater tubercle
   b. Distal portion of the infraspinatus tendon
   c. Intracapsular portion of the tendon of the long head of the biceps brachii muscle
   d. Near the insertion of the teres minor onto the greater tubercle
   e. Tendon of the subscapularis muscle near its insertion onto the lesser tubercle

4. Which of the following statements regarding bacterial polysaccharide capsules is *true?*

   a. Capsules allow the bacterium to evade the immune response by mimicking host cell antigens.
   b. Capsules allow bacteria to resist phagocytosis.
   c. Capsules are capable of destroying secretory IgA molecules.
   d. Capsules are limited to gram-positive bacteria.
   e. Capsules are the site of origin of flagella.

5. Light waves do *not* pass through which of the following before striking the retina?

   a. Vitreous humor
   b. Pupil
   c. Iris
   d. Cornea
   e. Lens

6. Which of the following is *not* a factor associated with the development of hepatocellular carcinoma (hepatoma)?

   a. Cirrhosis
   b. Aflatoxin exposure
   c. Hepatitis B infection
   d. Hereditary tyrosinemia
   e. Hepatitis A infection

7. Before a physician can release confidential communication about a competent, adult patient during a routine hospitalization, the patient is *not* required to consent to the release of information to which of the following?

   a. The patient's family
   b. The patient's attorney
   c. The patient's treatment team
   d. The patient's insurance carrier
   e. The patient's primary care physician

8. Which of the following statements is *not* an assumption regarding psychopathology proposed by family systems theory?

   a. Psychological problems are more likely the product of a conflict between family members.
   b. An individual's psychological symptoms may fulfill a meaningful function for the family.
   c. Psychopathology tends to occur when an individual becomes fixated at an immature level of psychosexual development.

    d. An individual's psychological symptoms are likely representative of a dysfunctional family system.

    e. The family should typically be the focus when psychological treatment for an individual is provided.

9. In the examination of a blood smear for malarial parasites, the crescent-shaped gametocyte is diagnostic for which type of malaria?

    a. *Plasmodium falciparum*

    b. *Plasmodium ovale*

    c. *Plasmodium malariae*

    d. *Plasmodium vivax*

    e. *Plasmodium bergheii*

10. All of the following statements about enzymatic digestion of lipids are true *except* which one?

    a. Pancreatic lipase hydrolyses triglycerides into monoglycerides and free fatty acids.

    b. The pH optimum for pancreatic lipase is pH 7-8, and the lipase acts at the lipid-water interface.

    c. The function of colipase is to potentiate formation of micelles of bile acids and triglycerides.

    d. Hydrolysis of phospholipids by phospholipase A_2 results in removal of one fatty acid molecule from the phospholipid.

    e. Hydrolysis of cholesterol ester into free cholesterol allows cholesterol to be absorbed as the free sterol.

11. Viruses may evade the immune response by all *except* which of the following mechanisms?

    a. Antigenic variation

    b. Blocking production of interferon

    c. Blocking sensation of viral antigen

    d. Opsonization of specific antibody

    e. Cytolysis of lymphoid cells

12. If a mutation in the gene encoding beta-2 microglobulin prevented the expression of this polypeptide, the likely effect would be which of the following?

    a. Prevention of the synthesis of the Transporter in Antigen Processing (TAP) 1 and 2 proteins

    b. Prevention of expression of Class I MHC

    c. Prevention of expression of Class II MHC

    d. Prevention of the synthesis of the cytosolic protease complex (proteasome) involved in generating peptides from cytosolic proteins

    e. None of the above, since beta-2 microglobulin is not encoded within the MHC complex

13. Which of the following statements describing the Watson-Crick model for DNA structure is *incorrect?*

    a. DNA has two grooves running helically along its length, one of which is wider than the other.

    b. The base-paired polynucleotide chains have antiparallel directions.

    c. The classic Watson-Crick hydrogen bonding between AT and GC pairs is found in Z-DNA.

    d. One turn of the double helix involves approximately 10 nucleotides and occurs every 34 angstroms.

    e. The helical structure is stabilized entirely by hydrogen bonding.

14. Which of the following is *not* true of carbon monoxide?

    a. It is a chemical type of asphyxiant.

    b. Its toxic properties are due to disruption of electron transport via cytochrome oxidase.

    c. It combines with hemoglobin to form carboxyhemoglobin.

    d. It reacts with hemoglobin in a similar manner as oxygen.

    e. It produces cherry-colored blood.

15. All *except* which of the following statements regarding indirect inguinal hernias is correct?

    a. Exit abdominal cavity via the deep inguinal ring

    b. Exit abdominal cavity medially to the inferior epigastric vessels

    c. More common in males than in females

    d. Occur more frequently than do direct hernias

    e. Follow the course of the inguinal canal

16. In humans, the primary metabolism of nitrogen in amino acids to urea involves which of the following?

    a. Amino acid oxidases and arginase

    b. Glutaminase and amino acid oxidases

    c. Transaminases and glutamate dehydrogenase

    d. Argininosuccinate lyase and cytosolic carbamoyl phosphate synthetase

    e. Glutamine synthetase and urease

17. Which of the following separates portions of the internal thoracic vessels from the parietal pleura?

    a. Internal intercostals

    b. External intercostals

    c. Transversus thoracis

    d. Subcostalis

    e. Costal cartilages

18. In Figure 1 of a peripheral nerve, which of the following does "A" represent?

    a. Epineurium

    b. Myelin sheath

    c. Perineurium

    d. Schwann cell cytoplasm

    e. Endoneurium

Figure 1

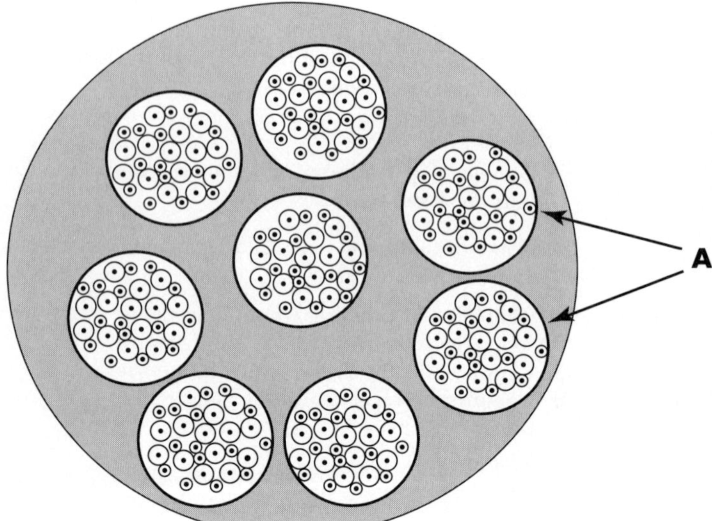

19. Which of the following produces a conductive hearing loss?

    a. Aging
    b. Childhood rubella
    c. Exposure to industrial noise
    d. Exposure to ototoxic antibiotics
    e. Otitis media

20. The motor nucleus of nerve V supplies all *except* which of the following muscles?

    a. Masseter
    b. Posterior belly of the digastric
    c. Temporalis
    d. Tensor tympani
    e. Tensor veli palatini

21. After discovering a sexual partner has AIDS, a patient with no previous psychiatric history requests HIV testing. At the onset of the interview the patient reveals an intention to commit suicide if the test is positive. Which of the following is the most ethical action for the physician to take?

    a. Initiate proceedings for involuntary, psychiatric hospitalization
    b. Conduct testing and report negative results regardless of the findings
    c. Refuse to conduct the HIV test and discontinue the interview
    d. Provide counseling and education about HIV/AIDS and postpone testing
    e. Provide counseling and education about HIV/AIDS and initiate testing

22. Which of the following statements is *true* of food poisoning caused by staphylococci?

    a. Both *Staphylococcus aureus* and *Staphylococcus epidermidis* may be implicated.
    b. The incubation period before symptoms begin is usually between 24 and 48 hours.
    c. Heating the suspected food prior to ingestion would prevent the food poisoning from occurring.
    d. Antibiotic therapy is usually not warranted.
    e. Poultry and poultry products are usually the reservoir of the causative organism.

23. Which of the following statements concerning hepatitis A is *not* correct?

    a. Hepatitis A is transmitted by the fecal-oral route.
    b. Hepatitis A has a 10% to 20% carrier state at the end of the acute infection.
    c. Hepatitis A typically has an incubation period of 15 to 45 days.
    d. Hepatitis A is caused by a member of the picornavirus group.
    e. Hepatitis A is rarely fatal in the acute infection.

24. What causes the increase in systolic pressure that occurs with aging?

    a. A decrease in diastolic pressure due to loss of connective tissue
    b. A decrease in stroke volume
    c. An increase in maximum aerobic capacity
    d. An increase in venomotor tone
    e. A decrease in arterial compliance

25. In the CD nomenclature for classifying lymphocytes, most cytotoxic T lymphocytes (CTLs) would be which of the following?

    a. $CD3^+$ $CD4^+$ $CD8^-$
    b. $CD3^+$ $CD4^-$ $CD8^+$
    c. $CD3^-$ $CD4^+$ $CD8^-$
    d. $CD3^+$ $CD4^+$ $CD8^+$
    e. $CD3^+$ $CD4^-$ $CD8^-$

26. Which of the following statements is *true* of progressing from the well-fed state (0 to 2 hour postprandial) to the fasting state (18 hour postprandial)?

    a. Glycogen synthesis in the liver increases to its maximum rate.
    b. There is a decrease in activity of the Cori cycle and the alanine cycle.
    c. Serum glucose drops below 50 mg/dl.
    d. There is an increase in the rate of production of ketone bodies.
    e. There is an increased reliance of the brain on free fatty acids as a fuel.

27. A number of structures in the inner ear are composed exclusively of extracellular matrix. Which of these structures is *not?*

    a. Vestibular membrane of Reissner
    b. Cupula
    c. Basilar membrane
    d. Otolithic membrane
    e. Tectorial membrane

28. Injury to the left side of the aortic arch may invoke all *except* which of the following?

    a. Vagus nerve
    b. Superior intercostal vein
    c. Recurrent laryngeal nerve
    d. Phrenic nerve
    e. Azygous vein

29. A 42-year-old patient reports a history of dissatisfaction with life and mild depression, which has lasted for 10 to 15 years. Although the patient describes a constant sense of sadness, functioning occupationally and interpersonally have not been problematic, and the patient denies symptoms of major depression or mania. Based on this limited information, what would the most likely diagnosis be?

    a. Generalized anxiety disorder
    b. Schizophrenia
    c. Panic disorder
    d. Dysthymia
    e. Bipolar disorder

30. What does a decrease in the ventilation/perfusion ratio ($\dot{V}_A/\dot{Q}$) cause alveolar P_{O_2} and alveolar P_{CO_2} to do?

    a. Increase, increase
    b. Decrease, increase
    c. Decrease, decrease
    d. Increase, decrease
    e. Increase, not change

31. If barometric pressure is 747 mm Hg and inspired air contains 80% N_2, what is the partial pressure of N_2 in the alveoli?

    a. 760
    b. 500
    c. 560
    d. 598
    e. 700

32. Which one of the following is a characteristic of the mitochondrial electron transport chain?

    a. Each of the three sites is directly associated with a non-heme iron protein.
    b. Glycerol 3-phosphate oxidation results in the pumping of protons at all three sites.
    c. Rotenone blocks electron flow between cytochrome b and cytochrome c_1
    d. Carbon monoxide and cyanide inhibit cytochrome oxidase.
    e. Each of the three sites contains one of the cytochrome proteins.

33. Vestibular output to the nuclei that control the extraocular muscles is found in which of the following?

    a. Central tegmental tract
    b. Dorsal longitudinal fasciculus
    c. Lateral vestibulospinal tract
    d. Medial lemniscus
    e. Medial longitudinal fasciculus

34. Megaloblastic anemia occurs when DNA synthesis is retarded in erythroblasts, due to an inadequate supply of nucleotide precursors. This is due to either a primary folate deficiency (dietary) or a folate deficiency secondary to another nutrient, which reduces the availability of single carbon units for purine and pyrimidine synthesis. Which of the following is the best explanation for the cause of the secondary deficiency?

    a. Methylcobalamin is needed to prevent all of the folate from becoming trapped in the methylfolate form.
    b. Dietary iron is needed as a cofactor to convert folate to its active form, tetrahydrofolate.
    c. Methylcobalamin is needed to convert methylfolate with other forms of folate to the single carbon unit in more oxidized states.
    d. Biotin is needed to recycle dihydrofolate back to tetrahydrofolate.
    e. Tetrahydrobiopterin is needed to convert homocysteine to methionine.

35. A 45-year-old patient has been developing seizures and headaches of increasing frequency and severity over the last 8 to 10 years. Because she was afraid of losing her driver's license, she has not seen a physician for the problem, since it occurred fairly infrequently. However, the seizures now are occurring several times per week. She finally saw her physician who, as part of the work-up, ordered skull x-ray examinations and a CT scan. The CT scan showed a space-occupying lesion over the convexity of the right cerebral hemisphere. The lesion seemed to be outside of the cerebral parenchyma but was definitely pressing onto it. On the plain film, the calvarium appeared eroded over the area where the lesion was found. When biopsied, the lesion showed a whorled appearance and was formed of large cells with round to oval nuclei and abundant cytoplasm. Psammoma bodies were present. Concerning this patient's tumor, which of the following statements is *incorrect?*

    a. These lesions are frequently malignant.
    b. These lesions are more frequently found in women than in men.
    c. These lesions tend to produce seizure disorders rather than neurologic deficits.
    d. If completely excised, the tumor will regrow.
    e. The histologic subtype has no bearing on the clinical course.

36. Which of the following antiarrhythmic drugs is associated with cinchonism?

    a. Lidocaine
    b. Verapamil
    c. Dopamine
    d. Nifedipine
    e. Quinidine

37. Chronic poisoning with which of the following most commonly causes peripheral neuropathy in adults but encephalopathy in children?

    a. Arsenic
    b. Lead
    c. Mercury
    d. Chromium
    e. Beryllium

38. Which of the changes listed below represent the effects of digitalis glycosides in patients with congestive heart failure?

	Stroke volume	Heart rate	Cardiac output	Peripheral vascular resistance
a.	increase	decrease	increase	increase
b.	decrease	increase	decrease	decrease
c.	increase	decrease	increase	decrease
d.	increase	decrease	no change	increase
e.	decrease	decrease	increase	decrease

39. Griseofulvin would be an appropriate antifungal therapy for the treatment of which of the following?

    a. Mucormycosis
    b. Candidiasis
    c. Tinea capitis
    d. Coccidioidomycosis
    e. Sporotrichosis

40. The cell bodies of the axons in the posterior spinocerebellar tract are in which of the following?

    a. Contralateral lamina II of Rexed
    b. Contralateral nucleus proprius
    c. Ipsilateral C1-C8 dorsal horn
    d. Ipsilateral lamina IX of Rexed
    e. Ipsilateral nucleus dorsalis of Clark

41. Which of the following has a blood-brain barrier?

    a. Area postrema
    b. Locus ceruleus
    c. Median eminence
    d. Neurohypophysis
    e. Pineal gland

42. The parents of a set of identical twins, age 17, inform a physician that one of the twins has been recently diagnosed as having schizophrenia. The parents ask the physician to comment on the likelihood that the other twin will also develop schizophrenia. What is the likelihood that the twin sibling is also schizophrenic?

    a. No greater than the risk in the general population
    b. Very unlikely (i.e., almost 0%)
    c. Highly likely (i.e., almost 100%)
    d. Probably between 35% to 50%
    e. Unknown, a genetic link for schizophrenia has not been supported by research

43. Large oral doses of which of the following may lower blood levels of cholesterol and lipoproteins?

    a. Vitamin D
    b. Nicotinic acid (niacin)
    c. Nicotinamide
    d. Thiamine
    e. Ascorbic acid

44. While conducting a mental status examination, a physician asks a patient "What does the following saying mean? People in glass houses shouldn't throw stones." This question is primarily a measure of which of the following?

    a. Memory
    b. Thought content
    c. Attention
    d. Vocabulary
    e. Abstraction

45. Sperm acquire the ability to fertilize an egg only after they are deposited in the female reproductive tract. What is the process that involves altering the sperm membrane in the female reproductive tract called?

    a. Spermiogenesis
    b. Spermatogenesis
    c. Luteinization
    d. Capacitation
    e. Differentiation

46. Which of the following is the most common form of joint disease?

    a. Osteoarthritis
    b. Rheumatoid arthritis
    c. Pigmented villonodular synovitis
    d. Gouty arthritis
    e. Infectious arthritis

47. A 4-year-old male child may have sexual impulses toward the opposite sex parent while simultaneously fantasizing about the elimination of the same sex parent. This phenomena, termed the Oedipus Complex, occurs in which Freudian stage of psychosexual development?

    a. Oral Stage
    b. Anal Stage
    c. Phallic Stage
    d. Latent Stage
    e. Genital Stage

48. In the kidney, what is the primary mechanism for reabsorbing phosphate?

    a. Cotransport with Na^+ in the proximal tubule
    b. Primary active transport in the collecting duct
    c. Passive paracellular diffusion down the electrical gradient in the last part of the proximal tubule
    d. Antiport with NH_4^+
    e. Antiport with H^+

49. Which of the following structures in Figure 2 is *not* composed of cells similar to the one depicted here?

    a. Proximal convoluted tubule (PCT) in kidney
    b. Striated ducts in sublingual glands
    c. Striated duct in submandibular gland
    d. Interlobular bile duct in liver
    e. Striated duct in parotid gland

Figure 2

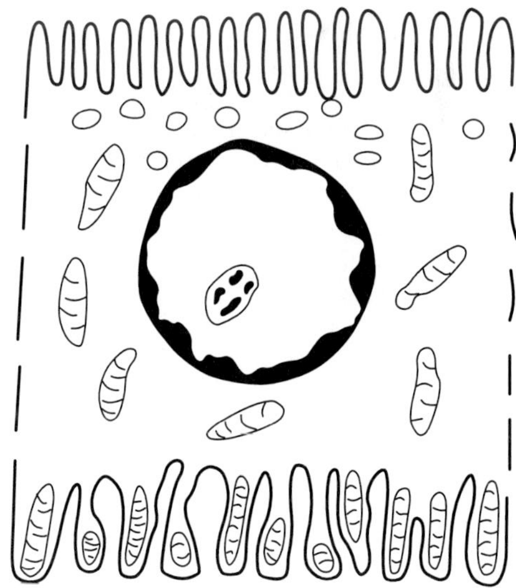

50. Which of the following structures does *not* contain baroreceptors?

    a. Carotid sinuses
    b. Aortic arch
    c. Cardiac ventricles
    d. Kidneys
    e. Skeletal muscle arterioles

51. In a positively skewed distribution, what is the measure of central tendency that is generally considered to be the best summary statistic?

    a. Mean
    b. Median
    c. Mode
    d. Range
    e. Variance

52. While grasping the fetal head in the region of the ear during a forceps delivery, which of the following is at risk?

    a. Trigeminal nerve
    b. Facial nerve
    c. Hypoglossal nerve
    d. Accessory nerve
    e. Greater occipital nerve

53. Nonspecific mechanisms that serve to protect humans against microbial invasion do *not* include which of the following?

    a. Cytokines
    b. Lactoferrin
    c. Mucus
    d. Immunoglobulins
    e. Lysozyme

54. The cutaneous mechanoreceptors include all *except* which of the following?

    a. Meissner's corpuscle
    b. Merkel's receptor
    c. Nuclear bag fibers
    d. Pacinian corpuscle
    e. Ruffini's endings

55. The spinal tract of cranial nerve V contains axons from all *except* which of the following cranial nerves?

    a. Facial nerve
    b. Glossopharyngeal nerve
    c. Oculomotor nerve
    d. Trigeminal nerve
    e. Vagus nerve

56. In control and prophylaxis of tuberculosis infection in the United States, which of the following is *not* true?

    a. Therapy for all infections is usually prolonged, for example, 6 to 9 months or longer.
    b. Vaccination with BCG is used as an immunoprophylaxis.
    c. Multiple antibiotics should be administered simultaneously to prevent development of resistance.
    d. Prophylaxis with isoniazid for 1 year is the usual regimen for individuals exposed to *Mycobacterium tuberculosis.*
    e. Control of *Mycobacterium bovis* infection in cattle herds reduces human exposure.

57. Surgical exploration of the adult superior mediastinum reveals that which of the following choices lies most anteriorly within this region?

    a. Trachea
    b. Brachiocephalic trunk
    c. Left common carotid artery
    d. Brachiocephalic veins
    e. Vagus nerves

58. Lymphatic capillaries (lacteals) serve as a preferential conveyance for which of the following, which are absorbed from the small intestine?

    a. Proteins
    b. Carbohydrates
    c. Lipids
    d. Steroids
    e. Immunoglobulins

59. Which heart valve is most commonly and severely affected in chronic rheumatic heart disease?

    a. Tricuspid
    b. Mitral
    c. Aortic
    d. Pulmonic
    e. All are affected about equally.

60. Which pair of phrases matches the type of adrenergic receptor with the appropriate second messenger system?

    a. $Alpha_1$ receptors, inositol triphosphate-diacylglycerol
    b. $Alpha_2$ receptors, inositol triphosphate-diacylglycerol
    c. $Beta_1$ receptors, calmodulin
    d. $Beta_1$ receptors, inositol triphosphate-diacylglycerol
    e. $Beta_2$ receptors, cyclic GMP

61. Figure 3 below is a schematic electron micrograph that depicts every significant morphologic structure in this cell. Which of the following spaces or lumina does *not* contain many, if any, of these cells?

    a. Right ventricle of heart
    b. Lumen of liver sinusoid
    c. Lumen of splenic sinus
    d. Lumen of renal arcuate artery
    e. Lumen of subcapsular sinus of lymph node

Figure 3

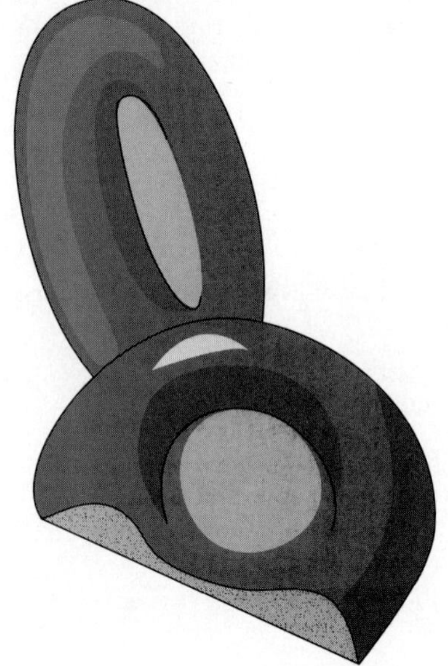

62. Which of the following is *not* thought to have central pattern generators that initiate a complex pattern of chained reflexes?

    a. Chewing
    b. Coughing
    c. Knee jerk
    d. Locomotion
    e. Swallowing

63. Which of the following is *not* associated with non-dream sleep?

    a. Bedwetting (nocturnal enuresis)
    b. Lowered arousal threshold
    c. Night terrors
    d. Penile tumescence
    e. Sleep walking (somnambulism)

64. Which of the agents used in the treatment of Parkinsonism, is an antiviral that may potentiate dopaminergic function by influencing the synthesis, release, or reuptake of dopamine?

    a. Carbidopa
    b. Bromocriptine
    c. Amantadine
    d. L-DOPA
    e. Trihexyphenidyl

65. Which of the following is the most likely cell type in the liver to be initially damaged when obstructive jaundice occurs?

    a. Kupffer cell
    b. Hepatocyte
    c. Sinusoidal endothelial cell
    d. Epithelial cell of canal of Hering
    e. Fibroblast in connective tissue of portal tract (triad)

66. Which agent, when given intravenously, is the drug of choice for stopping continuous seizure activity, especially tonic-clonic status epilepticus?

    a. Triazolam
    b. Diazepam
    c. Clomipramine
    d. Naloxone
    e. Fluphenazine

67. When two individuals are faced with similar stressors, one individual may react pathologically, whereas, the other individual may cope in a healthy manner. Which theory below explains this discrepancy by stating that the two individuals had a different personal threshold for stress based on their child rearing experiences, physical health, genetics, and social environment?

    a. Double bind theory
    b. Downward drift hypothesis
    c. Social causation theory
    d. Attribution theory
    e. Vulnerability theory

68. All *except* which of the following enzymes are found in macrophages?

    a. Lipase
    b. Interleukin-1
    c. Transforming growth factor (TGF)
    d. Acid phosphatase
    e. Collagenase

69. Which ganglion contains cell bodies of special sensory fibers carrying taste from the anterior two-thirds of the tongue?

    a. Superior cervical ganglion
    b. Otic ganglion
    c. Pterygopalatine ganglion
    d. Ciliary ganglion
    e. Geniculate ganglion

70. Increasing stimulus intensity to a slow adapting receptor will lead to an increase in all *except* which of the following?

    a. Number of action potentials
    b. Receptive field for that receptor
    c. Receptor potential amplitude
    d. Subjective sensation of the intensity of the stimulation

71. A patient with a stroke affecting the left internal capsule might be expected to have which of the following?

    a. A Babinski's reflex in the left foot
    b. Fasciculations in the right arm and leg
    c. Hyperactive deep tendon reflexes in the right arm and leg
    d. Increased tone in the left arm
    e. Telegraphic speech

72. Which of the following is *not* a characteristic of lipopolysaccharides (endotoxin)?

    a. Contain lipid A
    b. Contain a core polysaccharide
    c. Are pyrogenic
    d. Are heat labile
    e. Can activate the complement cascade by the alternate pathway

73. The duration of an isometric twitch of ocular muscle is about 25 milliseconds, compared to 200 milliseconds for the soleus muscle. What properties does ocular muscle have relative to soleus muscle?

    a. Mostly small diameter fibers with low glycolytic capacity
    b. Many mitochondria
    c. A high capillary density
    d. Mostly large diameter fibers with high glycolytic capacity
    e. Very little sarcoplasmic reticulum

74. Why does extracellular fluid (ECF) volume increase in response to an increase in dietary Na^+ intake?

    a. Increased plasma osmolality suppresses thirst.
    b. Aldosterone secretion increases.
    c. K^+ shifts from the ECF to the intracellular fluid.
    d. Na^+ intake exceeds excretion for about 3 days.
    e. Water shifts from the interstitial fluid to the plasma.

75. Systemic administration of a muscarinic stimulator such as carbachol would be expected to produce which of the following?

    a. Mydriasis, dry mouth, urinary retention, hypotension
    b. Increase in mean blood pressure, decrease in heart rate and mydriasis
    c. Relaxation of the trigone muscle of the bladder, increase in gastrointestinal activity, increase in blood flow to skeletal muscle
    d. Salivation, sweating, and mydriasis
    e. Bronchodilation, increased bronchial secretion, bradycardia

76. Which of the following drugs may be used to treat bipolar affective disorder (manic-depressive disorder) when mania is mild?

    a. Imipramine
    b. Diazepam
    c. Clomipramine
    d. Lithium
    e. Doxepin

77. Which of the following is a hepatitis virus with double-stranded DNA?

    a. Hepatitis A
    b. Hepatitis B
    c. Hepatitis C
    d. Hepatitis D
    e. Hepatitis E

78. Cerebrospinal fluid flows directly from the 4th ventricle into which of the following?

    a. Cisterna magna
    b. Cisterna pontis
    c. Interpeduncular cistern
    d. Quadrigeminal cistern
    e. Suprasellar cistern

79. Which of the following statements is *true?*

    a. NADH reducing equivalents are used mainly in biosynthetic reactions.
    b. A flavoprotein is an intermediate electron transport chain carrier between NADH and ubiquinone.
    c. Both of the "high energy" phosphate linkages of ATP are added during oxidative phosphorylation.
    d. NADH is used as the primary electron carrier in electron transport.
    e. Cyanide blocks the transfer of electrons from NADH to ubiquinone.

80. Which agent is an active spasmolytic and is thought to act as a GABA agonist at $GABA_B$ receptors?

    a. Dantrolene
    b. Vecuronium
    c. Baclofen
    d. Atracurium
    e. Glycine

81. Which of the following cells is *not* capable of undergoing mitosis in the adult?

    a. Proerythroblasts
    b. Basophilic erythroblasts
    c. Polychromatophilic erythroblasts
    d. Reticulocytes
    e. Neutrophilic myelocytes

82. Which of the following statements concerning diphtheria toxin is *true?*

    a. Diphtheria toxin causes ADP-ribosylation of a membrane-bound G-protein leading to chloride secretion.
    b. Diphtheria toxin inactivates elongation factor 2.
    c. Diphtheria toxin is an adenylate cyclase that interferes with neutrophil chemotaxis.
    d. Diphtheria toxin is a protein synthesis inhibitor that may play a role in bacterial adhesion.
    e. Diphtheria toxin is an enterotoxin.

83. In most tissues, severe hypoxia causes coagulation necrosis. In which of the following tissues is liquifactive necrosis the result of severe hypoxia rather than coagulation necrosis?

    a. Brain
    b. Pancreas
    c. Large intestine
    d. Liver
    e. Kidney

84. Determining the concentration of a hormone by radioimmunoassay (RIA) depends on which of the following?

    a. Determination of the concentration of the unknown hormone by spectrophotometry
    b. Serial dilution of the unknown sample for production of a standard curve
    c. Competition for antibody binding between the hormone in the unknown and added radioactive hormone
    d. Binding of radioactive iodine to the hormone in the unknown sample
    e. A greater affinity for antibody binding of the hormone in the unknown sample compared to the standard

85. Cardiac muscle cells *cannot* be modified to form which of the following?

    a. Multipolar neurons
    b. Sinoatrial (SA) node cells
    c. Purkinje fibers
    d. Atrioventricular (AV) node cells
    e. Bundle of His cells

86. Which of the following statements concerning osteoid osteoma is *incorrect?*

    a. It occurs in the third and fourth decades of life.
    b. It occurs more frequently in males.
    c. It is usually found in the appendicular skeleton.
    d. Growth is generally without symptoms.
    e. It is readily cured by conservative surgery.

87. Which of the following is *not* true concerning the pupillary light reflex pathway?

    a. Axons in the brachium of the superior colliculus synapse in the pretectal area.
    b. Axons from the pretectal area decussate in the anterior commissure.
    c. Axons from the nucleus of Edinger-Westphal terminate in the ciliary ganglion.
    d. Ganglion cell axons terminate in the pretectal area.
    e. Postganglionic parasympathetic axons originate from neurons in the ciliary ganglion.

88. Which of the effects listed below represent likely side effects of chronic antihypertensive treatment with propranolol?

	Exercise tolerance	Airway resistance	HDL cholesterol
a.	decrease	decrease	decrease
b.	decrease	increase	decrease
c.	increase	increase	decrease
d.	increase	decrease	increase
e.	decrease	increase	increase

89. Which of the following is *not* a characteristic of pulmonary surfactant?

    a. Surfactant consists primarily of phosphatidycholine and protein.
    b. Surfactant is more effective in lowering surface tension in small alveoli than in large alveoli.
    c. Surfactant forms a lipid bilayer on the surface of the alveoli.
    d. Surfactant is synthesized primarily by the endothelium of pulmonary capillaries.
    e. Surfactant increases pulmonary compliance by reducing surface tension.

90. Of the following, which does *not* cause atrophy?

    a. Destruction of the brachial plexus
    b. Aging
    c. Sudden occlusion of a coronary artery
    d. Casting of a broken leg
    e. Castration

91. Of the following tissues, which one has the fewest cells and the most intracellular substance per unit volume?

    a. Simple columnar epithelium
    b. Dense, irregular connective tissue
    c. Smooth muscle
    d. Myelinated nerve
    e. Stratified, squamous, nonkeratinized epithelium

92. Ventricular depolarization corresponds to what part of the electrocardiogram?

    a. P wave
    b. QRS complex
    c. T wave
    d. ST segment
    e. P-P interval

93. Extensive accumulation of rER are *not* found in which of the following cell types?

    a. Plasma cells
    b. Neurons
    c. Osteoblasts
    d. Young chondrocytes
    e. Primitive mesenchymal cells

94. Which of the following is *not* correct?

    a. Ketoconazole, an imidazole derivative, is clinically useful in a variety of systemic fungal diseases. It is given orally for systemic disease.
    b. Amphotericin B is used for deep (systemic) mycotic infections. It is given intravenously when used for systemic disease.
    c. Flucytosine is used for systemic mycotic infections. It is given orally when used for systemic disease.
    d. Griseofulvin is used to treat mycoses of the skin, and it is given orally to treat skin and nail infections.
    e. Nystatin is used for topical infections of skin and mucous membranes. It is also given orally to treat systemic mycotic infections.

95. A number of important skin diseases are characterized by the presence of bullae (blisters). Of this group, which is characterized by formation of the bulla by separation of the stratum spinosum and the basal layer forming a blister with an intact basal layer as its floor?

    a. Pemphigus vulgaria
    b. Bullous pemphigoid
    c. Junctional epidermolysis bullosa
    d. Dermatitis herpetiformis
    e. Dermolytic epidermolysis bullosa

96. Which of the following malignancies is least likely to involve or metastasize to the spleen?

    a. Lymphocytic leukemia
    b. Granulocytic leukemia
    c. Hodgkin's disease
    d. Non-Hodgkin's lymphoma
    e. Carcinoma of the breast

97. What is the primary mechanism regulating the secretion of bile salts?

    a. Decreased parasympathetic stimulation
    b. Increased sympathetic stimulation
    c. Secretion of cholecystokinin
    d. Release of motilin from the gastric mucosa
    e. Negative feedback from hepatic portal venous bile salt concentration

98. The arterial supply to the gallbladder arises most frequently as a branch of which of the following?

    a. Left hepatic artery
    b. Right hepatic artery
    c. Left gastric artery
    d. Proper hepatic artery
    e. Celiac trunk

99. What is the correct order of action of these enzymes in prokaryotic lagging strand DNA replication?

    1. DNA polymerase I
    2. DNA ligase
    3. Helicase
    4. Primase
    5. DNA polymerase III

    a. 5, 1, 2, 4, 3
    b. 3, 4, 5, 1, 2
    c. 1, 2, 5, 3, 4
    d. 4, 3, 5, 1, 2
    e. 1, 5, 2, 4, 3

100. Processing of eukaryotic 45S ribosomal precursor RNA includes which of the following?

    a. Addition of poly A to the 3′ end
    b. Action of spliceosomes
    c. Capping the 5′ end with inverted 7-methyl guanosine triphosphate
    d. Endonuclease processing to produce 28S and 18S RNA
    e. Production of transfer RNA

101. Which of the following does *not* require GTP during prokaryotic protein synthesis?

    a. Binding of aminoacyl-tRNA to ribosomes with EF-T$_u$
    b. Polypeptide chain initiation with IF-1, IF-2, and IF-3
    c. Peptidyl-tRNA translocation with EF-G
    d. Aminoacylation of tRNA by aminoacyl tRNA synthetase
    e. Polypeptide chain termination by RF-1, RF-2, and RF-3.

102. A patient is diagnosed with anemia. The levels of folic acid in red cells are normal, but serum levels of vitamin B$_{12}$ are below normal. Oral absorption of vitamin B$_{12}$ is impaired, but the oral absorption of a complex between vitamin B$_{12}$ and intrinsic factor is normal. What is the most likely cause of the patient's anemia?

    a. Iron deficiency leading to microcytic, hypochromic anemia
    b. Folic acid deficiency leading to megaloblastic anemia
    c. Drug-induced hemolytic anemia
    d. Malabsorption of vitamin B$_{12}$ due to a receptor-transport defect in the small intestine
    e. Malabsorption of vitamin B$_{12}$ due to lack of production of intrinsic factor

103. Human to human contact is a primary mode of transmission of which of the following diseases?

    a. Toxoplasmosis
    b. Bancroftian filariasis
    c. Chagas' disease
    d. Taeniasis
    e. Trichomoniasis

104. Birds and bats have been shown to be important in the ecology of which of the following dimorphic fungi?

    a. *Sporothrix schenckii*
    b. *Histoplasma capsulatum*
    c. *Coccidioides immitis*
    d. *Candida albicans*
    e. *Aspergillus fumigatus*

105. Cross-dependence does *not* occur between which of the following pairs?

    a. Midazolam-phenobarbital
    b. Midazolam-buspirone
    c. Triazolam-ethanol
    d. Diazepam-thiopental
    e. Phenobarbital-ethanol

106. A worker in a smelting plant developed symptoms of stomatitis, bleeding gums, tremor, and emotional depression. What is the most likely cause of these symptoms?

    a. Inorganic lead poisoning
    b. Phosphorus (white)
    c. Nitroglycerin
    d. Elemental mercury
    e. Picric acid

107. A dissection of an aortic aneurism (dissecting hematoma) has been separated into two morphological forms, type A and type B. What is the distinction between these two forms?

    a. Type A becomes double barreled and thus is a self-healing lesion.
    b. Type A never involves the abdominal aorta.
    c. Type A involves the ascending aorta.
    d. Type A extends to the iliac arteries.
    e. Type A is exclusive to patients with Marfan's syndrome.

108. Von Willibrand's disease is caused by an abnormality or deficiency of the Von Willibrand factor, which is necessary for platelet function and stablization of factor VIII. In what cells is Von Willibrand factor synthesized, other than megakaryocytes?

    a. Macrophages
    b. Endothelium
    c. Lymphocytes
    d. Plasma cells
    e. Fibroblasts

109. Which mechanism is used to shuttle NADH equivalents from the cytoplasm into the mitochondrion?

    a. The Cori cycle in the liver only
    b. Diffusion of protons into the mitochondrion
    c. Active transport coupled with hydrolysis of ATP
    d. The use of a malate-alpha-ketoglutarate transporter
    e. Facilitated diffusion via the NADH transporter protein

110. Which of the following statements concerning *Campylobacter jejuni* is *not* correct?

    a. *Campylobacter jejuni* causes as much enteric disease in humans as *Salmonella* and *Shigella*.
    b. All age groups are affected.
    c. Human to human spread through the fecal-oral route can occur.
    d. Significant human infection has been attributed to ingestion of contaminated milk, water, or food.
    e. *Campylobacter jejuni* causes an opportunistic and often fatal septicemia.

111. Which of the following statements is true for chlortetracycline but is *not* true for chloramphenicol?

    a. Can be tolerated in higher dosage levels in infants
    b. Structurally related to phenylalanine
    c. Mechanism of action involves competitive antagonism of *p*-aminobenzoic acid (PABA)
    d. May cause dental mottling in young children
    e. Broad-spectrum antibiotic

112. Which of the following drugs inhibits the iodide "trapping" (i.e., uptake) mechanism of the thyroid gland?

    a. Perchlorate
    b. Propylthiouracil
    c. Probenecid
    d. Colchicine
    e. Estrogen

113. At normal plasma ADH concentration, urine osmolality increases if there is an increase in which of the following?

    a. Plasma aldosterone concentration
    b. Urine flow
    c. Renal medullary blood flow
    d. NaCl reabsorption by the loop of Henle
    e. Plasma angiotensin II concentration

114. The cranial nerve that exits the brain in the preolivary sulcus is which of the following?

    a. Abducens nerve
    b. Hypoglossal nerve
    c. Oculomotor nerve
    d. Trochlear nerve
    e. Vagus nerve

115. *Chlamydia trachomatis* differs from *Neisseria gonorrhoeae* in that infection by the former can do which of the following?

    a. Cause urethritis
    b. Cause pneumonia
    c. Cause neonatal conjunctivitis
    d. Frequently be asymptomatic
    e. Cause pelvic inflammatory disease

116. Which one of the following second generation antidepressant drugs is most likely to exhibit some antipsychotic activity?

    a. Trazodone
    b. Fluoxetine
    c. Amoxapine
    d. Amitriptyline
    e. Imipramine

117. Major symptoms of toxicity of triclyic antidepressant overdosage include all *except* which of the following?

    a. Coma
    b. Cardiac arrhythmias
    c. Renal dysfunction
    d. Agitation or delirium
    e. Respiratory depression

118. The autonomic plexus of nerve fibers associated with the internal carotid artery consists of which of the following?

    a. Postganglionic sympathetic fibers
    b. Preganglionic sympathetic fibers
    c. Preganglionic parasympathetic fibers
    d. Postganglionic parasympathetic fibers
    e. General somatic afferent fibers

119. All *except* which of the following fiber groups can be found in a cutaneous nerve?

    a. A-alpha fibers
    b. A-beta fibers
    c. A-delta fibers
    d. C fibers
    e. D fibers

120. A patient with an inability to identify objects visually but an ability to identify them by sound or touch has which of the following?

    a. Broca's aphasia
    b. Conduction aphasia
    c. Transcortical sensory aphasia
    d. Visual agnosia
    e. Wernicke's aphasia

121. Ingestion of large amounts of rhubarb may result in symptoms of poisoning by which of the following agents?

    a. Phenol (carbolic acid)
    b. Muscarine
    c. Formaldehyde
    d. Oxalic acid
    e. Boric acid

122. What is the primary mechanism of chloride reabsorption by the latter part of the proximal tubule?

    a. Primary active transport via a Cl^- ATPase
    b. Coupling of Na^+ and Cl^- at the basolateral cell membrane
    c. Passive diffusion, driven by the concentration gradient for Cl^-
    d. Secondary active cotransport of $2Na^+$, $1K^+$, and $1Cl^-$ across the luminal membrane
    e. Exchange for lactic acid

123. Why is mean arterial pressure (MAP) increased during exercise?

    a. The baroreceptors do not function during exercise.
    b. Increased blood flow to the muscle increases MAP.
    c. Increased activity of the muscle pump raises arterial pressure.
    d. Cardiac output increases more than total peripheral resistance decreases.
    e. Cardiac contractility is decreased.

124. All of the listed chromosomal abnormalities cause developmental abnormalities and may be associated with mental retardation as well. Which abnormality also has a high incidence in the development of Wilm's tumor of the kidney?

    a. 47(XY, +18)
    b. 47(XY, +21)
    c. 47(XY, +13)
    d. 46(XY, 5p−)
    e. 46(XY, 11p−)

125. The process by which haploid sperm cells differentiate is called spermiogenesis. Spermiogenesis consists of four phases. Which phase is *not* a component of spermiogenesis?

    a. Golgi
    b. Cap
    c. Mitotic
    d. Acrosome
    e. Maturation

126. Cross striations in skeletal muscle cells are a major histologic feature of this type of cell. When a skeletal muscle cell relaxes, which of the following does *not* occur?

    a. A band remains the same width.
    b. I band decreases in width.
    c. Z band remains the same width.
    d. H band increases in width.
    e. The sarcomere increases in width.

127. Patients with Parkinson's disease may exhibit all *except* which of the following?

    a. Bradykinesia
    b. Cogwheel rigidity
    c. Hypotonia
    d. Resting tremor
    e. Shuffling gait

128. Axons in the tectospinal tract have their cell bodies in which of the following?

    a. Central caudal nucleus
    b. Medial geniculate nucleus
    c. Red nucleus
    d. Superior colliculus
    e. Trochlear nucleus

129. All *except* which of the following muscles is under voluntary control?

    a. Levator ani
    b. Bulbospongiosus in the female
    c. Ischiocavernosus in the male
    d. Superficial transverse perinei
    e. Sphincter ani internus

130. What is the characteristic histologic change seen in any stage of a syphilis infection?

    a. Acute inflammation with liquifactive necrosis
    b. Tuberculoid granulomata within the stromal connective tissue
    c. Diffuse lymphocytic infiltrate within the lesion
    d. Endoarteritis with prominent plasma cell infiltrate
    e. Large colonies of visable organisms within the lesion

131. In a healthy subject, exercise caused stroke volume to increase from 100 to 125 milliliters, with no change in end-diastolic ventricular volume. This change in stroke volume is an example of which of the following?

    a. Starling's law of the heart
    b. A cardiac effect of increased parasympathetic activity
    c. A cardiac effect of decreased sympathetic activity
    d. An increase in ventricular contractility
    e. A decrease in ventricular contractility

132. The hepatic veins are typically tributaries in which of the following?

    a. Portal vein
    b. Inferior mesenteric vein
    c. Inferior vena cava
    d. Azygos vein
    e. Middle colic vein

133. In delayed-type hypersensitivity, which of the following statements is *not* true?

    a. The onset following antigen challenge is usually 24 to 48 hours.
    b. The effector cells are $CD4^+$ T cells and/or macrophages.
    c. The effector molecules are cytokines, particularly interferon-gamma and tumor necrosis factor.
    d. It may be transferred to animals by lymphocytes.
    e. The pathologic lesion includes vascular dilation and local smooth muscle contraction.

134. All *except* which of the following statements regarding the pelvic splanchic nerves is correct?

    a. Motor fibers arise in spinal cord segments S2, S3, and S4.
    b. Motor fibers innervate the descending colon.
    c. GVE (general visceral efferent) fibers innervate the sigmoid colon.
    d. They give rise to the inferior rectal nerves.
    e. They carry afferent nerve fibers.

135. When does most of the filling in the ventricle occur?

    a. The first third of diastole
    b. The last third of diastole
    c. Isovolumetric contraction
    d. Isovolumetric relaxation
    e. The period of rapid ventricular ejection

136. Which of the following conditions is not a predisposing condition for development of the Budd-Chiari syndrome (hepatic vein thrombosis)?

    a. Polycythemia vera
    b. Pregnancy
    c. Oral contraceptives
    d. Hepatocellular carcinoma
    e. Chronic lymphocytic leukemia

137. Which of the following statements concerning acute myelogenous leukemia is *not* true?

    a. The peripheral white count may be normal.
    b. Untreated, the disease is usually fatal in less than 2 months.
    c. The major clinical problems are neutropenia, anemia, and thrombocytopenia.
    d. Discrete tumor masses may form in bones, soft tissues, and lymph nodes.
    e. The disease often terminates in Richter's syndrome.

138. A mechanism of gene transfer between bacteria, which is dependent on bacteriophages, is known as which of the following?

    a. Conjugation
    b. Transduction
    c. Transfection
    d. Transformation
    e. Lysogeny

139. Thirst *cannot* be caused by which of the following?

    a. Decreased extracellular fluid volume
    b. Decreased osmotic pressure
    c. Diabetes insipidus
    d. Heavy salt intake
    e. Hemorrhage

140. Alpha motor neurons innervating muscles of the hand are found in which of the following?

    a. Anterior horn from C5-T1
    b. Dorsal horn from C5-T1
    c. Lissauer's tract in the cervical cord
    d. Nucleus proprius
    e. Substantia gelatinosa

141. The most posterior structure situated deep to the flexor retinaculum is which of the following?

    a. Flexor digitorum longus
    b. Flexor hallucis longus
    c. Posterior tibial artery
    d. Tibial nerve
    e. Tibialis posterior

142. The Epidemiologic Catchment Area Study (ECA), published in 1991, is to date the largest and the most respected investigation conducted to determine the prevalence of psychiatric disorders in America. According to the ECA, what are the most most common psychiatric conditions across the lifespan in America?

    a. Dysthymia and somatization
    b. Schizophrenia and mania
    c. Phobias and alcohol abuse
    d. Antisocial personality and drug abuse
    e. Major depression and panic

143. Which of the following is *not* an action of propranolol?

    a. It is useful in ventricular arrhythmias.
    b. It causes depression of cardiac pacemaker activity.
    c. It has a blockade of catecholamine-induced bronchial dilation.
    d. It has a positive inotropic effect.
    e. It causes the reduction of catecholamine-induced hyperglycemia.

144. Which of the following is *not* a true statement regarding nodular hyperplasia of the prostate?

    a. Nodular hyperplasia occurs predominantly in the preprostatic region, proximal to the veru montanum.
    b. Nodular hyperplasia is probably mediated by dihydrotestosterone.
    c. Nodular hyperplasia docs not occur in eunuchs.
    d. Nodular hyperplasia is a premalignant condition.
    e. Nodular hyperplasia will occur in 75% to 90% of males by the eighth decade of life.

145. Which of the following nematodes is *not* indigenous to the United States?

    a. *Necator americanus*
    b. *Enterobius vermicularis*
    c. *Trichuris trichiura*
    d. *Wuchereria bancrofti*
    e. *Trichinella spiralis*

146. When does the aortic valve open?

    a. When the isovolumetric relaxation period ends
    b. When the left ventricular pressure exceeds aortic pressure
    c. When the left ventricular pressure decreases below left atrial pressure
    d. When the right ventricle begins to fill
    e. When the aortic diastolic arterial pressure exceeds left ventricular pressure

147. Which of the following statements is *true* of increased sympathetic nervous activity?

    a. It increases the duration of systole.
    b. It dilates the arterioles in most organs.
    c. It increases the rate of depolarization of the SA nodal pacemaker potential.
    d. It decreases ventricular contractility.
    e. It inhibits renin secretion from the juxtaglomerular cells.

148. Which of the following statements concerning squamous cell carcinoma in sun-exposed skin is *not* true?

    a. It tends to be raised lesions with rolled pearly edges.
    b. It tends to be histologically well differentiated.
    c. Often it is in an area with a precursor actinic keratosis.
    d. It readily metastasizes to regional lymph nodes.
    e. It is rare in people with black skin.

149. What is one way norepinephrine increases cardiac contractility?

    a. It inhibits membrane-bound adenylyl cyclase.
    b. It opens slow Ca^{2+} channels in the cell membrane.
    c. It decreases the rate of pumping of Ca^{2+} into the sarcoplasmic reticulum.
    d. It stimulates synthesis of actin.
    e. It increases the rate of depolarization of the SA nodal cells.

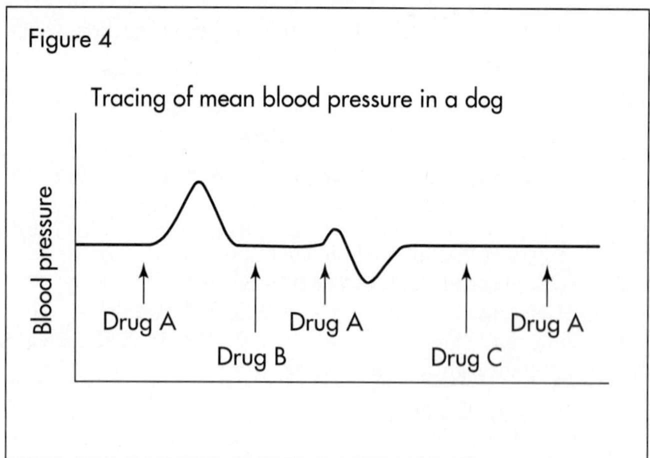

150. Drugs A, B, and C are sympathetic agonists or antagonists. From the schematic tracing of their effects on blood pressure, you conclude that drug A could be which of the following?

   a. Epinephrine
   b. Isoproterenol
   c. Phenylephrine
   d. Terbutaline
   e. Clonidine

151. Drugs A, B, and C are sympathetic agonists or antagonists. From the schematic tracing of their blood pressure effects, you conclude that drug B could be which of the following?

   a. Phentolamine
   b. Scopolamine
   c. Propranolol
   d. Hexamethonium
   e. Timolol

152. Drugs A, B, and C are sympathetic agonists or antagonists. From the schematic tracing of their effects on blood pressure drug C (assume that drug B remains active throughout the duration of the experiment) could be which of the following?

   a. Acetylcholine
   b. Prazosin
   c. Phenylephrine
   d. Timolol
   e. Phentolamine

153. Drugs A, B, and C are sympathetic agonists or antagonists. From the schematic tracing of their effects on blood pressure and knowing that drug C may precipitate an attack of myocardial failure in patients with myocardial disease, drug C is likely to be which of the following?

   a. An alpha-adrenergic blocking agent
   b. A ganglionic blocking agent
   c. A selective muscarinic antagonist
   d. A selective beta$_2$ blocker
   e. A nonselective beta blocker

154. Muscles of the anterior compartment of the leg, which act as dorsiflexors of the foot, include all *except* which of the following?

   a. Extensor digitorum longus
   b. Extensor hallucis longus
   c. Peroneus longus
   d. Peroneus tertius
   e. Tibialis anterior

155. Lysozyme is secreted by all *except* one of the following?

   a. Lacrimal gland
   b. Chief cells in the stomach
   c. Serous cells in the submaxillary gland (submandibular gland)
   d. Paneth cells
   e. Neutrophils

156. One source of sensory input *not* used in the regulation of normal posture is which of the following?

   a. Auditory system
   b. Muscle and joint receptors in the limbs
   c. Receptors in cervical ligaments and neck muscles
   d. Vestibular system
   e. Visual system

157. Which of the following is *not* a risk factor for the development of atherosclerosis?

   a. Hyperlipidemia
   b. Hypertension
   c. Diabetes
   d. Cigarette smoking
   e. Mönckeberg's arteriosclerosis

158. The cranial nerve that exits the brainstem between the superior cerebellar and posterior cerebral arteries is known as which of the following?

   a. Abducens nerve
   b. Facial nerve
   c. Glossopharyngeal nerve
   d. Oculomotor nerve
   e. Trochlear nerve

159. In a resting skeletal muscle cell, the Nernst potential for K^+ was observed to be -90 mV, and the resting membrane potential was -80 mV. What is the likely explanation for the difference between these two potentials?

   a. The cell membrane has a lower permeability to K^+ than to Na^+ or Cl^-
   b. Cl^- diffuses into the cell due to the electrical gradient.
   c. K^+ is actively transported out of the cell.
   d. Na^+ diffuses into the cell.
   e. The difference represents the pacemaker potential.

160. Clearance measurements in a healthy adult revealed that inulin clearance = 92 ml/min and creatinine clearance = 110 ml/min. After administration of the drug cimetidine, inulin clearance was unchanged, but creatinine clearance decreased to 92 ml/min. This change in creatinine clearance can be accounted for by which of the following factors?

    a. An increase in the volume of plasma cleared of creatinine
    b. Inhibition of renal tubular creatinine secretion by cimetidine
    c. Net renal absorption of cimetidine
    d. An increase in renal blood flow
    e. An increase in glomerular capillary hydrostatic pressure

161. A 58-year-old male patient presents with a 4-year history of decreased libido and cold intolerance. He has had progressive visual impairment and headache in the last 4 months. Examination reveals that he has coarse skin, enlargement of the bones of the face and hands, and a subnormal body temperature. There is a bitemporal hemianopsia. The signs and symptoms in this patient are most likely due to which of the following?

    a. Diabetes insipidus
    b. Gonadotrophin-secreting tumor
    c. Hyperthyroidism
    d. Primary hypothyroidism
    e. Pituitary growth hormone secreting tumor

162. Placement of sutures during a sacrospinous colpopexy is done at least 2 finger breadths posteromedially to the ischial spine in order to avoid which vessels?

    a. Internal pudendal vessels
    b. Superior gluteal vessels
    c. Obturator vessels
    d. Lateral sacral vessels
    e. Uterine vessels

163. In Class II MHC-associated antigen presentation, which of the following principal steps is *not* relevant?

    a. Antigen-presenting cells internalize native protein antigens from the extracellular environment.
    b. Peptides that bind to Class II molecules are proteolytically generated in the cytoplasm and delivered to the cell surface.
    c. Exocytic vesicles are the sites where the binding of peptides with Class II molecules occurs.
    d. Expression of the peptide-MHC Class II complex occurs on the cell surface.
    e. Complexes are recognized by T cells specific to the peptide and self-MHC molecule.

164. The decibel range for average conversational speech in a noisy office is which of the following?

    a. 10 to 20 decibels
    b. 60 to 70 decibels
    c. 100 to 110 decibels
    d. 140 to 150 decibels
    e. 180 to 200 decibels

165. Many of the axons of the ascending reticular activating systems that terminate in the thalamus synapse in which of the following?

    a. Anterior nucleus
    b. Dorsomedial nucleus
    c. Intralaminar nuclei
    d. Nucleus basalis of Meynert
    e. Septal nucleus

166. All *except* which of the following has lymphatic drainage to the lumbar (lateral aortic) lymph nodes?

    a. Ureters
    b. Testes
    c. Descending colon
    d. Ascending colon
    e. Uterine tubes

167. Which of the following statements concerning colorectal carcinoma is *not* correct?

    a. Adenocarcinomas largely arise from adenomatous polyps.
    b. Diet is a significant risk factor in colorectal carcinoma.
    c. Loss of multiple supressor genes is required to develop colon cancer.
    d. Chronic ulcerative colitis is a predisposing condition for colon cancer.
    e. Cancer of the left colon is generally asymptomatic.

168. A number of intestinal diseases are associated with malabsorption. Which of the following diseases is characterized by large numbers of macrophages which contain masses of PAS positive bacilli, in the lamina propria mucosae?

    a. Tropical sprue
    b. Whipple's disease
    c. Non-tropical sprue
    d. Protein losing enteropathy
    e. Bacterial overgrowth syndrome

169. Which of the following is *true* concerning the mechanism of action of antifungal agents?

    a. The polyenes bind to the sterols of the cell membrane.
    b. The imidazole derivatives bind to the sterols of the cell membrane.
    c. The imidazole derivatives inhibit the growth of fungal cells by interfering with cell wall synthesis.
    d. Flucytosine inhibits the growth of fungal cells by interfering with ergosterol synthesis.
    e. Griseofulvin inhibits fungal protein synthesis.

170. Parasympathetic stimulation of the salivary glands results in which of the following?

    a. Decreased blood flow to the glands
    b. Decreased $HCO_3{}^-$ secretion in saliva
    c. Increased reabsorption of Na^+ from the saliva
    d. Increased secretion of amylase and mucin
    e. Inhibition of secretion of saliva

171. Chloracne is a characteristic effect following exposure to which of the following?

    a. Chlordecone
    b. Chlordane
    c. Polychlorinated biphenyls
    d. Chloramphenicol
    e. Methylmercuric chloride

172. Some human diseases are mediated by antibodies against fixed cell and tissue antigens. These diseases do not include which of the following?

    a. Myasthenia gravis
    b. Goodpasture's syndrome
    c. Grave's disease
    d. Rheumatoid arthritis
    e. insulin-resistant diabetes mellitus

173. Which is a unique feature of the left lung?

    a. Lingula
    b. Oblique fissure
    c. Apex
    d. Horizontal fissure
    e. Middle lobe

174. Which of the following statements does *not* pertain to the T cell receptor?

    a. It contains both an alpha chain and a beta chain or a gamma and delta chain.
    b. The polypeptides of the T cell receptor contain both a constant (C) region and a variable (V) region.
    c. A single T cell receptor confers specificity for both antigen and MHC.
    d. T cell antigen recognition requires the simultaneous binding of two independent receptors, one to foreign antigen and the other to self-MHC.
    e. There are both transmembrane and cytoplasmic domains.

175. Second order axons carrying pain information from the big toe decussate in which of the following?

    a. Anterior commissure
    b. Anterior medullary velum
    c. Anterior white commissure
    d. Decussation of the medial lemniscus
    e. Posterior commissure

176. Which of the following is *true* for restriction fragment length polymorphism (RFLP) analysis?

    a. The term polymorphism refers to the production of different restriction enzymes by the cell.
    b. The different length of the restriction fragments is due to the creation of new restriction sites by mutations.
    c. The different length of the restriction fragments is due to deletion mutations.
    d. Western blotting is used to detect the products of restriction digestion.
    e. An RFLP will identify a point mutation occurring at a restriction site within the coding sequences of a gene.

177. Which of the sequences listed below represents the relative antihypertensive effectiveness of diuretic drugs (+ least, + + + most effective)

	Loop diuretics	Potassium-sparing diuretics	Thiazide diuretics
a.	+++	++	+
b.	+++	+	++
c.	++	+	+++
d.	++	+++	+
e.	+	++	+++

178. The induced fit model of enzyme action states which of the following?
    a. Binding of inhibitor to an allosteric site brings about a conformational change to fit the shape of the inhibitor.
    b. Binding of substrate changes the shape of the active site to fit the shape of the substrate.
    c. D-isomers of optically active substrates are converted to L-isomers so that they will bind correctly.
    d. Is also known as cooperativity and requires enzymes with more than one subunit.
    e. The transition state is induced in the substrate prior to binding to the active site.

EXTENDED MATCHING QUESTIONS

Directions for Questions 179 through 200: Each set of questions has several lettered options, followed by several numbered items. For each numbered item, select ONE lettered option that is most closely associated with it. Each lettered option may be used once, more than once, or not at all.

Questions 179 and 180

    a. Loss of arylsulfatase A activity results in accumulation of sulfatides.
    b. Loss of beta-glucosidase results in accumulation of glucosylceramide.
    c. Deficiency of beta-hexosaminodase A causes accumulation of GM_2 ganglioside.
    d. Deficiency of phosphorylase causes painful cramps on exercise.
    e. This is the inability to degrade sphingomyelin to ceramide.

For each disease listed select the correct description.

179. Niemann-Pick disease.

180. McArdle's disease

Questions 181 and 182

- **a.** Peyer's patches
- **b.** IgG
- **c.** IgE
- **d.** Plasmacytes
- **e.** Small lymphocytes
- **f.** Activated mast cells
- **g.** IgA
- **h.** Large lymphocytes

Match each cell type with its description.

181. Converts arachidonic acid into the three main leukotrienes, LTC_4, LTD_4, and LTE

182. Epithelial cells of organs such as the intestine express F_c receptors for dimeric forms of this secretory immunoglobulin.

Questions 183 and 184

- **a.** Hemoglobin H
- **b.** Hemoglobin A_2
- **c.** Fetal hemoglobin
- **d.** Lepore hemoglobin
- **e.** Bart's hemoglobin

For each of the descriptions below, choose the most appropriate type of hemoglobin.

183. Contains a delta-beta hybrid globin

184. Tetramers composed only of gamma globin

Questions 185 and 186

- **a.** Sensorimotor
- **b.** Preoperational Thought
- **c.** Concrete Operations
- **d.** Formal Operations
- **e.** Deductive Reasoning

For each of the following concepts, select the associated stage of cognitive developing according to Jean Piaget.

185. Object Permanence

186. Conservation

Questions 187 through 189

- **a.** *Neisseria gonorrhoeae*
- **b.** *Neisseria meningitidis*
- **c.** *Treponema pallidum*
- **d.** *Chlamydia trachomatis*
- **e.** *Haemophilus influenzae*
- **f.** *Haemophilus ducreyi*

Match each bacteria with its description.

187. An obligate intracellular bacterium that is a leading cause of sexually transmitted disease

188. A gram-negative diplococcus that is the leading cause of pelvic inflammatory disease

189. The most frequent cause of meningitis in unimmunized children under 5 years of age

Questions 190 through 194

- **a.** Triiodothyronine (T_3)
- **b.** Thyroxine (T_4)
- **c.** Thyroxin-binding globulin
- **d.** Thyroid-stimulating hormone
- **e.** Thyroglobulin

For each of the lettered options listing factors related to thyroid function, select the numbered item with which it is most closely associated.

190. Effects mediated by nuclear receptor

191. Secretion inhibited by increased plasma T_3 and T_4

192. Produced by thyrotropes of anterior pituitary gland

193. Principal biologically active form of thyroid hormone

194. Main component of colloid

Questions 195 and 196

- **a.** Fatty acyl CoA
- **b.** Malate shuttle
- **c.** Citrate lyase
- **d.** Acetyl CoA carboxylase
- **e.** Glycerol kinase

For each statement below, pick the most appropriate metabolite or enzyme from the list provided.

195. Absence in adipose tissue prevents synthesis of triacylglycerols when serum insulin levels are low

196. Provides a mechanism to shuttle acetyl CoA from the mitochondria to the cytosol

Questions 197 and 198

- **a.** Orotic aciduria
- **b.** Purine nucleoside phosphorylase deficiency
- **c.** Adenosine deaminase deficiency
- **d.** Lesch-Nyhan syndrome
- **e.** Gout

For each metabolic situation below, choose the disease that applies.

197. Results in increased levels of PRPP coupled with decreased IMP and GMP

198. Inhibition of ribonucleotide reductase by increased concentration of dATP

Questions 199 and 200.

- **a.** Blocking
- **b.** Circumstantiality
- **c.** Perseveration
- **d.** Flight of Ideas
- **e.** Mutism

For each of the following patient examples select the most appropriate term to describe the patient's behavior.

199. During an interview a patient stops speaking abruptly before completing a thought and after a long silence has no recall of what he/she was previously saying.

200. While providing historical information, a patient tends to discuss excessive details regarding events, but eventually provides the answer to the question asked.

Categories and Answers for Exam 1

Question Number	Answer	Check Here if Correct	Category 1	Category 2	Category 3
1	A	☐	Pathology	Immune System	Immune Response
2	A	☐	Pharmacology	Autocoids & Diuretics	General Properties
3	D	☐	Pharmacology	Autonomic Nervous System	Main Effects
4	C	☐	Biochemistry	Nitrogen Metabolism	Synthesis
5	C	☐	Microbiology	Bacteriology	Diseases
6	B	☐	Anatomy	Pelvis & Perineum	Clinical Anatomy
7	E	☐	Pharmacology	Immune System	Side Effects
8	C	☐	Neuroscience	Central Nervous System	Normal Anatomy
9	E	☐	Pharmacology	General Principles	Pharmacodynamics
10	D	☐	Pharmacology	Endocrine System	Side Effects
11	A	☐	Microbiology	Bacteriology	Normal Anatomy
12	E	☐	Microbiology	Bacteriology	Structure
13	A	☐	Histology	Cells & Tissues	Pathogenesis
14	C	☐	Physiology	Cardiovascular System	Microcirculation
15	A	☐	Pathology	Cardiovascular System	Diseases
16	A	☐	Physiology	Cells & Tissues	Signaling
17	C	☐	Pathology	Liver & Pancreas	Pathogenesis
18	C	☐	Anatomy	Back & Spinal Cord	Normal Anatomy
19	A	☐	Pharmacology	Endocrine System	General Properties
20	A	☐	Microbiology	Bacteriology	Diseases
21	C	☐	Anatomy	Pelvis & Perineum	Clinical Anatomy
22	B	☐	Physiology	Urinary System	Circulation
23	A	☐	Anatomy	Lower Limb	Normal Anatomy
24	B	☐	Biochemistry	Enzymes	Inhibition
25	E	☐	Physiology	Cardiovascular System	General Properties
26	B	☐	Neuroscience	Motor System & Reflexes	Normal Anatomy
27	A	☐	Pathology	Female Reproductive System	General Properties
28	C	☐	Pathology	Female Reproductive System	Pathophysiology
29	D	☐	Physiology	Musculoskeletal System	Metabolism
30	D	☐	Biochemistry	Intermediary Metabolism	Glycolysis & Gluconeogenesis
31	D	☐	Pharmacology	Autonomic Nervous System	Interactions
32	B	☐	Microbiology	Virology	General Properties
33	B	☐	Neuroscience	Central Nervous System	Normal Anatomy
34	A	☐	Biochemistry	Amino Acids & Proteins	Structure
35	A	☐	Histology	Cells & Tissues	Normal Tissues
36	B	☐	Biochemistry	Endocrine System	Signaling
37	E	☐	Neuroscience	Central Nervous System	Normal Anatomy
38	C	☐	Microbiology	Immune System	Immune System Cells
39	B	☐	Microbiology	Bacteriology	Structure
40	D	☐	Histology	Gastrointestinal System	Normal Tissues
41	C	☐	Microbiology	Bacteriology	General Properties
42	E	☐	Neuroscience	Back & Spinal Cord	Normal Anatomy
43	E	☐	Neuroscience	Motor Systems & Reflexes	Lesions
44	E	☐	Histology	Eye	Normal Tissues
45	E	☐	Pathology	Liver & Pancreas	Diseases
46	C	☐	Neuroscience	Central Nervous System	Lesions
47	C	☐	Biochemistry	Intermediary Metabolism	Transport
48	E	☐	Biochemistry	Amino Acids & Proteins	Structure
49	C	☐	Pharmacology	Central Nervous System	Clinical Uses
50	D	☐	Microbiology	Parasitology	Laboratory Diagnosis

Categories and Answers for Exam 1

Question Number	Answer	Check Here if Correct	Category 1	Category 2	Category 3
51	D	☐	Histology	Cells & Tissues	Bones, Joints, & Soft Tissues
52	E	☐	Anatomy	Pelvis & Perineum	Normal Anatomy
53	A	☐	Neuroscience	Central Nervous System	Lesions
54	D	☐	Neuroscience	Central Nervous System	Diseases
55	C	☐	Histology	Molecular Genetics	Genetics
56	B	☐	Physiology	Cells & Tissues	Transport
57	C	☐	Biochemistry	Intermediary Metabolism	Glycolysis & Gluconeogenesis
58	A	☐	Neuroscience	Motor Systems & Reflexes	Normal Anatomy
59	E	☐	Pathology	Immune System	Diseases
60	E	☐	Anatomy	Pelvis & Perineum	Normal Anatomy
61	C	☐	Microbiology	Bacteriology	Epidemiology
62	C	☐	Biochemistry	Molecular Genetics	Synthesis
63	D	☐	Microbiology	Immune System	Immune System Cells
64	B	☐	Physiology	Cardiovascular System	Circulation
65	B	☐	Neuroscience	Central Nervous System	Normal Function
66	E	☐	Physiology	Cells & Tissues	Transport
67	D	☐	Anatomy	Abdomen	Normal Anatomy
68	D	☐	Microbiology	Bacteriology	Laboratory Diagnosis
69	E	☐	Anatomy	Head & Neck	Normal Anatomy
70	D	☐	Anatomy	Head & Neck	Normal Anatomy
71	A	☐	Physiology	Cells & Tissues	Transport
72	B	☐	Microbiology	Immune System	Genetics
73	E	☐	Pathology	Gastrointestinal System	Diseases
74	C	☐	Pharmacology	Central Nervous System	Main Effects
75	B	☐	Neuroscience	Autonomic Nervous System	Normal Anatomy
76	E	☐	Pharmacology	Autocoids & Diuretics	Clinical Uses
77	E	☐	Pathology	Immune System	Diseases
78	D	☐	Pathology	Musculoskeletal System	Bones, Joints, & Soft Tissues
79	B	☐	Neuroscience	Central Nervous System	Normal Anatomy
80	D	☐	Neuroscience	Head & Neck	Normal Function
81	D	☐	Pharmacology	Immune System	Clinical Uses
82	B	☐	Pharmacology	Immune System	Clinical Uses
83	D	☐	Pharmacology	Cardiovascular System	General Properties
84	A	☐	Biochemistry	Molecular Genetics	Recombinant DNA
85	B	☐	Biochemistry	Liver & Pancreas	Metabolism
86	E	☐	Pharmacology	Central Nervous System	Toxicology
87	A	☐	Pharmacology	Central Nervous System	Toxicology
88	C	☐	Pharmacology	Central Nervous System	Toxicology
89	B	☐	Histology	Gastrointestinal System	Normal Tissues
90	B	☐	Pharmacology	Endocrine System	Pharmacokinetics
91	D	☐	Pharmacology	Cardiovascular System	Side Effects
92	A	☐	Pathology	Gastrointestinal System	Neoplasia
93	C	☐	Histology	Musculoskeletal System	Normal Tissues
94	A	☐	Neuroscience	Head & Neck	Lesions
95	B	☐	Physiology	Respiratory System	Circulation
96	C	☐	Neuroscience	Head & Neck	Normal Anatomy
97	D	☐	Anatomy	Head & Neck	Normal Anatomy
98	C	☐	Pathology	Liver & Pancreas	Diseases
99	D	☐	Microbiology	Immune System	Immune System Cells
100	A	☐	Histology	Respiratory System	Normal Tissues

Categories and Answers for Exam 1

Question Number	Answer	Check Here If Correct	Category 1	Category 2	Category 3
101	B	☐	Physiology	Musculoskeletal System	Normal Function
102	D	☐	Histology	Eye	Normal Function
103	A	☐	Neuroscience	Autonomic Nervous System	Normal Anatomy
104	A	☐	Neuroscience	Central Nervous System	Normal Anatomy
105	D	☐	Anatomy	Head & Neck	Normal Anatomy
106	E	☐	Microbiology	Parasitology	Epidemiology
107	B	☐	Pharmacology	Central Nervous System	Clinical Uses
108	C	☐	Pharmacology	Chemotherapy	Interactions
109	C	☐	Physiology	Urinary System	Acid-Base Balance
110	E	☐	Histology	Cells & Tissues	General Properties
111	A	☐	Histology	Cells & Tissues	Structure
112	D	☐	Pathology	Liver & Pancreas	Diseases
113	E	☐	Pathology	Molecular Genetics	Neoplasia
114	A	☐	Anatomy	Thorax	Normal Anatomy
115	B	☐	Physiology	Cardiovascular System	Microcirculation
116	E	☐	Pathology	Immune System	Diseases
117	B	☐	Neuroscience	Back & Spinal Cord	Lesions
118	A	☐	Pathology	Urinary System	Normal Anatomy
119	E	☐	Microbiology	Virology	Epidemiology
120	D	☐	Histology	Urinary System	Pathophysiology
121	C	☐	Pharmacology	Blood & Lymphs	General Properties
122	D	☐	Physiology	Musculoskeletal System	Normal Function
123	E	☐	Microbiology	Bacteriology	Diseases
124	D	☐	Pharmacology	Chemotherapy	General Properties
125	A	☐	Pathology	General Principles	Diseases
126	D	☐	Physiology	Respiratory System	General Properties
127	C	☐	Pharmacology	Urinary System	Main Effects
128	C	☐	Physiology	Cardiovascular System	Circulation
129	A	☐	Biochemistry	Molecular Genetics	Structure
130	B	☐	Physiology	Respiratory System	General Properties
131	E	☐	Pathology	Molecular Genetics	Diseases
132	D	☐	Anatomy	Back & Spinal Cord	Normal Anatomy
133	A	☐	Physiology	Musculoskeletal System	Normal Function
134	C	☐	Pathology	General Principles	Neoplasia
135	E	☐	Pathology	Respiratory System	Epidemiology
136	E	☐	Neuroscience	Peripheral Nervous System	Normal Function
137	B	☐	Physiology	Cardiovascular System	Microcirculation
138	E	☐	Anatomy	Lower Limb	Normal Anatomy
139	E	☐	Neuroscience	Motor Systems & Reflexes	Normal Anatomy
140	D	☐	Biochemistry	Intermediary Metabolism	Energy & Oxidation
141	D	☐	Neuroscience	Central Nervous System	Normal Anatomy
142	E	☐	Neuroscience	Central Nervous System	Lesions
143	A	☐	Physiology	Cardiovascular System	Regulation
144	C	☐	Biochemistry	Molecular Genetics	Structure
145	A	☐	Pathology	Gastrointestinal System	Diseases
146	E	☐	Pathology	Respiratory System	Pathophysiology
147	A	☐	Anatomy	Upper Limb	Normal Anatomy
148	E	☐	Pathology	Endocrine System	Pathophysiology
149	A	☐	Microbiology	Bacteriology	Pathogenesis
150	A	☐	Neuroscience	Back & Spinal Cord	Normal Anatomy

Categories and Answers for Exam 1

Question Number	Answer	Check Here if Correct	Category 1	Category 2	Category 3
151	C	☐	Pathology	Forensic Medicine	Laboratory Diagnosis
152	D	☐	Microbiology	Bacteriology	Structure
153	B	☐	Biochemistry	Molecular Genetics	Mutation
154	D	☐	Histology	Urinary System	Normal Tissues
155	C	☐	Biochemistry	Enzymes	Regulation
156	A	☐	Anatomy	Head & Neck	Normal Anatomy
157	E	☐	Physiology	Urinary System	Regulation
158	A	☐	Pharmacology	Central Nervous System	Side Effects
159	D	☐	Biochemistry	Molecular Genetics	Synthesis
160	B	☐	Pharmacology	Chemotherapy	General Properties
161	A	☐	Neuroscience	Motor Systems & Reflexes	Normal Function
162	E	☐	Pathology	General Principles	Cell Injury & Cell Death
163	A	☐	Microbiology	Bacteriology	Structure
164	C	☐	Biochemistry	Lipids & Steroids	Synthesis
165	A	☐	Histology	Gastrointestinal System	Normal Anatomy
166	A	☐	Physiology	Cardiovascular System	The Heart as a Pump
167	C	☐	Pharmacology	Central Nervous System	Side Effects
168	B	☐	Microbiology	Bacteriology	General Properties
169	A	☐	Pathology	Endocrine System	Pathophysiology
170	C	☐	Pharmacology	Central Nervous System	Clinical Uses
171	C	☐	Microbiology	Immune System	Immune System Cells
172	C	☐	Pharmacology	Central Nervous System	Toxicology
173	B	☐	Physiology	Musculoskeletal System	Normal Tissues
174	D	☐	Histology	Cardiovascular System	Secretion
175	B	☐	Histology	Male Reproductive System	Semen
176	C	☐	Physiology	Cardiovascular System	The Heart as a Pump
177	A	☐	Physiology	Respiratory System	Regulation
178	C	☐	Neuroscience	Autonomic Nervous System	Normal Function
179	B	☐	Pharmacology	Cardiovascular System	Side Effects
180	A	☐	Pathology	Musculoskeletal System	Diseases
181	B	☐	Histology	Cells & Tissues	Normal Tissues
182	D	☐	Physiology	Gastrointestinal System	Secretion
183	C	☐	Physiology	Gastrointestinal System	Secretion
184	A	☐	Physiology	Gastrointestinal System	Secretion
185	A	☐	Physiology	Gastrointestinal System	Secretion
186	A	☐	Physiology	Gastrointestinal System	Secretion
187	B	☐	Physiology	Gastrointestinal System	Secretion
188	A	☐	Physiology	Gastrointestinal System	Secretion
189	G	☐	Microbiology	Immune System	Cytokines
190	A	☐	Microbiology	Immune System	Cytokines
191	F	☐	Microbiology	Immune System	Cytokines
192	D	☐	Pathology	Virology	Cell Injury & Cell Death
193	B	☐	Pathology	Bacteriology	Cell Injury & Cell Death
194	B	☐	Microbiology	Immune System	Cytokines
195	F	☐	Microbiology	Immune System	Cytokines
196	G	☐	Microbiology	Immune System	Cytokines
197	G	☐	Neuroscience	Head & Neck	Normal Function
198	A	☐	Neuroscience	Head & Neck	Lesions
199	M	☐	Neuroscience	Motor Systems & Reflexes	Normal Anatomy
200	K	☐	Neuroscience	Head & Neck	Normal Anatomy

Answers and Explanations to Exam 1

1. **Answer a:**

   Although it is produced during complement activation, C5a is not part of the attack complex that is formed of complement components Cb5 through C9.

   b: The classical pathway of complement activation produces C5a.

   c: The alternate pathway of complement activation produces C5a.

   d: C5a is thought to be a major mediator of chemotaxis of neutrophils in acute inflammation. It is also an attractant of eosinophils, monocytes, and basophils.

   e: Although C5a is involved in attracting neutrophils to an area of inflammation, it is not involved in the induction of adhesion molecules on the surface of endothelial cells. TNFa and IL-1 are the major cytokines involved in that process.

2. **Answer a:**

   Epinephrine is an effective and rapidly acting bronchodilator. The effect lasts for 60 to 90 minutes, therefore it is not suitable for prophylactic treatment.

   b: Theophylline is used for prophylaxis between attacks.

   c: Methylprednisolone is used for prophylaxis between attacks.

   d: Cromolyn sodium is used for prophylaxis between attacks.

   e: Methotrexate is used for prophylaxis between attacks.

3. **Answer d:**

   Cocaine competitively blocks the uptake of catecholamines into the nerve terminal.

   a: Tyramine releases norepinephrine.

   b: Clonidine is an $alpha_2$ agonist

   c: Isoproterenol is a nonspecific beta agonist.

   e: Oxymetazoline is an alpha agonist.

4. **Answer c:**

   The inability to convert phenylalanine to tyrosine causes a buildup of phenylalanine and a shunting of phenylalanine skeletons into harmful metabolites. It also makes tyrosine a required amino acid.

   a: Phenylpyruvate, phenyllactate, and phenylacetate are normally produced in low amounts by normal intakes of phenylalanine, because phenylalanine hydroxylase can convert any excess to tyrosine to be further metabolized. A low phenylalanine diet is required in phenylalanine hydroxylase deficiency to reduce the shunting of phenylalanine skeletons into these harmful metabolites.

   b: Phenylalanine hydroxylase catalyzes the formation of tyrosine from phenylalanine.

   d: Phenylalanine hydroxylase requires a cofactor, tetrahydrobiopterin, which is a pterin-containing cofactor synthesized by the body from GTP.

   e: PKU is treated by a controlled diet alone, in which the phenylalanine is kept present but at low concentrations. The effectiveness of the diet is monitored by measuring blood phenylalanine concentrations.

5. **Answer c:**

    Rickettsia prowazekii, a nonspirochete, is the etiologic agent of louse-borne typhus fever.

    a: Tick-borne relapsing fever is caused by *Borrelia* species, which are spirochetes.

    b: Louse-borne relapsing fever is caused by *Borrelia recurrentis,* a spirochete.

    d: Lyme disease is caused by *Borrelia burgdorferi,* a spirochete.

    e: Syphilis is caused by *Treponema pallidum,* a spirochete.

6. **Answer b:**

    The ureter crosses the pelvic brim very near the bifurcation of the common iliac artery. In this location the ureter lies immediately posteromedial to the infundibulopelvic ligament (suspensory ligament of the ovary).

    a: The sympathetic chain ganglia are located much more medially and deep to the psoas muscle.

    c: The obturator nerve is located on the lateral pelvic wall, inferior to the infundibulopelvic ligament.

    d: The inferior epigastric vessels are located on the deep surface of the lower anterior abdominal wall.

    e: The uterine artery arises from the internal iliac artery more inferiorly within the pelvis.

7. **Answer e:**

    Ibuprofen's main toxic effects are on the GI system and kidneys; it also causes agranulocytosis.

    a: True. Aspirin has been shown to cause GI disturbances.

    b: True. Phenacetin is nephrotoxic.

    c: True. Acetaminophen is hepatotoxic.

    d: True. Indomethorin causes agranulocytosis.

8. **Answer c:**

    The major sensory input layer of the cerebral cortex is layer IV. It is so large in the occipital lobe that it was named the line of Gennari.

    a: Layer I is not the major sensory layer.

    b: Layer II is not the major sensory layer.

    d: Layer V is not the major sensory layer.

    e: Layer VI is not the major sensory layer.

9. **Answer e:**

    Thyroid hormone binds to specific response elements of DNA, stimulating the transcription of genes.

    a: Beta-adrenergic agonists act via cAMP.

    b: Muscarinic agonists decrease the level of cAMP.

    c: ACTH's second messenger is cAMP.

    d: Action of PTH on bone cells involves a cAMP.

10. **Answer d:**

    Large doses of corticosteroids may cause psychosis.

    a: Growth hormone does not evoke psychosis.

    b: Deoxycorticosterone is a mineralocorticoid.

    c: Potassium iodide does not evoke psychosis.

    e: Calcitriol does not evoke psychosis.

11. **Answer a:**

    Mannose is present in the epithelial receptor for this organism, and the organism does not adhere in its presence because of competition from extracellular mannose.

    b: There is no evidence that mannose forms a bridge between fimbrial structures to facilitate adherence to the epithelial cell.

    c: Mannose may be present on the cell surface, but unless it is part of the epithelial cell receptor, it would not prevent adherence.

    d: If mannose were not present in the receptor, adherence would not take place in the presence or absence of mannose.

    e: Adherence has nothing to do with mannose as a growth factor.

12. **Answer e:**

    Bacterial capsules or slime layers are evasins and allow bacteria to resist phagocytosis.

    a: Capsules or slime layers do not contain bacterial endotoxin.

    b: Capsules or slime layers do not contain beta-lactamases.

    c: Capsules or slime layers do not contain enzymes that degrade host cell membranes.

    d: Capsules or slime layers may be immunogenic, but this is not why they are considered virulence factors.

13. **Answer a:**

    The lens is composed largely of anucleate lens fibers (specialized epithelial cells that are filled with proteins called crystallins). Hence, the lens is normally composed of organic material.

    b: Dentin possesses approximately 70% inorganic material.

    c: Endochondral bone and intramembranous bone are tissues comprised of a substantial amount of hydroxyapatite crystals (inorganic material). The percentage varies from 50% to 85% depending on the function of the osseous tissue.

    d: Cementum is generally considered to be the softest of the calcified tissues. It is comprised of approximately 50% hydroxyapatite crystals.

    e: Enamel is, without question, the hardest of the calcified tissues. The tissue composition is 96% hydroxyapatite crystals.

14. **Answer c:**

    A decrease in plasma protein concentration means a decrease in plasma oncotic (colloid osmotic) pressure and increased filtration of water into the interstitium.

    a: An increase in plasma protein will draw fluid into the capillaries.

    b: The opposite is true; an increase in capillary permeability may cause edema.

    d: For edema to occur due to changes in venous pressure, the pressure must increase.

15. **Answer a:**

    Takayasu's arteritis is an uncommon vasculitis that involves the major branches of the aorta in patients generally under the age of 50. Sometimes it is referred to as "pulseless disease."

    b: Takayasu's arteritis primarily involves major branches of the aorta, rather than medium sinew muscular arteries.

    c: Takayasu's arteritis primarily involves major branches of the aorta, rather than small muscular arteries.

    d: Takayasu's arteritis primarily involves major branches of the aorta, rather than capillaries.

    e: Takayasu's arteritis primarily involves major branches of the aorta, rather than veins.

16. **Answer a:**

    Peptide hormones like vasopressin act via cell membrane receptors and use cyclic AMP as an intracellular second messenger.

    b: Cortisol and other steroid hormones diffuse through the lipid portion of the cell membrane and bind to nuclear receptors; they do not use the cAMP second messenger system.

    c: The steps are out of sequence; after vasopressin interacts with a cell membrane (not nuclear) receptor, G proteins then activate adenylyl cyclase.

    d: Phosphodiesterase catalyzes the conversion of cAMP to a noncyclic form of AMP, a step that occurs later in the pathway; diphosphoinositol is involved in a different second messenger pathway.

    e: Steps are out of order; G protein is activated when a peptide hormone binds to the cell membrane receptor and activates adenylyl cyclase.

17. **Answer c:**

    During enzymatic injury to the adipose tissue surrounding the pancreas, free fatty acids are released by the action of lipases. The free fatty acids that are released will form calcium and magnesium soaps, which are insoluble and precipitate out. The insoluble precipitate thus ties up calcium from the plasma.

18. **Answer c:**

    A small branch from each vertebral artery unites with its counterpart to form the anterior spinal artery, which extends the entire length of the spinal cord.

    a: The lumbar arteries provide small branches, known as radicular arteries, which communicate with anterior and posterior spinal arteries as well as supply the vertebrae and meningeal coverings.

    b: Radicular branches of the posterior intercostal arteries communicate with the spinal arteries and also supply the vertebrea and meninges.

    d: Branches of the posterior inferior cerebellar arteries unite to form the posterior spinal artery.

    e: Radicular arteries arise as branches of the vertebral, posterior intercostal, lumbar, and lateral sacral arteries.

19. **Answer a:**

    The half-life of oxytocin is 5 minutes.

    b: True. Oxytocin is optimally administered via intravenous drip.

    c: True. High doses of oxytocin produce uterine tetany.

    d: True. Oxytocin is used to promote milk "let down."

    e: True. Oxytocin is used to control post-partum uterine hemorrhage.

20. **Answer a:**

Typhoid fever is caused by *Salmonella typhi*.

    b: Rocky Mountain spotted fever is caused by *Rickettsia rickettsii*.

    c: Ehrlichiosis is caused by the rickettsiae *Ehrlichia sennetsu* and *Ehrlichia chaffeensis*.

    d: Q fever is caused by the *rickettsia, Coxiella burnetii*.

    e: Bacillary angiomatosis is caused by the *rickettsia, Rochalimaea*.

21. **Answer c:**

The pudendal nerve innervates most of the labial region, although branches of the ilioinguinal nerve also contribute to their innervation.

    a: Although branches of the ilioinguinal nerve reach the labia, those of the iliohypogastric nerve do not.

    b: The pudendal nerve innervates most of the labia, but the iliohypogastric does not extend far enough inferiorly to reach the labia.

    d: Although the pudendal nerve innervates most of the labia, the latter also receive innervation from one of the branches of the first lumbar nerve.

    e: The pelvic splanchnic nerves are not involved with the innervation of the labia.

22. **Answer b:**

The calculation of net ultrafiltration pressure is:

$$(GCp - BSp) - (GC\pi - BS\pi) = (40 - 8) - (23 - 0) = 9 \text{ mm Hg}$$

23. **Answer a:**

The gastrocnemius muscle will produce flexion of the knee joint as well as plantarflexion at the ankle joint.

    b: The piriformis produces lateral rotation and abduction of the femur at the hip.

    c: The iliacus crosses only the hip joint and produces flexion of the same when it contracts.

    d: Although this muscle originates within the pelvis, its contraction results in lateral or external rotation of the femur at the hip joint.

    e: The vastus intermedius, one member of the quadriceps group, only crosses the knee joint and is responsible, in part, for extension of the leg at the latter.

24. **Answer b:**

Because they lower the concentration of active enzyme, noncompetitive inhibitors decrease the V_{max}.

    a: The only way to increase the V_{max} is to increase the amount of active enzyme. The Km is increased by competitive inhibitors.

    c: A decrease in the Km amounts to an increase in affinity for substrate and an increase in the reaction rate at a given concentration of substrate.

    d: Competitive inhibitors cause an increase in Km (decreased affinity), without affecting the V_{max}.

    e: Noncompetitive inhibitors are reversible by definition. Irreversible inhibitors have the same effect in that they remove active enzyme, but because the effect is permanent, they are not considered noncompetitive.

25. **Answer e:**

Resistance is inversely proportional to the fourth power of the radius. For A, radius = 3 mm, for B, radius = 1 mm so:

$$\frac{(\text{Resistance A})}{(\text{Resistance B})} = \frac{1^4}{3^4} = \frac{1}{81}$$

    a: The resistance is inversely proportional to the fourth power of the radius.

    b: The resistance is inversely proportional to the fourth power of the radius.

    c: The resistance is inversely proportional to the fourth power of the radius.

    d: The resistance is inversely proportional to the fourth power of the radius.

26. **Answer b:**

Spindle primary sensory axons (1A) convey data about length and velocity of stretch.

    a: Spindle primary sensory axons do not convey data about muscle tension.

    c: Spindle primary sensory axons do not report cerebellar commands to muscles.

    d: Spindle primary sensory axons do not synapse with Renshaw cells in the cord.

    e: Spindle primary sensory axons do not terminate upon dorsal column neurons.

27. **Answer a:**

     Fibrocystic change is extremely common and 60% to 80% of adult women will develop it to some degree. Because it is a nearly universal condition, current terminology refers to it as a change in the breast, not a disease.

     b: True. Non proliferative fibrocystic change has no increased risk for the development of carcinoma.

     c: True. Proliferative fibrocystic change has an increased risk of about 1.5 × for the development of carcinoma.

     d: True. Atypical proliferation increase the risk for cancer by a factor of about 5.

     e: True. Proliferative lesions are bilateral and multifocal. Risk of subsequent development of cancer is equal in both breasts.

28. **Answer c:**

     This is a case of polycystic ovary syndrome previously termed Stein-Leventhal syndrome. Once considered unusual, it is now recognized as one of the more frequent causes of infertility. The pathogenesis is not completely known but the data currently available suggest that a circular chain of events is occurring. First, excess ovarian-produced androgen is converted to estrone by the peripheral adipose tissue. The excess circulating estrogens stimulate the hypothalamus to release gonadotropin-releasing hormone (GnRH) and inhibit the secretion of FSH. Next, the GnRH acts on the pituitary to produce LH. The combination of high LH and low FSH is characteristic of this syndrome. The increase in LH causes the ovarian theca cells to produce excess androgen, which brings the process full circle. The next effect is suppression of ovulation, abnormal maturation of the ovarian follicles, and production of follicular cysts.

29. **Answer d:**

     Preformed ATP and phosphocreatine provide a source of energy that can be used rapidly but is soon exhausted. Aerobic metabolism provides energy for prolonged exercise.

     a: Oxidation of fatty acids supports prolonged exercise; creatine phosphate stores are rapidly exhausted.

     b: Oxidation of fatty acids supports prolonged exercise; anaerobic glycolysis (a relatively short-term source of energy) is used as long as glycogen is available.

     c: Glycogenesis requires energy; amino acids are oxidized in prolonged exercise, but fatty acids are the main source of energy.

     e: Preformed ATP and creatine phosphate are used for brief bursts of exercise. Preformed creatine phosphate is rapidly exhausted, and oxidation of fatty acids primarily supports prolonged exercise.

30. **Answer d:**

     Aldolase B converts fructose 1-phosphate to glyceraldehyde and dihydroxyacetone phosphate. Hereditary fructose intolerance results when this enzyme is genetically deficient.

     a: Fructose carbons enter normal glycolysis as dihydroxyacetone phosphate and glyceraldehyde 3-phosphate.

     b: Fructose is converted directly into fructose 1-phosphate by fructokinase. It is glucose that is converted to fructose 6-phosphate.

     c: Galactose, not fructose, is converted to a UDP intermediate that is then epimerized to UDP-glucose.

     e: Phosphofructokinase does not act on free fructose. It acts to phosphorylate fructose 6-phosphate, which is derived from glucose 6-phosphate.

31. **Answer d:**

     Stimulation of nicotinic receptors in the adrenal medulla is not inhibited by atropine (muscarinic blocker) and results in the release of catecholamines, mediated by nicotinic receptors.

     a: Nonselective cholinergic agonists do not stimulate alpha receptors.

     b: The release of nitric oxide, which is blocked by atropine, would decrease blood pressure.

     c: Nonselective cholinergic agonists do not stimulate the myocardium, and they have negative effects.

     e: Nonselective cholinergic agonists do not stimulate beta receptors.

32. **Answer b:**

     Agents of slow virus infections are resistant to disinfection by formaldehyde, ultraviolet irradiation, and heating to 80° C.

     a: Slow viruses possess protein but may not possess nucleic acids.

     c: Slow virus infections are characterized by spongiform encephalopathy.

     d: Individuals at highest risk include surgeons and transplant and brain surgery patients.

     e: Slow viruses are filterable infectious agents.

33. **Answer b:**

Beta activity is the background brainwave type of a normal awake person.

a: Alpha activity is not the background brainwave type of a normal awake person.

c: Delta activity is not the background brainwave type of a normal awake person.

d: Gamma activity does not exist.

e: Theta activity is not the background brainwave type of a normal awake person.

34. **Answer a:**

Serine, like threonine, contains a hydroxyl group on its side chain.

b: Only cysteine, with its free sulfhydryl group, can form disulfide bonds.

c: The polar side chain of serine prevents its participation in hydrophobic interactions.

d: Histidine and tryptophan have nitrogen-containing ring structures, but serine does not.

e: The hydroxyl group of serine does not ionize in the normal physiologic pH range and, therefore, would not acquire a charge.

35. **Answer a:**

Excepting the capsule and trabecula, the stroma of the lymph node (including the medulla) is composed almost exclusively of type III collagen fibers (also known as reticular fibers).

b: Aponeuroses are composed of alternating sheets of dense regular connective tissue, which are arranged perpendicular to one another, layer upon layer.

c: The lamina propria of the duodenum, as well as the rest of the GI tract, is characterized by a preponderance of type I collagen fibers.

d: The submucosa of the esophagus and the remainder of the GI tract is composed, in large part, of type I collagen.

e: Type I collagen is the major fiber type in the tunica adventitia.

36. **Answer b:**

Pro-opiomelanocortin is produced in the pituitary as a 285 amino acid precursor, which is processed differently in different locations of the pituitary. Processing gives rise to nine peptides, which function either as hormones, neurotransmitters, or neuromodulators. Adrenocorticotropic hormone is a 39 amino acid that, as its name suggests, stimulates the synthesis and release of adrenal steroids by increasing the conversion of cholesterol to pregnenolone.

a: C-peptide (connecting peptide) is derived from proinsulin by proteolytic cleavage just prior to insulin release from the B cells of the pancreatic islets of Langerhans. C-peptide has no known physiologic function, but its presence in the blood stream can help to distinguish secreted insulin from exogenously administered insulin.

c: Glucagon is derived from a proglucagon precursor in the A cells of the pancreatic islets.

d: Parathyroid hormone (PTH) is derived from prepro-PTH, a 115 amino acid precursor that contains a 25 amino acid signal sequence and a 6 amino acid prosequence. A C-fragment is also produced from PTH, but it differs from that of insulin in that it is produced during the inactivation of PTH in the serum and it is named for the carboxy terminal end of the PTH molecule.

e: Somatostatin is derived from a large (MW ~11,500) prosomatostatin polypeptide in the D cells of the pancreatic islets.

37. **Answer e:**

The suprachiasmatic nucleus is the anatomical substrate for the timing of circadian rhythms.

a: The Arcuate nucleus is not the correct substrate.

b: The Habendar nucleus is not the correct substrate.

c: The lateral mammilary nucleus is not the correct substrate.

d: The nucleus proprius is not the correct substrate.

38. **Answer c:**

Following activation of T cells, there is a sustained **increase** in cytosolic calcium from membrane-sequestered intracellular stores.

a: True. Phosphatidylinositol-phospholipase C-gamma 1 catalyzed hydrolysis of phosphatidylinositol 4,5-bisphosphate does occur.

b: True. Increased levels of cytoplasmic inositol 1,4,5-triphosphate and diacylglycerol do occur.

d: True. Activation of protein kinase C does occur.

e: True. Activation by calmodulin or kinases other than protein kinase C and phosphatases does occur.

39. **Answer b:**

Cell walls of gram-positive bacteria may have lipoteichoic or teichoic acids in their cell wall.

a: Both gram-positive and gram-negative bacteria have peptidoglycan in their cell walls.

c: Only gram-negative bacteria have polysaccharide in their cell walls.

d: Gram-negative bacteria have Lipid A in their cell walls.

e: Only gram-negative bacteria have O antigens in their cell walls.

40. **Answer d:**
Ciliated epithelial cells do not line the small intestine or any other portion of the GI tract.

a: Enterocytes are typical absorptive cells found in abundant supply in the small intestine.

b: Goblet cells are located in the intestinal epithelium but not the stomach.

c: Paneth cells line crypts primarily in the small intestine.

e: Stem cells are located near the bases of the crypts of Lieberkühn in the small intestine.

41. **Answer c:**
121° C is effective in killing both vegetative bacterial cells and spores.

a: 95° C is less than the boiling temperature of water and would probably be marginally effective in killing vegetative cells, but not spores.

b: 102° C is just above the boiling temperature of water and will kill most vegetative cells, but not spores.

d: 212° F is the boiling temperature of water and will kill vegetative cells, but not spores.

e: 225° F will kill vegetative cells, but not spores.

42. **Answer e:**
The substantia gelatinosa is lamina II of the dorsal horn.

a: The intermediolateral cell column is in lamina VII from T1-L2.

b: The nucleus dorsalis of Clark is in lamina VII.

c: The sacral parasympathetic nucleus is in lamina VII from S2-S4.

d: Spinal border cells are in lamina VII from L2-S3 and give rise to the ventral spinocerebellar tract.

43. **Answer e:**
The ophthalmic division of the trigeminal nerve supplies the nociceptors in the cornea. Loss of these fibers would interrupt the pathway for the corneal reflex.

a: A peripheral lesion of the trigerminal nerve does not cause cough.

b: A peripheral lesion of the trigerminal nerve does not cause dysphonia.

c: A peripheral lesion of the trigerminal nerve does not cause dysphagia.

d: The trigeminal nerve provides general sensation to the tongue, but taste is carried by cranial nerves VII, IX, and X.

44. **Answer e:**
Melanocytes are not present in the sensory retina. They are present in the choroid, ciliary body, and iris. The only melanosomes that exist in the sensory retina are found in pigment epithelial cells.

a: Ganglion cells in layer 8 of the retina are an example of multipolar neurons.

b: Pigment cells in layer 1 of the retina are epithelioid in nature.

c: Nerve cells in layer 6 of the retina are an example of bipolar neurons.

d: Arterioles in layers 8 and 9 of the retina possess smooth muscle cells.

45. **Answer e:**
The overall 5-year survival rate in carcinoma of the pancreas is about 3%. The 1-year survival rate is about 20%. Less than 15% of tumors are resectable at the time of diagnosis.

46. **Answer c:**
The left middle cerebral artery supplies the primary motor cortex and Broca's speech area in the dominant hemisphere. A lesion of Broca's area on the dominant side may leave a patient unable to speak or able to speak a few substantive words in a telegraphic manner, since it is so difficult to get out whole sentences. His hyperreflexia and spasticity of the right arm indicate that his lesion is in the left hemisphere, since the corticospinal tract decussates.

a: A stroke of the anterior spinal artery at the appropriate cervical level could account for the paralysis of his upper arm but probably also would have affected the foot. This lesion could not have accounted for his Broca's aphasia.

b: A stroke in the left anterior cerebral artery would have affected his right foot and probably spared his right arm and speech areas.

d: A stroke in the right anterior cerebral artery would have affected his left foot, spared his right arm, and not affected his speech.

e: A stroke in the right middle cerebral artery would have affected his left arm. If the speech area were on this side, it would be affected. However, since he is a right-handed person, there is only a small chance that his speech center is not in his dominant (left) hemisphere.

47. **Answer c:**

By preventing the flow of protons through the ATP synthetase stalk, ATP synthesis is inhibited. Because the protons cannot complete the circuit, they build up a steep gradient, and electron transport is inhibited by the law of mass action.

a: Antimycin A is the drug that blocks electron flow between cytochromes b and c.

b: Dinitrophenol serves as an uncoupler by permitting the free diffusion of protons back into the matrix circumventing ATP synthetase. This permits the uninterrupted flow of electrons, which pump the protons out while ATP synthetase remains inactive in producing ATP.

d: Atractyloside will inhibit the adenine nucleotide carrier and ultimately will inhibit ATP synthesis due to depletion of the ADP pool.

e: Amytal and rotenone inhibit the oxidation of NADH by NADH dehydrogenase and will inhibit oxidative phosphorylation indirectly by blocking proton pumping.

48. **Answer e:**

The association between side chains in the linear sequence of amino acids is spontaneous and causes folding to occur as the polypeptide is synthesized on the ribosome.

a: Although ionic or other interactions between the side chains can affect the stability of the helix, the primary stabilization is derived from a regular pattern of hydrogen bonding between donor and acceptor groups in peptide bonds.

b: Although adjacent cysteine residues could form a disulfide bond, the more likely interaction will be between cysteines that are separated by a significant distance in the primary structure and are brought together by folding into the native conformation.

c: Quarternary structure is the reversible association of monomeric subunits and, therefore, cannot be stabilized by covalent bonds. Weak bonds, such as hydrogen bonds, electrostatic (salt bridge) bonds, hydrophobic forces, and van der Waals interactions, contribute to stabilization of quaternary structure.

d: Denaturation involves a gradual unfolding of the native conformation and, in its early stages, can be reversed. When unfolding permits molecules to interact and aggregate, the process becomes irreversible.

49. **Answer c:**

Succinylcholine, a depolarizing neuromuscular blocker, is frequently used for muscle relaxation in surgery.

a: Tubocurarine is not a depolarizing muscle relaxant.

b: Tetrodotoxin is a sodium channel blocker and is not used in therapy.

d: Methacholine is a muscarinic agonist.

e: Bethanecol is a muscarinic agonist.

50. **Answer d:**

An anal impression smear is used to diagnose pinworm infection (*Enterobius vermicularis*).

a: Enterobius eggs are rarely seen in stool specimens, nor are adult worms.

b: Enterobius is not found in the blood.

c: Enterobius is not found in spinal fluid.

e: Skin snips are sometimes done to aid in the diagnosis of Leishmania infections, not in the diagnosis of pinworm.

51. **Answer d:**

Haversion systems are not a component of cancellous (spongy) bone. They *are* found in compact bone.

a: Osteoblasts are present in both spongy and compact bone.

b: Osteoclasts are present in both spongy and compact bone.

c: Osteocytes, as well as the spaces in which their cell bodies reside (lacunae), are present in both spongy and compact bone.

e: Lacunae are present in both spongy and compact bone.

52. **Answer e:**

The arterial supply of the testes is derived from the testicular arteries, which are paired branches of the abdominal aorta.

a: Most of the arterial supply to the pelvic viscera is derived from branches of the internal iliac artery.

b: Branches of the internal iliac arteries do gain access to the gluteal region via the greater sciatic foramen.

c: The labia majora receive their arterial supply, in part, from the posterior labial arteries, which are derived from the internal pudendal artery, a branch of the internal iliac artery.

d: The iliacus and psoas muscles receive a portion of their arterial supply from branches of the internal iliac artery.

53. **Answer a:**

   The arcuate fasciculus connects Broca's speech area with Wernicke's speech area. Characteristics of a lesion in the arcuate fasciculus include normal, spontaneous, and fluent speech but with impaired repetition, frequent paraphasias, and frequent word-finding pauses.

   b: The cingulum underlies the cingulate gyrus. It is not associated with these symptoms.
   c: The corpus callosum connects the two cerebral hemispheres. A lesion in the corpus callosum does not produce these symptoms.
   d: The inferior occipitofrontal fasciculus connects the frontal lobe with the occipital lobe.
   e: The uncinate fasciculus connects the orbital frontal gyri and parts of the inferior and middle frontal gyri with the anterior portion of the temporal lobe.

54. **Answer d:**

   Children with petit mal seizures do not have an aura that precedes their seizure.

   a: True. Petit mal seizures last 30 seconds or less.
   b: True. There is immediate mental clearing after a seizure.
   c: True. The EEG is normal between seizures.
   e: True. Petit mal seizures usually have a childhood onset.

55. **Answer c:**

   Prophase begins when chromosomes become visible. Each chromosome consists of two chromatids.

   a: The cell cycle refers to two phases, the interphase and mitosis. Chromatids are held together by centromeres, a synonym for kinetochores.
   b: The synthesis phase is that part of interphase when DNA replicates. Chromatids are held together by kinetochores, a synonym for centromeres.
   d: In interphase, chromosomes are invisible. The term "diplotene" is a stage (phase) of the meiotic I prophase.
   e: In metaphase, chromosomes line up on the equatorial plate. The term "leptotene" is a stage (phase) of the meiotic I prophase.

56. **Answer b:**

   As a result of the electrogenic exchange of 3 Na^+ for 2 K^+, the Na^+ pump contributes a small portion of the resting membrane potential.

   a: The pump is electrogenic (transports 3 Na^+ in exchange for 2 K^+).
   c: K^+ binds extracellularly for transport into the cell.
   d: Na^+ is transported actively from the intracellular fluid out of the cell.
   e: Na^+ binds at an intracellular site for extrusion from the cell.

57. **Answer c:**

   NADH (as well as acetyl CoA) has been shown to have a stimulatory effect on the PDC kinase, which inactivates the PDC by catalyzing its phosphorylation.

   a: Coenzyme A is a coenzyme that accepts the two carbon acetyl group from lipoic acid after the decarboxylation of pyruvate. It does not stimulate the kinase enzyme that inactivates the PDC.
   b: Thiamine pyrophosphate binds the substrate, pyruvate, and helps to catalyze its decarboxylation, but it has no effect on the PDC kinase.
   d: Insulin stimulates the dephosphorylation of the PDC by PDC phosphatase, causing its reactivation.
   e. Lipoic acid is a covalently bound prosthetic group that accepts the acetyl group from thiamine pyrophosphate and donates it to Coenzyme A to produce acetyl CoA.

58. **Answer a:**

   A motor unit is defined as an alpha motor neuron and the set of extrafusal muscle fibers that it innervates.

   b: A motor unit is not a corticospinal cell and all the alpha motor neurons it innervates.
   c: A motor unit is not a corticocerebellar neuron and its reticulospinal branches.
   d: A motor unit is not a large muscle fiber and all the alpha motor neurons contacting it.
   e: A motor unit is not a one gamma motor neuron and all the intrafusal fibers it innervates.

59. **Answer e:**

   Circulating immune complexes are deposited in the postcapillary venule walls. The immune complexes fix complement and with the release of C5a and C3a attract neutrophils to the site. The neutrophils are activated and then release toxic materials that cause endothelial injury. Neutrophils also migrate through the wall of the venule and form loose aggregates around the vessel. The leukocytes are themselves short lived and fragmented, hence the name leukocytoclastic.

60. **Answer e:**

The ischioanal fossa is not continuous with the superficial perineal space since the latter terminates at the posterior margin of the urogenital diaphragm.

a: The ischioanal fossa does typically contain an abundance of adipose tissue.

b: The pudendal canal is located along the inferior margin of the obturator internus muscle, which forms the lateral wall of the ischioanal fossa.

c: The inferior rectal nerves are derived from the pudendal nerve within the ischioanal fossa.

d: The inferior rectal arteries represent branches of the internal pudendal vessels and travel in a lateral to medial direction within the ischioanal fossa.

61. **Answer c:**

Vibrio cholerae has recently become much more prevalent as a diarrheal pathogen world-wide.

a: Bacteremia and sepsis are not part of the pathogenesis of cholera.

b: Cholera is wide-spread and not limited to the Nile River Valley.

d: Antibiotic therapy is of secondary value. Fluid and electrolyte replacement are essential.

e: *Vibrio cholerae* is not a normal inhabitant of the human bowel.

62. **Answer c:**

The repressor is the protein produced by the regulatory gene.

a: The promoter is not a protein, but a region of the gene (or operon) where RNA polymerase binds to initiate transcription.

b: The operator is not a protein, but a region of the promoter where the repressor binds, thus blocking the movement of RNA polymerase into the gene.

d: The enhancer is found in eukaryotes only and is a region of DNA that binds regulatory proteins that then interact with promoter regions to affect the rate of transcription.

e: The inducer is generally not a protein, but a metabolite that combines with the repressor to inactivate it, thus allowing RNA polymerase to bind to the promoter.

63. **Answer d:**

Depletion of donor bone marrow T lymphocytes reduces graft-versus-host disease, although in humans, depletion of T lymphocytes also reduces the efficiency of engraftment.

a, b, c: Depletion of host bone marrow B lymphocytes or T lymphocytes, or depletion of donor bone marrow B lymphocytes, has little or no effect on reducing graft-versus-host disease.

64. **Answer b:**

The skeletal muscle pump increases venous return as a result of muscle contraction squeezing the peripheral veins that contain valves directing flow toward the heart.

a: Dilation of the peripheral veins will decrease venous pressure and decrease flow toward the heart.

c: The opposite is true: increasing respiratory rate will increase venous return ("respiratory pump").

d: The opposite is true: increasing blood volume will increase venous return.

e: Decreased sympathetic stimulation of the veins will result in venous dilation and decrease flow toward the heart.

65. **Answer b:**

Microglia do not contribute to the regeneration of peripheral axons after the axons have been cut.

a: True. Microglia contribute to the phagocytosis of cellular debris at sites of CNS injury.

c: True. Microglia contribute to the release of cytokines in response to CNS injury.

d: True. Microglia contribute to the scar tissue formation in the CNS.

e: True. Microglia contribute to the stimulation of astroglial proliferation.

66. **Answer e:**

A more water-soluble solute will penetrate the lipid bilayer of the cell membrane less readily than a lipid-soluble solute.

a: Concentration gradients provide the force driving passive diffusion.

b: An increase in lipid solubility will allow the solute to penetrate the lipid bilayer of the cell membrane more readily.

c: A thinner membrane provides less barrier to diffusion than a thicker membrane.

d: More surface area will allow more diffusion to occur.

67. **Answer d:**
     The spleen occupies an intraperitoneal location.

     a: The ureters occupy a retroperitoneal location.
     b: The suprarenal glands occupy a retroperitoneal location on the posterior abdominal wall.
     c: The celiac ganglion is located retroperitoneally near the origin of the celiac trunk on the posterior abdominal wall.
     e: Although it once had a mesentery during embryonic development, the descending colon has come to occupy a retroperitoneal location.

68. **Answer d:**
     Catalase is produced by members of the genus staphylococcus but not by members of the streptococci or enterococci genera.

     a: Resistance to novobiocin does not differentiate staphylococci from streptococci and enterococci.
     b: Sensitivity to bacitracin serves to differentiate Group A beta-hemolytic streptococci from other beta-hemolytic streptococci.
     c: Ability to coagulate plasma differentiates *Staphylococcus aureus* from other staphylococci.
     e: There are overlapping hemolytic patterns between these groups that would not allow them to be distinguished from one another.

69. **Answer e:**
     The superior belly of the omohyoid muscle forms the anterior boundary of the carotid triangle of the neck.

     a: The sternomastoid muscle forms the posterior boundary of the carotid triangle of the neck.
     b: The trapezius muscle forms the posterior boundary of the posterior triangle of the neck.
     c: The mandible does not contribute to the boundaries of the anterior triangle of the neck.
     d: The posterior belly of the digastric muscle forms the superior boundary of the carotid triangle of the neck.

70. **Answer d:**
     The ophthalmic artery enters the orbital cavity, together with the optic nerve, via the optic foramen.

     a: The ophthalmic artery arises as a branch of the internal carotid artery.
     b: The central artery of the retina arises as a branch of the ophthalmic artery.

c: After entering the orbit, the ophthalmic artery passes from the lateral aspect of the optic nerve to its medial side by crossing superiorly to the nerve.
     e: The lacrimal branch of the ophthalmic artery supplies the lacrimal gland near the superolateral aspect of orbital margin.

71. **Answer a:**
     Intestinal and renal tubular cells contain Na^+ and glucose cotransport carriers in the luminal membrane that effect active transport of glucose across this membrane.

     b: The mechanism is secondary active cotransport with Na^+.
     c: The mechanism is secondary active cotransport with Na^+.
     d: The mechanism is secondary active cotransport with Na^+.
     e: The mechanism is secondary active cotransport with Na^+.

72. **Answer b:**
     Allelic exclusion is characteristic of both B and T lymphocyte receptors for antigens.

     a: Allelic exclusion does not allow deletion of allelic genes by homologous chromosomes.
     c: Allelic exclusion does not occur in B lymphocytes, but does occur in T lymphocytes.
     d: Allelic exclusion does not allow dual specificity.
     e: Allelic exclusion does not allow for production of both kappa and lambda light chains to be produced by a single B lymphocyte.

73. **Answer e:**
     This is a fairly classic description of ulcerative colitis. It has a number of clinical similarities to Crohn's disease, but the lack of involvement of the small bowel and left colon, coupled with inflammation that is limited to the mucosa, are good discriminators in this case. Crohn's disease can involve anyplace in the GI tract from the mouth to the anus. Ulcerative colitis is limited to the colon. In unusual instances, the terminal ileum may show some nonspecific inflammatory changes on the basis of toxic "washback" from the colon.

     a: The patient suffers from ulcerative colitis. Uveitis is a potential complication.
     b: The patient suffers from ulcerative colitis. Ankylosing spondylitis is a potential complication.

c: The patient suffers from ulcerative colitis. Sclerosing cholangitis is a potential complication.

d: The patient suffers from ulcerative colitis. Toxic megacolon is a potential complication.

74. **Answer c:**

Methylphenidate is a mild central nervous system stimulant slightly less active than d-amphetamine.

a: Phenytoin is an antiepileptic drug.
b: Diazepam is a sedative/hypnotic.
d: Amitriptyline is an antidepressant.
e: Dextropropoxyphene is a weak opiate agonist.

75. **Answer b:**

The Edinger-Westphal nucleus provides preganglionic parasympathetic axons that terminate in the ciliary ganglion.

a: The inferior salivatory nucleus provides preganglionic parasympathetic axons that terminate in the otic ganglion.
c: Nucleus solitarius is not a parasympathetic nucleus.
d: Nucleus ambiguus is not a parasympathetic nucleus.
e: The superior salivatory nucleus is a parasympathetic nucleus whose axons terminate in the pterygopalatine and submandibular ganglia.

76. **Answer e:**

Anti-inflammatory treatment may reduce the requirement of oral corticosteroid dose in patients with asthma.

a: The systemic effect of administering methotrexate via aerosol is important.
b: Methotrexate is not a bronchodilator, it is an anti-inflammatory.
c: Methotrexate is given as a "low dose pulse therapy" once in a week. Its anti-inflammatory effect may reduce the requirement of oral corticosteroid dose.
d: Methotrexate does not potentiate the effect of beta agonist and theophylline.

77. **Answer e:**

Patients with Hodgkin's disease have a deficiency in T-lymphocyte function, which often can be found early in the course of the disease if sensitive methods of testing are used. The degree of anergy increases as the disease progresses. The chemotherapeutic agents used in treatment also depress cellular immunity, which only exascerbates the problem. Typically, humoral immunity remains intact until late in the course of the disease.

a: Acquired agammaglobulinemia is not common in Hodgkin's disease.
b: Hypocomplementemis is not common in Hodgkin's disease
c: Increased serum IgM is not common in Hodgkin's disease
d: Absent serum IgA is not common in Hodgkin's disease.

78. **Answer d:**

Patients with osteopetrosis have an extremely attenuated marrow cavity, because of the retention of the primary spongiosum. As a result of this, the space for hematopoetic bone marrow is markedly reduced. These patients often have multiple foci of extramedullary hematopoesis as compensation for the lack of functional bone marrow.

a: Cartilaginous tumors are not associated with osteopetrosis.
b: Osteosarcoma is not associated with osteopetrosis.
c: Synthesis of abnormal type I collagen is not associated with osteopetrosis.
d: The foci of heterotopic bone formation are not associated with osteopetrosis.

79. **Answer b:**

The tectum is the roof of the mesencephalon. It is made up of the colliculi.

a: The tectum is not part of the diencephalon.
c: The tectum is not part of the myelencephalon.
d: The tectum is not part of the prosencephalon.
e: The tectum is not part of the thalamus.

80. **Answer d:**

The nucleus solitarius is not involved in the transmission of somatic afferent sensation.

a: Visceral afferent sensation from cranial nerve X is related through nucleus solitarius.
b: Visceral afferent sensation from cranial nerve IX from the carotid sinus and cranial nerve X from the aortic arch relay through nucleus solitarius for blood pressure control.
c: The nucleus solitarius is involved in respiration.
e: The nucleus solitarius is the origin of second order neurons in the taste pathway.

81. **Answer d:**
    Cyclosporine is used only for immunosuppressive therapy; it inhibits the gene transcription of IL-2, IL-3, IFN-γ.

    a: Vincristine is used in cancer chemotherapy.
    b: Cyclophosphamide is used in cancer chemotherapy.
    c: Methotrexate is used in cancer chemotherapy.
    d: Dacarbanine is used in cancer chemotherapy.

82. **Answer b:**
    Colchicine quickly relieves pain and inflammation by inhibiting phagocytosis.

    a: Methotrexate is not the drug of choice in gout, because immunological processes are not the main mechanisms in gout.
    c: Probenecid is the drug of choice, if serum uric acid levels are extremely high.
    d: Even though high dose aspirin may alleviate some of the symptoms, low dose aspirin elevates serum uric acid levels.
    e: Discontinuation of allopurinol will not solve the problem.

83. **Answer d:**
    The two glycosides differ significantly in their half-lives (168 hours for digitoxin and 40 hours for digoxin).

    a: The therapeutic index for digoxin and digitoxin are similar.
    b: The site of action on the heart for the drugs is similar.
    c: Both drugs can cause nausea and vomiting.
    e: Both digoxin and digitoxin are usually administered orally.

84. **Answer a:**
    Bacteria are *transformed* with plasmic vectors and are *transfected* with bacteriophage vectors.

    b: Although the process is very inefficient, intact (undegraded) circular plasmid DNA is taken up by bacterial cells.
    c: Antibiotic genes (selectable markers) in plasmids help to identify the host cells that contain the vector, since they will grow to form a colony on antibiotic-containing medium. Host cells without a plasmid fail to grow.

    d: The central portion of the bacteriophage chromosome is not essential to its role as a recombinant DNA vector and is removed during the ligation procedure.
    e: The recombinant DNA insert is ligated with linearized plasmid DNA at both ends, restoring the circular DNA of the plasmid.

85. **Answer b:**
    UDP-glucuronyl transferase adds two glucuronic moieties to bilirubin, converting it from a lipid-soluble molecule to a water-soluble molecule.

    a: Biliverdin is converted directly to bilirubin in a reaction that uses one NADPH.
    c: Direct-reacting bilirubin, as measured by the van den Bergh reaction, is the water soluble, or conjugated form, which is produced by UDP-glucuronyl transferase. Absence of this enzyme will, therefore, increase the amount of indirect-reacting bilirubin.
    d: Bilirubin is converted to urobilinogen in the small intestines, but the enzymes are located in the bacterial flora.
    e. Analogous to bilirubin, bile acids are produced in the liver, are conjugated with water-soluble molecules, and are secreted in the bile. However, although bilirubin is a breakdown product of heme, all bile acids are synthesized from cholesterol.

86. **Answer e:**
    There is no pointer among the symptoms toward any of the drugs listed.

    a: Morphine overdose would exhibit characteristic CNS symptoms.
    b: Phenytoin would have blocked convulsions.
    c: Diphenhydramine would have produced sedation.
    d: Chlorpromazine would have produced CNS symptoms.

87. **Answer a:**
    Morphine would have produced miosis and decreased rate of respiration.

    b: Phenytoin does not produce mydriasis.
    c: Diphenhydramine does not produce mydriasis.
    d: Chlorpromazine does not produce mydriasis.
    e: Guanethidine may produce mydriasis.

88. **Answer c:**

In the case of status epilepticus, intravenous diazepam is the right choice of drug.

a: Status epilepticus needs immediate treatment regardless of the cause.
b: Nalorphine is only effective in opiate overdose.
d: There is no time to wait for the effect of intramuscular phenytoin.
e: Physostigmine intramuscularly has no relevancy to this emergency situation.

89. **Answer b:**

The dental papilla is derived from mesoderm and, hence, is not a component of the enamel organ.

a: The external (outer) enamel epithelium is a component of the enamel organ.
c: The stellate reticulum is a component of the enamel organ.
d: The internal (inner) enamel epithelium is a component of the enamel organ.
e: The stratum intermedium is a component of the enamel organ.

90. **Answer b:**

Isophane (NPH) insulin is an intermediate acting insulin preparation with a delayed onset of action.

a: This curve represents the effect of protamine zinc insulin; it has a more delayed onset and a longer duration than isophane insulin.
c: This curve represents regular insulin, with a quick onset, and a short action.

91. **Answer d:**

Lidocaine in sensitive patients may produce convulsions in moderately high therapeutic doses.

a: Quinidine does not produce convulsions.
b: Hydralazine does not produce convulsions.
c: Phenytoin is an anticonvulsive agent.
e: Bretylium does not produce convulsions.

92. **Answer a:**

Mixed tumors of salivary gland, better termed pleomorphic adenomas, are benign tumors of the salivary gland that take origin from a single line of parenchymal cells. The cell line of origin is either a ductular epithelial cell or a myoepithelial cell, which differentiates in two separate lines.

b: Only a single cell line is responsible for the development of these tumors. The older mixed tumor concept is no longer considered valid.

c: Although true "collision" tumors do occur, they are fleetingly rare and usually malignant.
d, e: These are completely benign tumors.

93. **Answer c:**

Spectrin is not a structural protein in skeletal muscle cells. It is an intermediate filament in erythrocytes.

a: Titin is a structural protein in skeletal muscle cells that helps to anchor protein filaments so they function as a coordinated unit.
b: C protein is a structural protein in skeletal muscle cells that helps to anchor protein filaments so they function as a coordinated unit.
d: Myomesin is a structural protein in skeletal muscle cells that helps to anchor protein filaments so they function as a coordinated unit.
e: Alpha-actin is a structural protein in skeletal muscle cells that helps to anchor protein filaments so they function as a coordinated unit.

94. **Answer a:**

The middle cerebral artery supplies the frontal eye fields (area 8) and the primary motor cortex. Lesions to these areas would cause the left gaze palsy and left hemiparesis.

b, c, d: Wrong combinations of palsy and hemiparesis.
e: Achromatopsia is caused by a small lesion to the V4 area of the occipital lobe. This areas is supplied by the posterior cerebral artery.

95. **Answer b:**

There is little effect of autonomic activity on the pulmonary vasculature.

a: Pulmonary resistance is lowest at functional residual capacity, and increases when lung volume changes away from FRC.
c: Increased blood flow and arterial pressure open more capillaries and widen those already open, so that resistance decreases as flow increases.
d: The pulmonary and systemic circuits both receive the same blood flow (equal cardiac output), yet the driving pressure in the pulmonary circuit is about $\frac{1}{10}$ the driving pressure in the systemic circuit. Therefore, pulmonary resistance must be only $\frac{1}{10}$ the systemic resistance.
e: Although the mechanism is unknown, alveolar hypoxia induces pulmonary vasoconstriction.

96. **Answer c:**
    All sensory information from the head, including taste, is relayed though the VPM nucleus.

    a: The anterior nucleus is a nucleus of the limbic system.
    b: The VA nucleus is a motor relay nucleus.
    d: The VPL nucleus is a sensory relay nucleus for body sensation.
    e: The VL nucleus is a motor relay nucleus.

97. **Answer d:**
    Fibers responsible for the secretomotor innervation of the lacrimal gland do not travel with the ophthalmic division of the trigeminal nerve.

    a: The preganglionic parasympathetic input to the lacrimal gland synapses in the pterygopalatine ganglion with postganglionic parasympathetic neurons.
    b: The facial nerve, prior to the origin of the greater petrosal nerve, carries preganglionic parasympathetic (secretomotor) fibers destined for the lacrimal gland after synapsing in the pterygopalatine ganglion.
    c: The maxillary division of the trigeminal nerve carries postganglionic parasympathetic (secretomotor) fibers destined for the lacrimal gland.
    e: The greater petrosal nerve arises from the facial nerve and carries preganglionic parasympathetic (secretomotor) fibers destined for the lacrimal gland after synapsing in the pterygopalatine ganglion.

98. **Answer c:**
    Alcoholic liver disease is responsible for about 60% to 70% of cases of cirrhosis. Viral hepatitis is a poor second being responsible for about 10% of cases. Estimates are that about 15% of alcoholics will develop liver cirrhosis.

    a: Viral hepatitis is the second most frequent cause of hepatic cirrhosis. It accounts for only about 10% of cases.
    b: Biliary disease is not a common cause of hepatic cirrhosis.
    d: Alpha$_1$-trypsin deficiency is not a common cause of hepatic cirrhosis.
    e: Hemachromatosis is not a common cause of hepatic cirrhosis.

99. **Answer d:**
    Natural killer lymphocytes bear CD16, an F_c receptor for IgG, and are important in antibody-dependent cellular cytotoxicity.

    a: B lymphocytes do not possess CD16.
    b: T helper lymphocytes do not possess CD16.
    c: T cytotoxic lymphocytes do not possess CD16.
    e: Natural killer lymphocytes bear CD16.

100. **Answer a:**
    There are no glands in the true vocal chords.

    b: The epiglottis is supported mainly by elastic cartilage.
    c: Respiratory epithelium does line the lumen adjacent to the false vocal chords.
    d: The vocalis ligament is composed mainly of elastic fibers.
    e: True vocal chords are created by an aggregation of skeletal muscle cells, except near the epithelial surface where elastic fibers are located.

101. **Answer b:**
    Important features of the cross-bridge cycle include charging of myosin by ATP at rest, activation by increasing Ca^{2+} concentration, and binding of a second ATP molecule to release myosin from actin.

    a: Myosin is activated by ATP binding; interaction of Ca^{2+} with tropomyosin is necessary for linkage of myosin to actin.
    c: Myosin is charged by ATP binding; ADP and PI are released from myosin.
    d: Ca^{2+} does not "inactivate;" the ion is necessary for actin-myosin interaction.
    e: ATP binds to myosin; tropomyosin is a regulatory protein governing actin-myosin interaction.

102. **Answer d:**
    The cornea is avascular and thus lacks arterioles and their capillary beds. Therefore there is no smooth muscle, which means that muscle is the one basic tissue absent in the cornea. Epithelium, connective tissue, and nervous tissue are present.

    a: Endothelium is a form of epithelial tissue, one of the three basic tissues that the cornea possesses.
    b: Fibrocytes (fibroblasts) are present in connective tissue, one of the three basic tissues that the cornea possesses.

c: Epithelial cells compose stratified squamous nonkeratinized epithelium, one of the three basic tissues that the cornea possesses.

e: The surface of the cornea is exquisitely sensitive to pain, which means that nerve cell processes are abundant. This, in turn, means that nerve dendrites exist. They represent a component of nervous tissue, one of the three basic tissues present in the cornea.

103. **Answer a:**

Acetylcholine is released by both the sympathetic and parasympathetic systems at the preganglionic nerve terminal.

b: Epinephrine is not released at the preganglionic nerve terminal.

c: Norepinephrine is released by the majority of the sympathetic postganglionic nerve terminals.

d: Serotonin is not released by the autonomic nervous system.

e: Substance P is not released by the autonomic nervous system.

104: **Answer a:**

Sexual differentiation of the brain in humans occurs at about 5 months in utero.

b, c, d, e: These times are way too late.

105. **Answer d:**

The pterygomaxillary fissure is a vertically placed passage located between the infratemporal fossa and the pterygopalatine fossa. In transmits the maxillary artery.

a: The sphenopalatine foramen leads from the pterygopalatine fossa into the nasal cavity. It transmits the sphenopalatine artery, the terminal part of the maxillary artery.

b: The superior orbital fissure does not communicate with the pterygopalatine fossa.

c: The pterygopalatine fossa communicates with the middle cranial fossa via the pterygoid canal, which transmits the nerve of the same name.

e: The pterygopalatine fossa communicates with the orbit via the inferior orbital fissure.

106. **Answer e:**

Giaridiasis is usually a water-borne pathogen but may be transmitted by ingestion of contaminated, uncooked vegetables or fruits, or person to person spread by fecal-oral or oral-anal routes.

a: *Leishmaniasis* is transmitted by the bite of the sand-fly.

b: *Falciparum malaria* is transmitted by the bite of the mosquito.

c: *African trypanosomiasis* is transmitted by the tsetse fly.

d: *American trypanosomiasis* is transmitted by the "kissing" bug.

107. **Answer b:**

Ethosuximide is the drug of choice when absence seizures occur alone. It has less toxic effects than valproate.

a: Valproic acid is very effective against absence seizures, but it is preferred only when the patient has concomitant generalized tonic-clonic attacks.

c: Trimethadione is effective in absence seizures, but rarely used because it causes serious sedation and numerous toxic effects.

d: Thiopental is a general anesthetic.

e: Carbamazepine is the drug of choice for partial seizures.

108. **Answer c:**

Methotrexate is a folic acid antagonist; its toxic effects on bone marrow and GI mucosa can be reversed by administration of leucovorin (citrovorum factor) while still leaving the tumor cells subject to its cytotoxic action.

a: Trimethoprim potentiates the effect of sulfonamides and inhibits protozoal dihydrofolate reductase (not the human enzyme).

b: Pyrimethamine inhibits protozoal dihydrofolate reductase. It is much less active on the human enzyme.

d: AraCTP is a metabolite of cytarabine that inhibits DNA polymerase.

e: FdUMP, a metabolite of 5-FU, inhibits the synthesis of thymine nucleotides.

109. **Answer c:**

Acidosis stimulates renal glutamine utilization and as a result, HCO_3^- generation.

a: Plasma P_{CO_2} increases in respiratory acidosis.

b: Hyperventilation is the respiratory response to metabolic acidosis.

d: Renal compensation requires 3 to 5 days to increase plasma bicarbonate concentration and stabilize a respiratory acidosis.

e: Renal compensation is accompanied by an increase in urinary NH_4^+ excretion.

110. **Answer e:**

Hepatocytes are neither structurally nor functionally identical. Nonetheless, they are all active as exocrine and endocrine cells. They synthesize and secrete albumin and fibrinogen, as well as bile. They also detoxify lipid-soluble drugs. As a result, they possess extensive rER and sER, a prominent Golgi complex, and numerous mitochondria. Hence, their chromatin is predominantly extended (euchromatic) in contrast to the cells referred to in the other foils.

a: Fibrocytes are relatively inactive compared to fibroblasts. Hence, fibrocyte nuclei are heterochromatic.

b: Unilocular adipocytes possess few organelles and thus are inactive. Therefore, their nuclei are heterochromatic.

c: Orthochromatophilic erythroblasts are mitotically inactive and have formed the great majority of hemoglobin that is present in the adult erythrocyte. Hence, their nuclei are heterochromatic.

d: Perineuronal oligodendrocytes, along with microglia, possess the most heterochromatic nuclei in the central nervous system. This suggests that these two cell types are relatively inactive in comparison with astrocytes and neurons.

111. **Answer a:**

A cell with numerous mitochondria is generally involved in transporting ions and water rather than actively secreting protein for export.

b: Abundant rER is the hallmark characteristic of cells that synthesize protein for export. Ribosomes, unassociated with endoplasmic reticulum, are typically linked to cells that synthesize proteins that are not exported.

c: A nucleus with abundant euchromatin is characteristic of any synthetically active cell that is vigorously engaged in carrying out its own unique functions, which may include protein synthesis and secretion.

d: A well-developed Golgi complex is characteristic of any synthetically active cell that is vigorously engaged in carrying out its own unique functions, which may include protein synthesis and secretion.

e: A large nucleolus or several well-defined nuclei is characteristic of any synthetically active cell that is vigorously engaged in carrying out its own unique functions, which may include protein synthesis and secretion.

112. **Answer d:**

Gallstones are the major predisposing cause of the development of acute cholecystitis. In 90% of cases, a gallstone has caused obstruction of the neck of the gallbladder or the cystic duct.

a: Trauma is not a major predisposing cause of acute cholecystitis.

b: Sepsis is not a major predisposing cause of acute cholecystitis.

c: Postpartum state is not a major predisposing cause of acute cholecystitis.

e: Hepatic steatosis is not a major predisposing cause of acute cholecystitis.

113. **Answer e:**

NF-1 is a tumor-suppressor gene that is found on chromosome 17q11. When one allele is missing or dysfunctional, the patient develops schwannomas of the peripheral nerves. On occasion, some of these may progress to neurofibrosarcoma.

a: WT-1 is found on chromosome 11p13. As long as patients have at least one functional allele, they are protected. If both alleles are absent or dysfunctional, the patient is liable to develop Wilm's tumor of the kidney.

b: Rb is found on chromosome 13q14. When it is homozygously absent or dysfunctional, the patient develops retinoblastoma.

c: P53 is found on chromosome 17p13.1. It is homozygously absent in 70% of cases of colon cancers and a somewhat lesser number of breast cancers.

d: DCC is located on chromosome 18q21. It is frequently homozygously missing in cases of colon carcinoma.

114. **Answer a:**

The coronary sulcus is a groove between the atria above and ventricles below. It contains the right coronary artery, a branch of the left coronary artery, and the coronary sinus.

b: The atria are not separated on the surface of the heart by a groove.

c: The anterior and posterior interventricular grooves distinguish the right and left ventricles on the surface of the heart.

d, e: The coronary sulcus completely encircles the heart.

115. **Answer b:**

$$\text{Net pressure} = (P_{cap} - P_{in}) - (\pi_{cap} - \pi_{in})$$
$$= +7 \text{ mm Hg}$$

116. **Answer e:**

Myesthenia gravis is an autoimmune disease in which antibody is formed against the acetylcholine receptor site of skeletal muscle. Demyelination of either the CNS or PNS is not a part of this disease.

a: True. Patients with myesthenia gravis have a positive tensilon test.

b: True. Patients with myesthenia gravis have thymic hyperplasia frequently.

c: True. Patients with myesthenia gravis are ususally female.

d: True. Patients with myesthenia gravis have early involvement of the extraocular muscles.

117. Answer b:

The fasciculus gracilis would be spared since the dorsal columns receive their blood supply from the posterior spinal arteries.

a, c, d, e: All of these would be affected since the anterior spinal artery supplies blood to the lateral and ventral funiculi.

118. Answer a:

Brunn's epithelial nests are formed by the pinching off of hyperplastic invaginations of urothelium into the lamina propria. They are extremely common. Cystitis cystica is found, for example, in 60% of adult bladders. They are not a premalignant lesion.

b: Brunn's epithelial nests are formed by the pinching off of hyperplastic invaginations of urothelium into the lamina propria.

c: Brunn's epithelial nests are examples of epithelial hyperplasia.

d: Brunn's epithelial nests may be found in any urothelial covered structure.

e: Cystitis cystica is a Brunn's epithelial nest with rencual space.

119. Answer e:

Transfection is the artificial infection of a cell with purified viral nucleic acid, which results in replication of the virus.

a: Viruses can be transmitted by fomites such as clothing.

b: Viruses can be transmitted through contact with infectious secretions such as saliva and semen.

c: Zoonotic viral infections in humans may result from contact with infected animals or insects (arboviruses).

d: Aerosols are common methods of transmission of viruses to humans.

120. Answer d:

A defect in the glomerular basement membrane leads to proteinuria. Since PCTs reabsorb protein, a defect in their ability to do this might also lead to proteinuria.

a: Distal convoluted tubules do not reabsorb significant amounts of protein and thus have nothing to do with proteinuria.

b: The function of the urethra is not related in any way to proteinuria.

c: The function of the urinary bladder is not related in any way to proteinuria.

e: The function of collecting ducts is not related in any way to proteinuria.

121. Answer c:

Plasmin creates a generalized lytic state, thus all protective thrombi and target thromboemboli are broken down.

a: True. Protamine is an antidote to heparin overdose.

b: True. Vitamin K is an antidote to warfarin overdose.

d: True. Heparin is not administered orally or intramuscularly.

e: True. Warfarin is a racemic mixture of two enantiomers that have different anticoagulant potencies.

122. Answer d:

By covering the myosin binding sites when Ca^{2+} concentration is low, interaction of actin with myosin is prevented.

a, b, c, e: Tropomyosin covers myosin binding sites on actin molecules, preventing actin-myosin interaction when the muscle is at rest.

123. Answer e:

Staphylococcus epidermidis is frequently associated with bacteremia in patients with indwelling vascular catheters.

a: *Streptococcus pyogenes* is an important cause of necrotizing fasciitis.

b: *Staphylococcus aureus* is an important cause of folliculitis.

c: *Streptococcus pyogenes* is an important cause of postinfectious glomerulonephritis.

d: *Staphylococcus saprophyticus* is an important cause of urinary tract infections in young women.

124. Answer d:

Ampicillin is a broad-spectrum, lactamase sensitive, and orally effective agent.

a: Ampicillin is well absorbed from the intramuscular site.

b: Ampicillin is lactamase sensitive.

c: Ampicillin is penicillinase sensitive.

e: Ampicillin is acid resistant and penicillinase sensitive.

125. **Answer a:**

Alcaptonuria is a rare, autosomal-recessive, inborn error of amino acid metabolism in which homogentisic acid oxidase is deficient. The result is that these patients excrete homogentisic acid in their urine. On standing, the urine darkens due to the oxidation of homogentisic acid into a dark brown to black pigment. Similar pigment may be deposited into cartilages, synovia, tendons, and the sclerae.

b: Tay-Sachs disease is an autosomal-recessive disorder in which the ganglioside GM2 is not degraded normally and is deposited in the lysosomes of CNS neurons.
c: Gaucher's disease is caused by a number of single base mutations involving the long arm of chromosome 1, causing a deficiency in glucocerebrosidase. This deficiency results in the accumulation of glucosylceramide in lysosomes, particularly those of the macrophages.
d: Niemann-Pick lipidoses are a group of disorders in which cholesterol, sphingomyelin, and other glycolipids accumulate in the lysosomes of macrophages in many organs such as the brain and liver.
e: Mucopolysaccharidoses are a heterogeneous group of largely autosomal recessive disorders in which glycosaminoglycans accumulate in the lysosomes.

126. **Answer d:**

As $\dot{V}_A/\dot{Q}$ increases, alveolar P_{CO_2} decreases and P_{O_2} increases, so that alveolar gas tends to resemble inspired air.

a, b, c, e: As $\dot{V}_A/\dot{Q}$ increases, the composition of alveolar gas becomes less like mixed venous blood and more like inspired air.

127. **Answer c:**

Lovastatin inhibits HMG-CoA reductase, the first committed step in sterol biosynthesis.

a: Clofibrate increases lipolysis of lipoprotein triglyceride.
b: Cholestyramine is a bile acid-binding resin.
d: Niacin inhibits VLDL secretion.
e: Enalapril is an ACE inhibitor.

128. **Answer c:**

Brain blood flow is autoregulated to maintain the supply of oxygen to the brain, regardless of the level of arterial pressure.

a: Increased sympathetic activity to intestinal vasculature decreases blood flow.

b: Skeletal muscle blood flow increases primarily due to metabolic vasodilation.
d: Contraction of skeletal muscle in the legs aids venous return to the heart.
e: Venous return is increased during inspiration.

129. **Answer a:**

The DNA from polyoma virus is 44% GC pairs, while the DNA from medical students is only 36% GC pairs. Since a higher percentage of GC will raise the melting temperature (T_m), the medical student DNA will melt at a lower temperature than the "Pollyanna" DNA.

b: In all DNA the adenine and thymine content is equal because of complimentary base pairing.
c: The melting curves will be different because the percentage of GC is different.
d: In all DNA the cytosine and guanine content is equal because of complimentary base pairing.
e: Molecular weight is not a function of base composition.

130. **Answer b:**

Decreasing ventilation causes alveolar gas to more closely resemble mixed venous blood, i.e., lowering P_{O_2} and raising P_{CO_2}.

a, c, d, e: A decrease in this ratio increases P_{CO_2} and decreases P_{O_2}.

131. **Answer e:**

Patients with xeroderma pigmentosum (pigmented dry skin) have a defect in an endonuclease that is necessary in the repair of DNA damaged by actinic (ultraviolet) light. It is the inability to repair damaged DNA that accounts for their increased incidence of ultraviolet exposure associated with skin malignancies.

a: Loss of the P53 tumor suppressor genes is not associated with xeroderma pigmentosa.
b: Activation of the *ras* oncogene is not associated with xeroderma pigmentosa.
c: Abnormal melanin synthesis is not associated with xeroderma pigmentosa.
d: Patients with xeroderma pigmentosa show sensitivity to ultraviolet, not infrared light.

132. **Answer d:**

Erector spinae, like all intrinsic muscles of the back, is innervated by the dorsal rami of spinal nerves.

a: The erector spinae muscle is located between the posterior and middle layers of the thoracolumbar fascia.

b: The iliocostalis is the most lateral of the three vertical columns comprising the erector spinae muscle.

c: The transversospinalis muscle represents the most deeply placed of the intrinsic back muscles.

e: The spinalis is the most medial component of the erector spinae muscle.

133. **Answer a:**

As a result, Ca^{2+} concentration increases in the sarcomere, and myosin and actin can form cross-bridges.

b: The Ca^{2+} pump acts to return Ca^{2+} to the sarcoplasmic reticulum, ending cross-bridge cycling and relaxing the muscle.

c: Acetylcholinesterase in the postsynaptic membrane terminates neuromuscular transmission by cleaving acetylcholine into acetate and choline.

d: Na^+ channels are not involved here.

e: The action potential is propagated in muscle cells by nonspecific ion channels that allow both K^+ and Na^+ to equilibrate along their electrochemical gradients when open.

134. **Answer c:**

Remember that tumor cells have been immortalized as part of their malignant transformation. Because of this, cells do not die as new cells are formed, as occurs in normal tissues. The net effect is that even though tumors often have a lesser mitotic rate than do normal tissues, there is a gain in total cell mass.

a, b: These may cause acute swelling in a tumor, usually as a late stage and accompanied by hemorrhage, but they are not responsible for the general increase of tumor mass over time.

d: Most tumors have a lower mitotic rate than do many normal tissues. Some leukemias and small cell carcinoma of the lung may have a rapid rate of proliferation, but that is not the norm.

e: Tumors often cause the laying down of excessive amounts of connective tissue (desmoplasia), but this causes the tumor to become hard to palpation rather than causing a significant increase in tumor bulk.

135. **Answer d, e:**

The overall increase in risk of developing lung cancer in smokers is 10 to 20 times that of the nonsmoking population.

a: For smokers the risk of developing lung cancer is far greater than $1\times$ the risk for non-smokers.

b: For smokers the risk of developing lung cancer is far greater than $2\times$ the risk for non-smokers.

c: For smokers the risk of developing lung cancer is far greater than $5\times$ the risk for non-smokers.

136. **Answer e:**

Substance P is released by the damaged nociceptors.

a: Bradykinin is released by the damaged tissue, and it activates and sensitizes the nociceptors to release substance P.

b: Histamine is released by the mast cell, when substance P causes it to degranulate.

c: Prostaglandins are released by damaged tissue.

d: Serotonin acts on the nociceptor nerve terminal to activate it.

137. **Answer b:**

With arteriolar vasoconstriction more energy is required for blood to flow through the arterioles, and therefore pressure in the capillaries is decreased.

a: With arteriolar vasoconstriction more energy is required for blood to flow through the arterioles, and therefore pressure in the capillaries is decreased.

c: Capillary hydrostatic pressure decreases with arteriolar constriction and therefore less fluid is filtered out.

d: Vasoconstriction will decrease blood flow.

e: A decrease in blood flow due to arteriolar constriction will decrease lymph flow.

138. **Answer e:**

Quadratus plantae is attached to the calcaneus and tendons of the flexor digitorum longus. It assists the long flexor by adjusting the pull of the latter's tendons during flexion.

a: The abductor digiti minimi is attached to the calcaneous, plantar aponeurosis, and base of the proximal phalanx of the first digit.

b: The adductor hallucis lies deep to the tendons of the flexor digitorum longus muscle.

c: The flexor hallucis brevis is attached to the base of the proximal phalanx of the first digit, as well as to the cuboid and lateral cuneiform bones.

d: The quadratus plantae attaches to the base of the fifth metatarsal and to the proximal phalanx of the fifth digit.

139. **Answer e:**
   The subthalamic fasciculus terminates in the globus pallidus.

   a: Ansa lenticularis terminates in VL and VA.
   b: The dentatothalamic tract terminates in the VL nucleus.
   c: The lenticular fasciculus joins with the thalamic fasciculus, which terminates in the VL and VL thalamic nuclei.
   d: The nigrothalamic tract terminates in the VL nucleus.

140. **Answer d:**
   A common intermediate, such as a metabolite that is the product of one reaction and the substrate for another, is the essential requirement for coupling of two reactions.

   a: The transition state is an intermediate form between the substrate(s) and product(s) of one reaction. This should not be confused with the need for a common intermediate between two separate reactions.
   b: If two reactions do not have a common intermediate, their standard free energy changes are irrelevant.
   c: The concept of coupling does not concern reaction rates.
   e: The activation energies of individual reactions are unrelated either to coupling or to the total free energy change.

141. **Answer d:**
   The fornix originates from neurons in the hippocampus and is part of the Papez circuit.

   a: The amygdala does not give rise to the fornix.
   b: The anterior nucleus of the thalamus is part of the Papez circuit but does not give rise to the fornix.
   c: The cingulate gyrus is part of the Papez circuit but does not give rise to the fornix.
   e: The subthalamic nucleus does not give rise to the fornix.

142. **Answer e:**
   Sudden and complete occlusion of the internal carotid artery can cause a large stroke, if there is an incomplete circle of Willis. If the occlusion takes place gradually in a patient with an incomplete circle of Willis, there is potential collateral circulation from reversal of flow through the ophthalmic artery, a branch of the external carotid artery.

   a: Autoregulation is not the best answer.
   b: Blood pressure is not the best answer.

   c: Blood volume is not the best answer.
   d: Race does not play a role.

143. **Answer a:**
   Even if arterial pressure does not change with the modest hemorrhage occurring with blood donation, a decrease in blood volume may be sensed by baroreceptors in the large veins and the heart, signaling a reflex increase in heart rate.

   b: A decrease in contractility will not directly affect heart rate.
   c: Hemorrhage will stimulate vasopressin secretion.
   d: The Frank-Starling law relates stroke volume to cardiac output.
   e: Increased parasympathetic stimulation will decrease heart rate.

144. **Answer c:**
   Polynucleotide sequences are written by convention from 5′ (left) to 3′ (right). Because strands run antiparallel, whether the compliment is DNA or an RNA, one must first assign the complimentary sequence and then turn it around (antiparallel) to represent the sequence correctly.

   a: This is correct base pairing, but was derived in the parallel orientation.
   b: This is the original sequence in the antiparallel orientation, but is not complimentary.
   d: This is the original sequence, and is therefore not complimentary nor is it antiparallel.
   e: This is the correct sequence, but it contains the RNA base uracil in place of thymine.

145. **Answer a:**
   Helicobacter pylori infection (infestation) of the gastric mucosa is associated with 90% to 100% of patients with duodenal ulcers and probably more than 70% of patients with gastric ulcers. Its exact involvement in the production of duodenal ulcers is not understood. Urease and protease production are suspected mechanisms in the development of gastric ulcers.

146. **Answer e:**
   Alveolar proteinosis is a disease of obscure pathogenesis in which granular, lipid-rich material is deposited in the alveoli. The alveolar epithelium is largely intact and no damage is done to the capillary bed. Inflammation is not a feature of this disease. In DAD both the alveolar epithelium and the alveolar capillary endothelium are damaged.

   a: High inspired concentrations of oxygen for a prolonged period of time are associated with the development of diffuse alveolar damage.

b: A severe crush injury of the lower extremity with development of hypovolemic shock is associated with the development of diffuse alveolar damage.

c: Treatment of metastatic neoplasm with Beomycin is associated with the development of diffuse alveolar damage.

d: Inhalation of paraquat while working in a field is associated with the development of diffuse alveolar damage.

147. **Answer a:**

Only rotational movement occurs between the radial head and the ulna, and this is limited to the vertical axis of the joint.

b: The humeroulnar joint is a hinge joint, and motion here is about its horizontal axis.

c: Movements at the humeroradial joint include rotation, flexion, and extension.

d: Movements at the radiocarpal joint include flexion, extension, abduction, and adduction.

e: The radioulnar joint's movement is restricted to the vertical axis of rotation.

148. **Answer e:**

Thirty percent of cases of diabetes insipidus are of unknown cause. The next most frequent cause is a result of brain tumors, particularly craniopharyngioma.

a: Brain tumors are the second most frequent cause of diabetes insipidus.

b: Trauma is not associated to a high degree with diabetes insipidus.

c: Hypophysectomy is not the most frequent cause of diabetes insipidus.

d: Granulomatous diseases are not the most frequent causes of diabetes insipidus.

149. **Answer a:**

Brucella does not produce an exotoxin.

b: Scalded skin syndrome is associated with an exotoxin produced by staphylococci.

c: Whooping cough is associated with an exotoxin produced by *Bordetella pertussis.*

d: Scarlet fever is associated with an exotoxin produced by streptococci.

e: Diphtheria is associated with the production of an exotoxin produced by *Corynebacterium diphtheriae.*

150. **Answer a:**

The cell bodies of all somatosensory receptors below the neck are in the dorsal root ganglia.

b: The dorsal horn of the spinal cord contains second order cell bodies.

c: Nucleus dorsalis of Clark contains second order cell bodies.

d: Lamina VII of Rexed does not contain cell bodies of somatosensory receptors.

e: Terminal ganglia do not contain cell bodies of somatosensory receptors.

151. **Answer c:**

An open charcoal fire in a closed space is a classic source of carbon monoxide poisoning.

a: Barbituates tend to be upscale drug problems and, though not impossible, are not likely in this scenario.

b: Alcohol might have played a part in lack of judgement but generally wouldn't be the single cause of death.

d: HIV is not a likely acute cause of death with the characteristics given.

e: Cocaine tends to be an upscale drug problem, and, though not impossible, is not likely in this scenario.

152. **Answer d:**

Bacteria do not have a nuclear membrane.

a: Bacteria possess ribosomes, albeit smaller than eukaryotic cells.

b: Bacteria possess mesosomes, invaginations of the cytoplasmic membrane.

c: Bacteria have cytoplasmic membranes, which provide many of the same functions as those in cells of higher plants and animals.

e: The DNA of bacteria is a single molecule of double-stranded DNA.

153. **Answer b:**

A deletion in the promoter would prevent RNA polymerase from initiating mRNA synthesis and create the equivalent of a gene deletion.

a: An insertion in the second exon may inactivate the protein by garbling the amino acid sequence, but a protein could still be produced and the domain coded by the first exon could still retain its function. Even if a nonsense mutation were introduced in the second exon due to the frameshift, a shortened protein would nevertheless be produced.

c: Nonsense mutations cause premature termination of the translation of mRNA into protein, but introns do not appear in mRNA, so a nonsense mutation in this region would be undefined.

d: Premature termination of the domain coded by the second exon would still allow expression of a protein with a functional domain from the first exon.

e: Unless it produced a nonsense mutation, a base substitution mutation in the first intron would allow expression of the protein. Also, since not all base substitutions are deleterious, it might have no effect at all.

154. **Answer d:**

Neither stratified cuboidal epithelium nor stereocilia are found in the urinary system.

a: Simple squamous epithelium forms the thin portions of loops of Henle.

b: Transitional epithelium lines minor and major calyces.

c: Simple cuboidal epithelium with a brush border (i.e., numerous long microvilli) lines proximal convoluted tubules.

e: The larger collecting ducts and especially the ducts of Bellini are lined by a simple columnar epithelium.

155. **Answer c:**

Allosteric ("other site") effectors are distinguished by the fact that they bind to the enzyme at a specific location away from the active site.

a: Coenzymes do not serve also as allosteric effectors for the same enzymes.

b: Allosteric effectors do not bind to the active site.

d: Inhibitors are not effectors. Inhibitors are drugs and effectors are metabolites.

e: Because a noncompetitive inhibitor will bind at a location away from the active site, it is often confused with an allosteric effector.

156. **Answer a:**

Nerve fibers innervating the thyrohyoid muscle are derived from the ventral ramus of C1, but travel initially with the hypoglossal nerve.

b: The sternohyoid receives its innervation via branches of the ansa cervicalis.

c: The sternothyroid receives its innervation via branches of the ansa cervicalis.

d: Both bellies of the omohyoid muscle receive their innervation via branches of the ansa cervicalis.

e: The cricothyroid muscle receives its innervation via the external laryngeal nerve.

157. **Answer e:**

The primary stimulus for secretion of ANP is stretching of the atria with increased blood volume.

a: Activation of arterial baroreceptors results in ADH and renin secretin but not ANP.

b: Increased activity of cardiac parasympathetic nerves will result in inhibition of ADH secretion.

c: Increases in plasma osmolality do not regulate ANP secretion.

d: Increases in plasma [angiotensin II] do not regulate ANP secretion.

158. **Answer a:**

The GI side effects (mostly nausea, vomiting) are attributed to the stimulation of an emetic center in the CNS, so there is no frequent side effect directly on the GI tract.

b: Dystonia is a complication of levodopa.

c: Nightmares are a possible complication of levodopa.

d: Chorea is sometimes observed as a complication of levodopa.

e: Psychosis is a possible side effect of levodopa.

159. **Answer d:**

RNA synthesis begins at a promoter site and is terminated at a chain termination signal, which has an inverted hyphenated repeat.

a: Pyrophosphate is produced by formation of the sugar phosphate ester and is subsequently cleaved into inorganic phosphate.

b: Either strand can serve as a template, but generally only one strand is a template within a given gene.

c: Chain growth *always* occurs at the 3′ end in synthesis of both RNA *and* DNA.

e: Unlike DNA, RNA does not undergo proofreading during synthesis.

160. **Answer b:**

Amoxicillin has a broader spectrum then penicillin, but is sensitive to penicillinase.

a: Methicillin does not have a broader spectrum than penicillin G and *is resistant* to penicillinase.

c: Although nafcillin has a broader spectrum of activity than penicillin G, it *is resistant* to penicillinase.

d: Benzathine penicillin is a penicillin G salt used in depot formulations. It is a natural, not a semisynthetic, compound.

e: Although oxacillin does have a broader spectrum than penicillin G, it *is resistant* to penicillinase.

161. **Answer a:**
Swallowing is not initiated by touching the anterior two thirds of the tongue.

b: Water touching the arytenoid cartilages induces a swallow.
c: Water touching the pharyngeal surface of the epiglottis induces a swallow. Prolonged contact with food or a tongue blade on the laryngeal surface of the epiglottis, however, can induce gagging.
d: Water touching the posterior pharyngeal wall induces a swallow.
e: Water touching the tonsillar pillars induces a swallow.

162. **Answer e:**
Myocardial necrosis following thrombosis of a coronary artery is an example of coagulation necrosis rather than apoptosis.

a: Endometrial cellular breakdown during the menstrual cycle is an example of apoptosis induced by the loss of a necessary tropic hormone.
b: Administration of cortisone causes lymphocytes to undergo apoptosis.
c: Atrophy of the prostate following castration is an example of apoptosis induced by the loss of a necessary tropic hormone.
d: Organogenesis in a fetus is the classic description of apoptosis. During organogenesis, populations of cells often are changed radically in the developing organ. Apoptosis is the mechanism involved in the removal of cells.

163. **Answer a:**
Endotoxin is not able to activate the complement cascade by the traditional pathway.

b: Endotoxin is capable of activating the complement cascade by the alternate pathway.
c: Endotoxin can activate the tumor necrosis factor.
d: Endotoxin can elicit fever production.
e: Endotoxin can activate interleukin-1 and prostaglandins.

164. **Answer c:**
Palmitate, as the primary product of fatty acid synthetase, serves as a precursor for many other long chain fatty acids such as stearate, palmitoleate, and oleate.

a: Oleic acid is produced by a fatty acyl CoA desaturase acting on stearate.
b: Odd-chain fatty acids in humans are obtained entirely in the diet, primarily in the form of propionate. Therefore pathways exist for their degradation but not their synthesis.
d: While the pathway for fatty acid oxidation is found in the mitochondrial matrix, the pathway for synthesis that is catalyzed entirely by Acetyl CoA carboxylase and fatty acid synthetase is located in the cytosol.
e: The greatest activity of fatty acid synthetase is in the liver (and lactating mammary glands) and is active to a lesser extent in adipose tissue and kidney.

165. **Answer a:**
Collagen fibers attach cementum to alveolar bone, which serves to simultaneously anchor the tooth in the socket and protect tooth structures from fracturing due to excessive occlusal forces.

b: Collagen fibers of the periodontal ligament do not attach enamel to cementum.
c: Collagen fibers of the periodontal ligament do not attach enamel to alveolar bone.
d: Collagen fibers of the periodontal ligament do not attach dentin to enamel.
e: Collagen fibers of the periodontal ligament do not attach dentin to alveolar bone.

166. **Answer a:**
An increase in stroke volume after lying down results from a shift of blood toward the heart, increasing venous return, cardiac filling and, therefore, stroke volume.

b: An increase in stroke volume with no change in end-diastolic ventricular volume represents an increased contractility.
c: Venoconstriction will increase venous return and cardiac output.
d: Systolic blood pressure increases when aortic compliance decreases.
e: Parasympathetic stimulation will decrease heart rate and therefore cardiac output.

167. **Answer c:**
Amoxapine is a metabolite of the antipsychotic drug, loxapine, retaining some of its antipsychotic effects, including one of its untoward effects, tardive dyskinesia.

a: Tardive dyskinesia is not a characteristic side effect of antidepressants such as fluoxetine.
b: Tardive dyskinesia is not a characteristic side effect of antidepressants such as tranylcypromine.
d: Tardive dyskinesia is not a characteristic side effect of antidepressants such as trazodone.
e: Tardive dyskinesia is not a characteristic side effect of antidepressants such as bupropion.

168. **Answer b:**

    Coxiella burnetii is an obligate intracellular bacterium.

    a: *Haemophilus influenzae* is a free-living bacterium.
    c: *Gardnerella vaginalis* is a free-living bacterium.
    d: *Bacteroides fragilis* is a free-living bacterium.
    e: *Clostridium perfringens* is a free-living bacterium.

169. **Answer a:**

    Grave's disease is an autoimmune disease in which it is thought that the TSH receptors of the follicular epithelium are stimulated by a cross-reacting antibody resulting in increased release of thyroid hormones. With chronic stimulation, the thyroid undergoes hyperplasia and becomes excessively vascular.

    b: True. Grave's disease is an autoimmune disease.
    c: True. Exophthalmus in Grave's disease is caused by an increase in mass of the extraocular muscles within the orbit.
    d: True. Grave's disease is 7 to 10× more common in women than in men.
    e: True. Grave's disease has a higher level of concordance in monozygotic twins than dizygotic twins.

170. **Answer c:**

    Carbamazepine is the drug of choice for partial seizures and also effective in trigemine neuralgia.

    a: Primidone is also effective in partial seizures, but carbamazepine is more effective.
    b: Ethosuximide is the drug of choice when absence seizures occur alone. It has less toxic effects than valproate.
    d: Valproic acid is very effective against absence seizures, but it is preferred only when the patient has concomitant generalized tonic-clonic attacks.
    e: Phenytoin is effective against partial seizures, but not the drug of choice because of its many adverse effects.

171. **Answer c:**

    Antibodies that recognize the antigen combining site of the heavy chain and light chain of an immunoglobulin molecule are called anti-idiotypic antibodies.

    a: Anti-allotypic antibodies do not recognize the antigen combining site of the heavy chain and light chain of an immunoglobulin molecule.
    b: Anti-alloreactive antibodies do not recognize the antigen combining site of the heavy chain and light chain of an immunoglobulin molecule.
    d: Anti-isotypic antibodies do not recognize the antigen combining site of the heavy chain and light chain of an immunoglobulin molecule.
    e: Anti-xenotypic antibodies do not recognize the antigen combining site of the heavy chain and light chain of an immunoglobulin molecule.

172. **Answer c:**

    Clozapine causes agranulocytosis in approximately 1% to 2% of the patients treated, but it is a rare toxic effect with all the other antipsychotic drugs currently used in therapy.

    a: Granulocytopenia is not a frequent toxic effect of thiothixene.
    b: Granulocytopenia is not a frequent toxic effect of thioridazine.
    d: Granulocytopenia is not a frequent toxic effect of haloperidol.
    e: Granulocytopenia is not a frequent toxic effect of trifluoperazine.

173. **Answer b:**

    The role of calmodulin in smooth muscle is to bind with Ca^{2+} and then active myosin cross-bridges.

    a: Smooth muscle has little or no sarcoplasmic reticulum; Ca^{2+} for contraction enters from the extracellular fluid.
    c: Troponin is not present in smooth muscle; calmodulin acts as the Ca^{2+} regulatory protein.
    d: Cross-bridge cycling is relatively slow in smooth muscle.
    e: Skeletal muscle responds only to neural stimulation; smooth muscle may also be activated by interaction of various hormones directly with receptors on the cell membrane.

174. **Answer d:**

    Cardiac muscle cells (myocardial fibers) in the atrium secrete natriuretic hormone.

    a: Endothelial cells in the endocardium do not secrete hormones.
    b: Simple columnar epithelial cells do not exist in the myocardium.
    c: Neuron cell bodies do not exist in the endocardium.
    e: Smooth muscle cells in the myocardium do not secrete hormones.

175. **Answer b:**
Bartholin's glands (also called greater vestibular glands) are found in the female reproductive system. Thus, this is the only possible answer since semen is a secretory product produced by males.

a: The prostate gland produces a major component of semen.
c: The seminal vesicles produce a major component of semen.
d: The testes produce a major component of seminal fluid.
e: Bulbourethral (Cowper's) glands secrete mucus, which contributes in a minor way to the seminal fluid.

176. **Answer c:**
Starling's law of the heart states that stroke volume increases with increased ventricular filling. Filling is proportional to end-diastolic volume.

a: Increased sympathetic activity increases contractility and may increase ejection fraction.
b: According to Starling's law, cardiac output is directly related to sarcomere length at the end of diastole.
d: Increasing stroke volume increases pulse pressure.
e: Stroke volume increases when venous return increases.

177. **Answer a:**
This is the Hering-Breuer reflex; it is thought to act when large changes in tidal volume occur in exercise.

b: Irritant receptors in the mucosa act via myelinated vagal fibers to induce bronchospasm.
c: J receptors thought to be located in the pulmonary capillaries induce rapid, shallow respiration.
d: This statement is correct but does not represent the Hering-Breuer reflex.
e: Activation of intercostal muscle spindles influences the strength of contraction primarily.

178. **Answer c:**
Stimulation of the $beta_1$-adrenergic receptor causes cardioacceleration, not cardiac slowing.

a: Bronchodilation is caused by stimulation of $beta_2$ receptors.
b: Calorigenesis is caused by stimulation of $beta_2$ receptors.
d: Intestinal relaxation is caused by stimulation of $beta_2$ receptors.
e: Vasodilation is caused by stimulation of $beta_2$ receptors.

179. **Answer b:**
ACE inhibitors cause hyperkalemia, not hypokalemia.

a: Syncope is a potential side effect of all ACE inhibitors.
c: Coughing is a potential side effect of all ACE inhibitors.
d: Neutropenia is a potential side effect of all ACE inhibitors.
e: Angioderma is a potential side effect of all ACE inhibitors.

180. **Answer a:**
In this group Duchenne's and Becker's muscular dystrophy are X-linked, the others are autosomal diseases. Both the Duchenne and Becker form involve the same genetic locus, but there are important clinical differences. Duchenne is invariably fatal by the patient's early twenties. Becker's muscular dystrophy is a mild form, and the patients frequently have a nearly normal life span.

b: Fasioscapulohumeral muscular dystrophy is an autosomal disease.
c: Becker's muscular dystrophy, although X-linked, is not the most common form. It is a mild form, with patient's typically enjoying a nearly normal life span.
d: Oculopharyngeal muscular dystrophy is an autosomal disease.
e: Limb girdle dystrophy is an autosomal disease.

181. **Answer b:**
The liver possesses no intralobular ducts and thus neither intercalated nor striated ducts.

a: The pancreas possesses intercalated, but not striated ducts.
c: The parotid possesses many intralobular ducts; intercalated ducts are longer than striated ducts.
d: The sublingual gland possesses a few intralobular ducts (more striated than intercalated).
e: The submandibular gland possesses many intralobular ducts; striated ducts are longer than intercalated ducts.

Answers 182 through 188

182. **Answer d:**
Chief cells secrete pepsinogen, which is converted to pepsin in the gastric lumen.

183. **Answer c:**
G cells in the pyloric glands secrete gastrin.

184, 185, 186. **Answer a:**
Parietal cells (oxyntic cells) are the gastric acid se-creting cells (Question 185); acid secretion is stimulated by histamine (Question 184) and gastrin (Question 188). Secretion of acid results in addition of HCO_3^- to the blood draining from the stomach, the "alkaline tide" (Question 186).

187. **Answer b:**
D cells in the antrum secrete somatostatin.

188. **Answer a:**
Parietal cells are stimulated by gastrin (see Answers 184 through 186).
Answer e:
Mucus cells secrete mucus and HCO_3^- into the gastric lumen; this choice was not used in the question.

Matching answers 189 through 191

189. **Answer g:**
TNF-alpha is the principal mediator of the host response to gram-negative bacteria and possibly other infectious microorganisms. Its principal source is lipopolysaccharide-activated mononuclear cells, but it is also produced by T cells.

190. **Answer a:**
Chaperones are a special class of accessory protein that regulates the delivery and binding of peptides to class II MHC molecules.

191. **Answer f:**
E-selectins (endothelial-leukocyte adhesion molecule-I) mediate the initial attachment of neutrophils to endothelial cells in venules of peripheral tissues.

Matching answers 192 and 193

192. **Answer d:**
In hepatitis B, viral proteins are present on the surface of infected hepatocytes. During the infection, cellular immunity develops and the infected cell is attacked and killed by the host lymphocytes.

193. **Answer b:**
Under proper conditions, *C. diphtheriae* releases a potent exotoxin that kills cells by interfering with protein synthesis.

Matching answers 194 through 196

194. **Answer b:**
Gamma interferon is produced by stimulated T lymphocytes and natural killer cells, and in addition to activating macrophages, is responsible for maintaining MHC class II expression on cell surfaces, and inhibits cell proliferation.

195. **Answer f:**
Interleukin-2 (IL-2), produced by activated $CD4^+$ T cells, induces proliferation of activated T cells, B cells, and natural killer cells, as well as stimulating immunoglobulin and lymphokine production.

196. **Answer g:**
Tumor necrosis factor-beta (lymphotoxin) is produced by lymphocytes and functions in target cell destruction.

Matching answers 197 through 200

197. **Answer g:**
The hypoglossal nucleus is a GSE nucleus that receives only crossed supranuclear innervation.

198. **Answer a:**
The abducens nucleus gives rise to the 6th nerve, which can be involved in an alternating hemiplegia.

199. **Answer m:**
The red nucleus receives axonal projections from the interpositus nucleus.

200. **Answer k:**
The nucleus ambiguus innervates muscles of the larynx and pharynx derived from gill arch IV.

Categories and Answers for Exam 2

Question Number	Answer	Check Here If Correct	Category 1	Category 2	Category 3
1	E	☐	Biochemistry	Molecular Genetics	Recombinant DNA
2	C	☐	Pharmacology	Central Nervous System	Main Effects
3	B	☐	Anatomy	Lower Limb	Normal Anatomy
4	B	☐	Histology	Blood & Lymph	Immune System Cells
5	B	☐	Pathology	Blood & Lymph	Diseases
6	C	☐	Biochemistry	Intermediary Metabolism	Energy & Oxidation
7	D	☐	Biochemistry	Intermediary Metabolism	Transport
8	C	☐	Anatomy	Pelvis & Perineum	Normal Anatomy
9	B	☐	Anatomy	Head & Neck	Normal Anatomy
10	C	☐	Physiology	Cardiovascular System	Microcirculation
11	C	☐	Microbiology	Bacteriology	Pathogenesis
12	B	☐	Microbiology	Bacteriology	Epidemiology
13	B	☐	Pathology	Urinary System	Diseases
14	D	☐	Neuroscience	Motor Systems & Reflexes	Normal Function
15	C	☐	Neuroscience	Central Nervous System	Normal Function
16	B	☐	Microbiology	Virology	Structure
17	C	☐	Anatomy	Pelvis & Perineum	Normal Anatomy
18	C	☐	Biochemistry	Molecular Genetics	Synthesis
19	D	☐	Anatomy	Pelvis & Perineum	Clinical Anatomy
20	C	☐	Physiology	Cardiovascular System	Microcirculation
21	C	☐	Anatomy	Pelvis & Perineum	Clinical Anatomy
22	D	☐	Behavioral Science	Life Cycle	Psychosocial Development
23	C	☐	Physiology	Respiratory System	Transport
24	C	☐	Neuroscience	Central Nervous System	Normal Anatomy
25	A	☐	Physiology	Cells & Tissues	Signaling
26	B	☐	Neuroscience	Head & Neck	Lesions
27	D	☐	Microbiology	Bacteriology	Pathogenesis
28	D	☐	Pathology	Endocrine System	Diseases
29	D	☐	Pharmacology	Endocrine System	Clinical Uses
30	E	☐	Behavioral Science	Life Cycle	Death & Dying
31	D	☐	Neuroscience	Neurotransmitters	Normal Function
32	E	☐	Pharmacology	Cardiovascular System	Main Effects
33	C	☐	Biochemistry	Lipids & Steroids	Energy & Oxidation
34	C	☐	Microbiology	Bacteriology	Pathogenesis
35	C	☐	Neuroscience	Central Nervous System	Normal Anatomy
36	A	☐	Histology	Immune System	Immune System Cells
37	C	☐	Microbiology	Virology	Pathogenesis
38	B	☐	Microbiology	Bacteriology	General Properties
39	A	☐	Pharmacology	Central Nervous System	Main Effects
40	C	☐	Pharmacology	Chemotherapy	General Properties
41	B	☐	Biochemistry	Amino Acids & Proteins	General Properties
42	D	☐	Pathology	Immune System	Diseases
43	C	☐	Neuroscience	Peripheral Nervous System	Normal Function
44	D	☐	Neuroscience	Central Nervous System	Normal Function
45	E	☐	Neuroscience	Neurotransmitters	Lesions
46	C	☐	Histology	Immune System	Immune System Cells
47	B	☐	Anatomy	Lower Limb	Normal Anatomy
48	D	☐	Physiology	Cardiovascular System	General Properties
49	C	☐	Physiology	Musculoskeletal System	Normal Function
50	D	☐	Histology	Cells & Tissues	Normal Tissues

Categories and Answers for Exam 2

Question Number	Answer	Check Here if Correct	Category 1	Category 2	Category 3
51	B	☐	Physiology	Urinary System	Acid-Base Balance
52	C	☐	Microbiology	Immune System	Complement
53	D	☐	Behavioral Science	Statistics	General Properties
54	D	☐	Pathology	Female Reproductive System	Diseases
55	D	☐	Microbiology	Bacteriology	Pathogenesis
56	D	☐	Neuroscience	Head & Neck	Lesions
57	C	☐	Pathology	Cardiovascular System	Diseases
58	B	☐	Physiology	Gastrointestinal System	Normal Function
59	B	☐	Physiology	Gastrointestinal System	Regulation
60	B	☐	Pathology	Musculoskeletal System	Neoplasia
61	D	☐	Anatomy	Pelvis & Perineum	Normal Anatomy
62	B	☐	Pathology	Endocrine System	Diseases
63	C	☐	Pharmacology	Chemotherapy	Main Effects
64	D	☐	Neuroscience	Central Nervous System	Normal Function
65	D	☐	Pharmacology	Chemotherapy	General Properties
66	E	☐	Pathology	Liver & Pancreas	Neoplasia
67	E	☐	Anatomy	Back & Spinal Cord	Clinical Anatomy
68	D	☐	Anatomy	Pelvis & Perineum	Normal Anatomy
69	B	☐	Behavioral Science	Interviewing	Physician-Patient Relationship
70	B	☐	Physiology	Urinary System	Regulation
71	A	☐	Biochemistry	Cells & Tissues	Diseases
72	B	☐	Histology	Female Reproductive System	Normal Anatomy
73	A	☐	Physiology	Cardiovascular System	General Properties
74	B	☐	Neuroscience	Central Nervous System	Lesions
75	B	☐	Pharmacology	General Principles	Pharmacokinetics
76	E	☐	Neuroscience	Peripheral Nervous System	Normal Anatomy
77	D	☐	Pathology	Cells & Tissues	Cell Injury & Cell Death
78	B	☐	Biochemistry	Molecular Genetics	Synthesis
79	A	☐	Pharmacology	Chemotherapy	Clinical Uses
80	B	☐	Pharmacology	Central Nervous System	Main Effects
81	A	☐	Neuroscience	Central Nervous System	Normal Anatomy
82	E	☐	Pharmacology	Chemotherapy	General Properties
83	B	☐	Pharmacology	Chemotherapy	Clinical Uses
84	C	☐	Pathology	Bacteriology	Diseases
85	D	☐	Neuroscience	Head & Neck	Lesions
86	A	☐	Neuroscience	Head & Neck	Normal Anatomy
87	C	☐	Physiology	Cells & Tissues	General Properties
88	E	☐	Neuroscience	Back & Spinal Cord	Normal Anatomy
89	B	☐	Microbiology	Bacteriology	Pathogenesis
90	B	☐	Histology	Immune System	Normal Tissues
91	D	☐	Pharmacology	Autocoids & Diuretics	Clinical Uses
92	D	☐	Physiology	Urinary System	Regulation
93	B	☐	Physiology	Urinary System	Circulation
94	C	☐	Pharmacology	Central Nervous System	Side Effects
95	D	☐	Pharmacology	Chemotherapy	Main Effects
96	B	☐	Biochemistry	Endocrine System	Signaling
97	A	☐	Histology	Chemotherapy	Normal Tissues
98	C	☐	Neuroscience	Central Nervous System	Normal Anatomy
99	E	☐	Anatomy	Lower Limb	Normal Anatomy
100	D	☐	Microbiology	Virology	Diseases

Categories and Answers for Exam 2

Question Number	Answer	Check Here if Correct	Category 1	Category 2	Category 3
101	D	☐	Anatomy	Lower Limb	Normal Anatomy
102	E	☐	Behavioral Science	Learning Theory	General Properties
103	A	☐	Behavioral Science	Professional Issues	Stress
104	B	☐	Microbiology	Virology	Structure
105	B	☐	Biochemistry	Amino Acids & Proteins	Structure
106	E	☐	Pharmacology	Endocrine System	Clinical Uses
107	D	☐	Neuroscience	Central Nervous System	Normal Function
108	E	☐	Microbiology	Bacteriology	Structure
109	E	☐	Biochemistry	Molecular Genetics	Mutation
110	D	☐	Pathology	Molecular Genetics	Diseases
111	B	☐	Anatomy	Head & Neck	Normal Anatomy
112	B	☐	Pharmacology	Cardiovascular System	Side Effects
113	A	☐	Neuroscience	Head & Neck	Normal Function
114	C	☐	Microbiology	Bacteriology	Structure
115	A	☐	Behavioral Science	Statistics	General Properties
116	D	☐	Anatomy	Upper Limb	Clinical Anatomy
117	B	☐	Biochemistry	Molecular Genetics	Mutation
118	B	☐	Histology	Blood & Lymph	Immune System
119	C	☐	Pathology	Immune System	Immune Response
120	B	☐	Pharmacology	Chemotherapy	General Properties
121	A	☐	Physiology	Respiratory System	Transport
122	C	☐	Anatomy	Upper Limb	Clinical Anatomy
123	A	☐	Behavioral Science	Interviewing	Cognitive Assessment
124	A	☐	Pharmacology	Autonomic Nervous System	Clinical Uses
125	C	☐	Pharmacology	Endocrine System	General Properties
126	C	☐	Neuroscience	Motor Systems & Reflexes	Lesions
127	A	☐	Biochemistry	Intermediary Metabolism	Energy & Oxidation
128	B	☐	Pathology	Molecular Genetics	Neoplasia
129	D	☐	Anatomy	Abdomen	Clinical Anatomy
130	B	☐	Behavioral Science	Interviewing	Assessment
131	B	☐	Histology	Female Reproductive System	Normal Anatomy
132	C	☐	Physiology	Cardiovascular System	Regulation
133	B	☐	Histology	Cells & Tissues	Normal Tissues
134	E	☐	Microbiology	Liver & Pancreas	Immune Response
135	D	☐	Pathology	Blood & Lymph	Pathophysiology
136	E	☐	Pathology	General Principles	Cell Injury & Cell Death
137	E	☐	Pathology	Urinary System	Diseases
138	A	☐	Pathology	Male Reproductive System	Pathophysiology
139	B	☐	Histology	Musculoskeletal System	Normal Anatomy
140	E	☐	Pathology	Liver & Pancreas	Laboratory Diagnosis
141	B	☐	Physiology	Cells & Tissues	Transport
142	E	☐	Pathology	Liver & Pancreas	Diseases
143	A	☐	Behavioral Science	Interviewing	Assessment
144	C	☐	Physiology	Cardiovascular System	The Heart as a Pump
145	B	☐	Biochemistry	Enzymes	General Properties
146	B	☐	Pathology	Central Nervous System	Diseases
147	C	☐	Physiology	Gastrointestinal System	Pathophysiology
148	E	☐	Histology	Cells & Tissues	Normal Function
149	A	☐	Anatomy	Upper Limb	Clinical Anatomy
150	C	☐	Neuroscience	Central Nervous System	Lesions

Categories and Answers for Exam 2

Question Number	Answer	Check Here if Correct	Category 1	Category 2	Category 3
151	A	☐	Neuroscience	Motor Systems & Reflexes	Normal Anatomy
152	B	☐	Pharmacology	Toxicology	Side Effects
153	B	☐	Histology	Eye	General Properties
154	C	☐	Histology	Urinary System	Normal Anatomy
155	E	☐	Neuroscience	Peripheral Nervous System	Normal Function
156	B	☐	Histology	Endocrine System	Secretion
157	A	☐	Histology	Cells & Tissues	General Properties
158	B	☐	Microbiology	Virology	Structure
159	D	☐	Pharmacology	Toxicology	Treatment
160	A	☐	Microbiology	Bacteriology	Diseases
161	D	☐	Microbiology	Bacteriology	Diseases
162	A	☐	Pharmacology	Cardiovascular System	Main Effects
163	D	☐	Microbiology	Bacteriology	Epidemiology
164	B	☐	Pharmacology	Central Nervous System	Side Effects
165	D	☐	Biochemistry	Nitrogen Metabolism	Synthesis
166	D	☐	Pathology	Gastrointestinal System	Diseases
167	C	☐	Pathology	Cardiovascular System	Diseases
168	E	☐	Pathology	Female Reproductive System	Diseases
169	C	☐	Microbiology	Virology	Epidemiology
170	C	☐	Neuroscience	Central Nervous System	Normal Anatomy
171	B	☐	Physiology	Cells & Tissues	Transport
172	A	☐	Biochemistry	Endocrine System	Diseases
173	D	☐	Neuroscience	Peripheral Nervous System	Normal Function
174	C	☐	Neuroscience	Central Nervous System	Normal Anatomy
175	C	☐	Physiology	Cells & Tissues	General Properties
176	C	☐	Neuroscience	Central Nervous System	Normal Anatomy
177	C	☐	Pharmacology	Toxicology	Side Effects
178	C	☐	Pharmacology	Toxicology	Side Effects
179	C	☐	Pharmacology	Toxicology	Diseases
180	E	☐	Pathology	Bacteriology	Diseases
181	F	☐	Microbiology	Bacteriology	Pathogenesis
182	C	☐	Microbiology	Bacteriology	Diseases
183	A	☐	Microbiology	Bacteriology	Diseases
184	D	☐	Microbiology	Bacteriology	Pathogenesis
185	B	☐	Microbiology	Bacteriology	Pathogenesis
186	C	☐	Behavioral Science	Psychopathology	Personality Disorders
187	E	☐	Behavioral Science	Psychopathology	Personality Disorders
188	C	☐	Pathology	Male Reproductive System	Lesions
189	A	☐	Pathology	Male Reproductive System	Lesions
190	A	☐	Behavioral Science	Forensic Medicine	Legal Decisions
191	C	☐	Behavioral Science	Forensic Medicine	Legal Decisions
192	H	☐	Microbiology	Virology	Diseases
193	I	☐	Microbiology	Virology	Structure
194	E	☐	Physiology	Enzymes	General Properties
195	A	☐	Physiology	Enzymes	General Properties
196	B	☐	Physiology	Enzymes	General Properties
197	B	☐	Physiology	Enzymes	General Properties
198	C	☐	Physiology	Female Reproductive System	Normal Function
199	C	☐	Physiology	Female Reproductive System	Normal Function
200	E	☐	Physiology	Female Reproductive System	Normal Function

Answers and Explanations to Exam 2

1. **Answer e:**

   Restriction endonucleases have a specificity for a certain type of base sequence called a palindrome (a sequence that reads the same from either end).

   a: Enzymes that digest polynucleotides from either the 5′ or the 3′ end are *exo*nucleases.
   b: Restriction endonucleases are specific for duplex (double-stranded) DNA.
   c: Restriction endonucleases are produced by bacteria, primarily to stop (restrict) the growth of bacterial viruses (or other foreign DNA such as plasmid DNA).
   d: Some endonucleases can digest double-stranded DNA at random locations, but restriction endonucleases recognize specific sequences and do not digest at any other site.

2. **Answer c:**

   Meperidine has significant antimuscarinic effects.

   a: Meperidine does not produce peripheral vasoconstriction.
   b: Meperidine does not cause catecholamine release.
   d: Most opioid agonists have sedative action, but meperidine can cause CNS excitation. This is probably not the cause of the changes described.
   e: This scenario shows an acute treatment.

3. **Answer b:**

   The dorsalis pedis artery is the continuation of the anterior tibial artery onto the dorsum of the foot.

   a: The pulse of the dorsalis pedis artery may be felt midway between the lateral and medial malleoli.
   c: The dorsalis pedis artery is the continuation of the anterior tibial artery as the latter passes anteriorly to the ankle joint.
   d: The lateral plantar artery arises as a branch of the posterior tibial artery.
   e: The dorsalis pedis artery lies immediately lateral to the tendon of the extensor hallucis longus muscle on the dorsum of the foot.

4. **Answer b:**

   The neutrophil nucleus is highly lobulated (polymorphonuclear), rather than round or oval (monomorphonuclear). Therefore the neutrophil is *not* a component of the MPS (RES).

   a: Neutrophils are highly motile.
   c: The primary function of neutrophils is to ingest and destroy invading microorganisms.
   d: Neutrophils play a central role in early stages of acute inflammatory responses.
   e: Neutrophils are a major constituent of pus.

5. **Answer b:**

This is a case of Bruton's disease (X-linked hypo-gammaglobulinemia). In these patients there is a selective block in the bone marrow in the maturation of B lymphocytes at the pre-B lymphocyte stage. The effect of this is that the peripheral lymphoid tissue is not populated with B lymphocytes and germinal centers do not form.

a: Granulomatous inflammation is not an integral part of this disease.

c: Since the mantle zone surrounds germinal centers that would be absent in this case, it would be at best indistinct and, there is no reason it should be hyperplastic.

d: Plasma cells are essentially absent, since the basic defect of these patients is in maturation of B-cells.

e: The lack of peripheral B lymphocytes causes hypoplasia of the peripheral lymphoid tissue, particularly the tonsils. Histologically the peripheral lymphoid tissue is abnormal and shows lack of germinal centers which are B cell dependent.

6. **Answer c:**

The equilibrium for the condensation of acetyl CoA and oxaloacetate lies strongly in the direction of citrate.

a: Three molecules of NADH and one molecule of $FADH_2$ (and one GTP) are produced for each turn of the TCA cycle.

b: Pyruvate carboxylase is not a TCA cycle enzyme, although it produces oxaloacetate, a TCA cycle component. There are three rate-limiting enzymes in the TCA cycle: citrate synthase, isocitrate dehydrogenase, and alpha ketoglutarate dehydrogenase.

d: Both malate and succinate are four carbon intermediates, indicating that the two carbons introduced by acetyl CoA have already been lost as CO_2. Carbon dioxide is formed at the steps catalyzed by isocitrate dehydrogenase and alpha ketoglutarate dehydrogenase.

e: Since erythrocytes have no mitochondria, the TCA cycle, which is localized entirely within the mitochondrial matrix, cannot supply any of their ATP.

7. **Answer d:**

The flow of protons down an electrochemical gradient from the intermembrane space to the matrix contains the energy for ATP synthetase to join inorganic phosphate to ADP.

a: Although a sodium ion gradient is maintained across the plasma membrane by pumping sodium ions out of the cell, there is no such gradient between the matrix and the cytosol.

b: One early theory of oxidative phosphorylation postulated the generation of a high-energy intermediate in the synthesis of ATP based on the substrate level phosphorylation catalyzed by phosphoglycerate kinase, but no such chemical intermediate has been discovered in the mitochondrion.

c: Electron transport occurs entirely within the matrix and provides the driving force for pumping protons out of the matrix to the intermembrane space.

e: Protons are pumped out not in.

8. **Answer c:**

The sphincter urethrae muscle is composed of skeletal muscle fibers and is therefore under voluntary control.

a: The fibers of the sphincter urethrae muscle surround the membranous urethra, the shortest portion of the male urethra.

b: Fibers of the sphincter urethrae muscle are situated within the deep perineal space.

d: The sphincter urethrae muscle is located between the superior and inferior fascia of the urogenital (UG) diaphragm.

e: The sphincter urethrae muscle receives its innervation via branches of the pudendal nerves.

9. **Answer b:**

The floor of the submental triangle is formed by the two mylohyoid muscles.

a: The hyoid bone forms the inferior border of the submental triangle.

c: The apex of the submental triangle is formed by the symphysis menti.

d: The anterior bellies of the digastric muscles form the lateral borders of the submental triangle.

e: The submental lymph nodes receive lymph from the tip of the tongue as well as from the skin of the chin, a portion of the lower lip, the incisors of the mandible, and the floor of the mouth.

10. **Answer c:**

    Decreased capillary hydrostatic pressure, because of both arteriolar constriction and decreased arterial pressure, will result in a shift of interstitial fluid into the blood.

    a: In some species, the spleen releases erythrocytes with hemorrhage.

    b: There is no change in plasma protein concentration because of the hemorrhage itself. A decrease in plasma protein concentration results in increased filtration of fluid out of the capillaries and would increase hematocrit.

    d: Neither of these changes will directly affect hematocrit.

    e: Hemorrhage by itself will not change plasma Na^+ concentration.

11. **Answer c:**

    Helicobacter pylori has not been shown to cause epiglottitis.

    a: *Helicobacter pylori* has been shown to be associated with gastritis.

    b: *Helicobacter pylori* has been implicated in gastric ulcers.

    d: *Helicobacter pylori* recently has been implicated duodenal ulcers.

    e: *Helicobacter pylori* has been implicated in gastric cancer.

12. **Answer b:**

    The infectious dose for *Shigella* is very low, usually <200 bacilli.

    a: Outbreaks are common in day-care centers, prisons, and homes for the mentally retarded.

    c: *Shigella sonnei* is the most common cause of shigellosis in the industrial world.

    d: The natural habitat of *Shigella* is limited to primates.

    e: Children from 6 months to 10 years of age have the highest attack rate.

13. **Answer b:**

    With functional failure, the liver is incapable of synthesizing many proteins in adequate amounts. Among these are serum albumin and a number of the coagulation factors. The expectation is that serum albumin would be reduced in amount, not increased.

    a: Hepatic failure can result in coagulopathy.

    c: Hepatic failure can result in hepatorenal syndrome.

    d: Hepatic failure can result in testicular atrophy.

    e: Hepatic failure can result in hyperbilirubinemia.

14. **Answer d:**

    Muscles generate increasing force by increasing the number of active motor units. The smallest motor neurons are recruited first (size principle), and if more force is needed, additional larger neurons are recruited.

    a: Motor units are of three types: (1) slow, fatigue resistant, (2) fast, fatigue resistant, and (3) fast, fatigable. Muscles do not generate more force by decreasing the fatigue resistance of the motor units.

    b: Muscles do not generate more force by decreasing the oxidative phosphorylation of muscle fibers.

    c: Motor units cannot be induced to increase their conduction velocity.

    e: Increasing the number of muscle spindles activated will not generate more force.

15. **Answer c:**

    The supraoptic nucleus synthesizes vasopressin. The paraventricular nucleus also makes some vasopressin, but this was not a choice.

    a: The dorsomedial nucleus is involved in the limbic system.

    b: The nucleus basalis of Meynert is thought to be involved in Alzheimer's disease.

    d: The subfornical organ is involved in water balance and is thought to be the site of action of angiotensin in the brain.

    e: The ventromedial nucleus of the hypothalamus does not make vasopressin.

16. **Answer b:**

    Hepatitis B virus has a genome that is a small, circular, partly double-stranded DNA of only 3,200 bases.

    a: Hepatitis A virus has a positive, single-stranded RNA genome of about 7,470 nucleotides.

    c: Hepatitis C virus has an RNA genome of 9,500 nucleotides.

    d: Hepatitis D virus has a very small RNA genome of 1,700 nucleotides.

    e: Hepatitis E virus contains a single-stranded RNA genome of approximately 7,500 bases.

17. **Answer c:**

    The coccygeus muscle lies on the pelvic surface of the sacrospinous ligament, and its fibers do not leave the pelvis.

    a: The pudendal nerve exits the pelvis and enters the gluteal region via the greater sciatic foramen.
    b: Fibers of the piriformis muscle are attached to the pelvic surface of the sacrum and exit the pelvis via the greater sciatic foramen.
    d: The sciatic nerve exits the pelvis via the greater sciatic foramen and enters the gluteal region inferior to the piriformis muscle.
    e: The inferior gluteal artery exits the pelvis and enters the gluteal region via the greater sciatic foramen.

18. **Answer c:**

    Signal peptides are cleaved off at the final destination of their parent protein, namely the endoplasmic reticulum.

    a: Signal peptides contain a high proportion of hydrophobic polypeptides, which are compatible with the hydrophobic environment of the cell membrane.
    b: Signal peptides are cleaved off *after* translocation across the cell membrane.
    d: Signal peptides are encoded by the mRNA at the amino-terminal end of the polypeptide and are thus added at the time of translation.
    e: Membrane anchored proteins, like secreted proteins, have a hydrophobic region that becomes embedded in the cell membrane. However, the anchors are never cleaved off of the protein as are the signal sequences.

19. **Answer d:**

    Extravasation into the ischioanal fossa is not possible, since the deep and superficial perineal fascia are united along the posterior margin of the urogenital diaphragm.

    a: Urine will extravasate into the superficial perineal space, which includes the scrotum.
    b: Urine will extravasate into the superficial perineal space surrounding the penis.
    c: Urine will extravasate into the superficial perineal space, which extends upward along the inferior aspect of the anterior abdominal wall.
    e: Extravasation of urine in such an injury will be limited to the superficial perineal space.

20. **Answer c:**

    In peripheral tissues CO_2 is a vasodilator, and the increase in tissue P_{CO_2} that occurs with increased muscle metabolism contributes to arteriolar vasodilation.

    a: Muscle blood flow is under sympathetic control.
    b: Angiotensin II is a vasoconstrictor.
    d: Autoregulation means flow remains constant as pressure changes.
    e: Lymph flow will increase during exercise due to increased filtration of fluid from capillaries and increased sympathetic activity to lymph vessels.

21. **Answer c:**

    Although the obturator artery most frequently arises from the internal iliac, it may arise from the inferior epigastric artery. In the latter instance, it lies close to the pectinate ligament, as it crosses the pelvic brim to enter the obturator canal.

    a: The obturator nerve enters the obturator canal posterior and inferior to the pectinate ligament.
    b: The internal pudendal artery is located near the ischial spine and as such is not at risk.
    d: The ureter is too far posterior and inferior to be at risk.
    e: The pudendal nerve is located near the ischial spine and as such is not at risk.

22. **Answer d:**

    Industry versus inferiority represents the phase often associated with the introduction to formalized learning and occurs most often between ages 6 and 11.

    a: During the first year of life the child's major task is focused on the development of basic trust.
    b: From ages 1 to 3, a child gains a sense of separateness from caretakers and will develop either a sense of autonomy or shame and doubt.
    c: Children between the ages of 3 and 5 were hypothesized by Erikson to be in a stage labeled "initiative versus guilt" in which the psychosocial outcome was largely determined by adult responses to the child's natural sexual curiosity.
    e: Coinciding with puberty, the Eriksonian stage from 11 to 20 years of age, is characterized by the adolescent's striving for a sense of identity.

23. Answer c:

Diffusion of O_2 between plasma and tissue is determined by the PO_2 difference, just as diffusion of solutes is generally determined by the solute concentration gradient.

a: The percent saturation is related to the amount of O_2 carried by hemoglobin, but it is not directly responsible for the rate of delivery of O_2 to the tissues.

b: There is no special significance to the difference between alveolar PO_2 and PCO_2.

d: O_2 must diffuse from the blood to the cells; the driving force is the difference between capillary PO_2 and mitochondrial PO_2, not the arteriovenous difference.

e: O_2 must diffuse from the blood to the cells; the driving force is the difference between capillary PO_2 and mitochondrial PO_2, not the total amount of O_2 in the blood.

24. Answer c:

These capillaries are not fenestrated and will not allow large molecules like albumin to pass freely into the brain.

a: These capillaries allow substances like anesthetics with high-lipid solubility to enter the brain rapidly.

b: These capillaries do not allow serum albumin to enter the brain unless they have been damaged.

d: These capillaries are surrounded by astrocyte foot processes.

e: These capillaries have many mitochondria when compared with other capillaries.

25. Answer a:

Amplification occurs at each step by synthesis of increasing numbers of the intermediate compounds in the pathway.

b: Hormones do not bind to cyclic AMP, they bind to the receptors.

c: Phosphodiesterase is an enzyme that hydrolyses cAMP.

d: Any effects on oxidative phosphorylation will be secondary to other changes induced by the binding of the hormone.

e: The second messenger systems participate in determining which hormonal effects are specific to the cell type that is activated.

26. Answer b:

The cranial nerve does not innervate the intestines.

a: The uvula will deviate to the well side.

c: Taste is carried by fibers of the IX nerve from the posterior third of the tongue.

d: The cranial nerve IX is important in the gag reflex.

e: The cranial nerve IX provides sensation to the pharynx, tonsils, and back of tongue.

27. Answer d:

Bordetella pertussis does not cause disease by invading tissues.

a: *Bordetella pertussis* does possess a hemagglutinin, which is believed to be important in attachment of the organism to epithelia.

b: *Bordetella pertussis* produces several exotoxins.

c: *Bordetella pertussis* is a gram-negative coccobacillus.

e: *Bordetella pertussis* is a highly contagious disease.

28. Answer d:

Hyperprolactinemia occurs in about 26% of patients with pituitary adenoma. Second to hyperprolactinemeia is secretion of no hormone, which occurs in about 17% of tumors.

a, b, c, e: Hypersecretions of growth hormone, ACTH, FSH and LH, or TSH are not the most common endocrinopathy-associated with pituitary adenoma.

29. Answer d:

Oxytocin is a polypeptide that is inactivated when given orally.

a: Its half life is 5 minutes, it is quickly metabolized by the kidney and the liver.

b: It initiates the "letdown" of milk but does not stimulate milk production.

c: The sensitivity of the uterus develops over the time of pregnancy.

e: Atropine does not block the effects of oxytocin.

30. Answer e:

Actualization is a concept most commonly linked to the writings of humanistic psychologists and refers to a drive basic to most humans, which motivates us towards growth, completeness, and fulfillment of the self throughout the lifespan.

a: From extensive interviews with dying patients, Elisabeth Kübler-Ross's research suggested that denial is the first stage many individuals experience when dealing with issues of death.

b: Anger often follows denial when a patient is attempting to cope with impending death. This stage is characterized by the patient asking questions focused on "Why me?"

c: Once denial and anger have passed, a patient will commonly enter the bargaining stage of coping with death in which thoughts are focused on a religious or magical intervention that will allow the patient to avoid or postpone death.

d: Acceptance is the final stage associated with death as a patient realizes their existence is near an end. However, not all patients will fully accept their death prior to its occurrence.

31. **Answer d:**

Glutamate is released by the parallel fibers of the granule cells of the cerebellum.

a: Acetylcholine is not released by the granule cells.

b: Aspartate is an excitatory neurotransmitter but is not released by granule cells.

c: GABA is a major inhibitory neurotransmitter in the cerebellum and is not released by granule cells.

e: Taurine is an excitatory neurotransmitter but is not released by the granule cells.

32. **Answer e:**

Glyceryl trinitrate, as well as the other nitrites used in therapy as vasodilators, do not cause the formation of a significant amount of methemoglobin.

a: True. Tolerance occurs with frequent, repeated administration.

b: True. Total coronary blood flow is not usually increased with glyceryl trinitrate.

c: True. Glyceryl trinitrate may cause reflex tachycardia.

d: True. Glyceryl trinitrate is most quickly absorbed through oral mucosa.

33. **Answer c:**

The requirement for ATP is the carboxylation of propionyl-CoA (note the similarity to the pyruvate carboxylase reaction) reduces the net ATP production.

a: Propionyl-CoA is completely metabolized by conversion to methylmalonyl-CoA, which is then converted to succinyl-CoA, a TCA cycle intermediate.

b: Methylmalonyl-CoA is completely metabolized to CO_2 and water, because all of its carbons enter the TCA cycle at succinyl-CoA.

d: The pyruvate dehydrogenase complex is inhibited by acetyl CoA (both by direct product inhibition and by stimulation of pyruvate dehydrogenase kinase) as well as by NADH, but not by intermediates of priopionyl-CoA metabolism.

e: Propionyl-CoA does not enter the TCA cycle at any point.

34. **Answer c:**

The host's cellular immune response to *Mycobacterium tuberculosis* causes clinical disease.

a: *Mycobacterium tuberculosis* may cause both localized and systemic infections.

b: Humans are the only natural reservoirs of *Mycobacterium tuberculosis*.

d: The lipid-rich cell wall does make *Mycobacterium tuberculosis* resistant to disinfectants.

e: *Mycobacterium tuberculosis* can inhibit phagosome-lysosome fusion, thereby preventing phagocytic destruction.

35. **Answer c:**

The olivocerebellar tract originates from the inferior olive and is the sole source of climbing fibers input to the cerebellum.

a: Anterior spinocerebellar axons provide mossy fiber input.

b: Cuneocerebellar axons provide mossy fiber input.

d: Posterior spinocerebellar axons provide mossy fiber input.

e: Trigeminocerebellar axons provide mossy fiber input.

36. **Answer a:**

One significant reasons why AIDS is such a devastating disease is that it kills helper T cells, a cell type crucial in mounting humoral and cellular immune responses.

b: B cells are not infected by the AIDS virus.

c: Mast cells are not infected by the AIDS virus.

d: Eosinophils are not infected by the AIDS virus.

e: Neutrophilic myelocytes are not infected by the AIDS virus.

37. **Answer c:**

HIV-1 infection results in decreased IL-1 production.

a: Cytotoxic T cell activity against virus-infected cells is decreased following HIV-1 infection.

b: There is increased release of tumor necrosis factor and other cytokines following HIV-1 infection.

d: Following HIV-1 infection, there is decreased microbicidal activity.

e: There is decreased antigen-specific antibody production following HIV-1 infection.

38. **Answer b:**

There is no known degradation of antibiotics by proteolytic enzymes in the periplasmic space.

a: Bacitracin is a good example of an antibiotic that may fail to penetrate through the outer membrane, and thus, causes resistance.

c: Vancomycin is an example of an antibiotic that may fail to penetrate and bind to its target site, rendering an organism resistant.

d: Hydrolysis of antibiotics, such as penicillin, renders bacteria resistant.

e: Point mutations in genes, such as those for the initial beta-lactamases, have even more widespread resistance.

39. **Answer a:**

The depth of anesthesia inhalation is most nearly proportional to the partial pressure of the agent at the place of action: the brain.

b: There is a connection, but not a closely proportional one.

c: The partial pressure of the agent in the alveoli is proportional to the concentration in the brain.

d: The concentration of the agent in the blood is proportional to the concentration in the brain.

e: The concentration of the agent in the alveoli is proportional to the concentration in the brain.

40. **Answer c:**

Cross resistance is when resistance to one agent is induced by another.

a: When drug resistance is transferred between micro-organisms, it is called transduction or transformation.

b: Drug resistance is not transferred between patients.

d: There is no term for drug resistance being transferred from bacteria to eukaryotes.

e: When a drug is transformed from plasmid to chromosome, it is called transposition.

41. **Answer b:**

Weaker binding of bisphosophoglycerate gives fetal hemoglobin a slightly greater affinity for hemoglobin, enabling it to "pull" oxygen from adult hemoglobin.

a: The common genetic disorders involve a variety of sites, e.g., the sickle cell mutation is on the surface of the molecule.

c: The saturation curve for myoglobin is hyperbolic, which is characteristic for proteins that do not demonstrate cooperativity.

d: The saturation curve for hemoglobin is sigmoidal, which is characteristic for proteins that demonstrate cooperativity.

e: All hemoproteins use the same form of heme, but the way in which the heme is bound can be slightly different. Myoglobin and hemoglobin bind heme nearly identically.

42. **Answer d:**

The immune effects of HIV infection are caused mainly by infection and destruction of the $CD4^+$ lymphocytes, the "helper" T lymphocytes. The stage of the HIV infection is often classified by the number of $CD4^+$ cells remaining as an absolute number. When the count falls below 200, the clinical manifestations of full-blown AIDS, such as *Pneumocystic carinii* pneumonia, Kaposi's sarcoma, and Cryptosporidium infection, are likely to occur.

a: One must be careful when using any kind of ratio unless the numbers that the ratio was calculated from are available. For example, it has been often stated that clinical AIDS is likely when the CD4/CD8 ratio is less than 0.8. However, such a ratio could be achieved by having a normal number of $CD4^+$ cells and an increase in $CD8^+$ cells. In such as case, a patient's immune state would be fully competent. Remembering that the relative numbers of lymphocytes circulating may be altered by a number of things, including common acute viral infections.

b: At greater than 500 $CD4^+$ lymphocytes per microliter of blood, a patient will not manifest the clinical symptoms of AIDS.

c: At 200 to 500 $CD4^+$ lymphocytes per microliter of blood, a patient may begin to manifest some symptoms, but unless the fall in count is rapid, the progression of the disease is usually not rapid.

e: Absolute monocytosis is not a predictor of progression in HIV infection.

43. **Answer c:**

Paradoxical cold results when a heat stimulus of 45° C is applied selectively to a cold spot on the skin. This heat stimulus is painful when applied to the whole skin, but when applied selectively to a single cold spot, it is experienced as cold, not hot. Thus, paradoxical cold is an example of labeled line coding. This means that regardless of how it is stimulated, a cold receptor always responds by eliciting the sensation of cold.

a: Paradoxical cold is not an adaptation response to prolonged cold exposure.
b: Paradoxical cold does not develop when there is destruction of the heat conservation center.
d: Paradoxical cold does not develop when thermal nociceptors are stimulated.
e: Paradoxical cold is not part of the thermoregulatory process.

44. **Answer d:**

The organum vasculosum is thought to play a role in reproduction, and this would not affect autoregulation.

a: When arterial P_{CO_2} is raised, arterioles dilate, and cerebral blood flow increases. Breathing 5% CO_2 increases cerebral blood flow by 50%.
b: With hypocarbia, there is vasoconstriction, and cerebral blood flow decreases.
c: Local transluminal pressure would affect autoregulation.
e: Breathing 100% O_2 lowers cerebral blood flow by about 13%; breathing 10% O_2 raises cerebral blood flow by 35%

45. **Answer e:**

As stated, it is currently thought that myasthenia gravis is an autoimmune process in which the acetylcholine receptors are lost.

a: Tryptophan hydroxylase is the enzyme used to convert tryptophan to 5-hydroxytryptophan. These are not related to myasthenia gravis.
b: Tyrosine hydroxylase is the enzyme necessary to convert tyrosine to L-DOPA. These are not related to myasthenia gravis.
c: Monoamine oxidase is the enzyme necessary to convert norepinephrine to VMA in the peripheral nervous system and to MHPG in the CNS. Monoamine oxidase also converts dopamine in the CNS to HVA or DOPAC. Monoamine oxidase converts serotonin to 5HIAA in the PNS. None of these are involved in myasthenia gravis.
d: Loss of dopamine in the substantia nigra is related to Parkinson's disease.

46. **Answer c:**

Type II pneumocytes are epithelial cells that line pulmonary alveoli and function to secrete surfactant, a protein that reduces the surface tension within alveoli and thus prevents alveoli from col-

lapsing. A component of the MPS in the respiratory system is the alveolar macrophage.

a: Langerhan's cells, components of the MPS, are located in the epidermis of thick and thin skin and function as antigen processors.
b: Histiocytes, which are connective tissue macrophages, are components of the MPS.
d: Mesangeal cells, which are renal macrophages, are components of the MPS.
e: Osteoclasts, which are multinucleated macrophages that resorb bone, are components of the MPS.

47. **Answer b:**

The superior gluteal artery, a branch of the internal pudendal artery, does participate in the formation of the cruciate anastomosis of the thigh.

a: The inferior gluteal artery, a branch of the internal pudendal artery, anastomoses with a branch of the profunda femoris artery to contribute to the cruciate anastomosis.
c: The lateral circumflex femoral artery contributes to the formation of the cruciate anastomosis of the thigh.
d: The cruciate anastomosis of the thigh is formed in part by a branch of the medial circumflex femoral artery.
e: The first perforating branch of the profunda femoris artery anastomoses with several vessels to form the cruciate anastomosis of the thigh.

48. **Answer d:**

Decreasing arterial compliance with age is responsible for systolic hypertension in the elderly.

a: Mean arterial pressure is independent of pulse pressure; changes in blood volume are accommodated primarily on the venous side of the circulation.
b: To the extent that heart rate determines cardiac output, these two factors influence mean arterial pressure but not pulse pressure.
c: Changes in ventricular contractility may influence stroke volume, but the length of systole does not affect pulse pressure.
e: End-systolic volume and heart rate do not affect pulse pressure.

49. **Answer c:**

Diffusion of Na^+ and K^+ down their electrochemical gradients depolarizes the sarcolemma.

a, b, d, e: The postsynaptic receptor is a chemically gated Na^+, K^+ channel.

50. **Answer d:**

    Thin skin, not thick skin, possesses pilosebaceous organs, which are composed of hairs and associated structures including sebaceous glands.

    a: Both thick and thin skin possess common sweat glands.
    b: Both thick and thin skin possess the reticular and papillary layers of the dermis.
    c: Both thick and thin skin possess dermal papillae.
    e: Langerhan's cells are present in both thin and thick skin.

51. **Answer b:**

    The pK for NH_4^+ is 9.2; it is a base and cannot accept protons at physiological pH.

    a: About half the excess H^+ in metabolic acidosis is buffered intracellularly.
    c: Carbonates in bone provide a large buffer pool for reaction with H^+.
    d: About half the excess H^+ in metabolic acidosis is buffered acutely by extracellular HCO_3^-.
    e: A small quantity of H^+ is buffered by plasma proteins.

52. **Answer c:**

    C5b binds to the cell membrane with the subsequent addition of C6, C7, C8, and C9.

    a, b, d, e: Only C5b binds to the cell membrane. C6, C7, C8, and C9 then bind in succession to the membrane-bound C5.

53. **Answer d:**

    The power of a statistical study represents the probability of rejecting the null hypothesis when an alternative hypothesis is true. Decreasing the level of alpha (i.e., 0.05 to 0.01) makes rejecting the null hypothesis less likely, which decreases power.

    a: A large effect size (i.e., the strength of the relationship between variables) makes extreme outcomes of the test statistic more likely increasing power.
    b: Larger samples permit the means for each sample to be more precise, enhance stability, and allow a researcher to make increasingly precise estimates elevating power.
    c: One-tailed tests allow the entire alpha to be placed in one rejection region, resulting in increased power as it is equivalent to having a higher alpha in the appropriate tail of the distribution.

    e: Balancing the research design by maintaining equal sample sizes allows the mean of each group to be adequately and consistently measured, resulting in a higher power.

54. **Answer d:**

    HPV 6 is associated with condyloma acuminatum rather than squamous cell carcinoma. In low-grade intraepithelial neoplasia, the HPV is episomal and replicates, killing the infected cells. In high-grade intraepithelial neoplasia, the HPV DNA is integrated into the host genome where specific viral oncogenes have transforming functions.

    a: True. Fifty percent of intraepithelial neoplasia cases regress to normal.
    b: True. Ten percent of intraepithelial neoplasia may progress to high-grade cervical intraepithelial neoplasia.
    c: True. Progression to carcinoma in situ would take more than 10 years.
    e: True. The patient should be examined culposcopically.

55. **Answer a:**

    Pathogenic strains of *Staphylococcus aureus* are usually beta-hemolytic on sheep blood agar.

    b: *Staphylococcus aureus* can produce beta-lactamases, which are able to inactivate penicillins.
    c: Capsules and other cell wall components do inhibit phagocytosis.
    d: *S. aureus* is coagulase positive.
    e: *Staphylococcus aureus* is the most frequent cause of pyogenic infections.

56. **Answer d:**

    This patient's findings are consistent with an acoustic neuroma of the VIII nerve. Cranial nerves VII and VIII exit the brainstem at the cerebellopontine angle. The tumor is beginning to encroach on the facial nerve, accounting for her left-sided muscle weakness. Her nausea and headache are due to the increased intracranial pressure in the posterior fossa.

    a: A stroke on the left vertebral artery would cause UMN signs on the right side. Additionally, the medial lemniscus would be affected, leading to loss of discriminitive touch on the right side, since these neurons have already crossed.

b: A stroke on the right posterior inferior cerebellar artery is on the wrong side, since her signs are on her left. Also, her hearing loss was gradual, indicative of a slow process not sudden onset as in a stroke.

c: Same as in B above.

e: A pinealoma might grow into the quadrigeminal cistern and press down on the inferior and superior colliculi. However, her hearing loss is only on one side and the inferior colliculus has input from both ears. This lesion would not account for her ataxia and falling to the left.

57. **Answer c:**

Polyarteritis nodosa is a disease of the small muscular arteries, and although the kidney is frequently involved in the disease, it is the larger vessels that are affected.

a: Fever is a symptom of polyarteritis nodosa.

b: Weight loss is a symptom of polyarteritis nodosa.

d: Hypertension is a symptom of polyarteritis nodosa.

e: Abdominal pain is a symptom of polyarteritis nodosa.

58. **Answer b:**

The major digestion products of lipids within the intestinal lumen are monoglycerides and fatty acids. These products are lipid soluble and cross the cell membrane by simple passive diffusion.

a: Solubilizing of fatty acids and monoglycerides by micelle formation allows the lipids to cross the unstirred aqueous boundary layer at the luminal membrane of the enterocyte.

c: The products of lipid digestion are lipid soluble and cross the cell membrane by simple passive diffusion.

d: Reconstitution of lipids into triglycerides allows their incorporation into chylomicrons and VLDLs for transport in the lymph.

e: Chylomicrons and very-low-density lipoproteins in the lymph, and fatty acids bound to albumin in the portal blood, are the main forms for transport of lipid in the circulation.

59. **Answer b:**

Parasympathetic stimulation of the enteric nervous system enhances activity of most GI functions.

a: In addition to acetylcholine and norepinephrine, VIP, ATP, serotonin, dopamine, substance P, and other neurotransmitters are present.

c: Increased sympathetic activity decreases GI function, and slows the movement of food.

d: Autonomic activity modulates the activity of the enteric nervous system.

e: The primary sympathetic neurotransmitter in the GI tract is norepinephrine.

60. **Answer b:**

A rhabdomyosarcoma is a malignant mesenchymal tumor of skeletal (striated) muscle origin. The suffix "sarcoma" denotes its malignancy and its mesenchymal origin. "Myo" refers to muscle and "Rhabdo" means rodlike.

a: Carcinomas are by definition of epithelial cell origin.

c: This is a benign tumor of skeletal muscle origin hence the suffix "-oma" rather than "sarcoma."

d: This is a benign tumor of smooth muscle origin ("leio" means smooth).

e: This is the malignant counterpart of the leiomyoma ("sarcoma").

61. **Answer d:**

The male homologue of the round ligament of the uterus is the gubernaculum of the testis.

a: The vas deferens is located lateral to the inferior epigastric vessels as the former passes through the anterior abdominal wall to enter the pelvic region.

b: The vas deferens dilates to form the ampulla of the vas deferens near the posterior aspect of the urinary bladder.

c: The duct of the vas deferens unites with that of the seminal vesicle to form the ejaculatory duct, which enters the prostatic urethra.

e: The muscular wall of the vas deferens is composed of smooth muscle and is thus under involuntary or autonomic control.

62. **Answer b:**

Waterhouse-Friderichsen syndrome is acute adrenal hemorrhage that probably represents a manifestation of the generalized Schwartzman reaction. It is typically associated with septisemia due to *Meningococcus* or *Pseuodomonas* and results in acute adrenal insufficiency that is often fatal.

a: Acute adrenal insufficiency associated with meningococcal septisemia is not associated with withdrawal of exogenous corticosteroid therapy.

c: Acute adrenal insufficiency associated with meningococcal septisemia is not caused by isolate ACTH deficiency.

d: Acute adrenal insufficiency associated with meningococcal septisemia is not caused by tuberculosis.

e: Acute adrenal insufficiency associated with meningococcal septisemia is not caused by oat cell carcinoma of the lung.

63. **Answer c:**

Neurotoxicity, which limits its therapeutic use to short courses, is characteristic for vincristine. It is cell-cycle dependent.

a: Busulfan is not neurotoxic and not cell-cycle dependent.

b: 5-fluorouracil is not neurotoxic but is cell-cycle dependent.

d: Actinomycin D is not neurotoxic but is cell-cycle dependent.

e: Etoposide (VP-16) is not neurotoxic and not cell-cycle dependent.

64. **Answer d:**

Rubbing or otherwise stimulating mechanoreceptors in the area of the pain reduces or even completely inhibits pain from the C-fibers according to the gate control theory.

a: Stimulating adjacent P-releasing C-fibers will only make the pain worse.

b: Stimulating glutamate-releasing A-delta fibers will make the pain worse.

c: The high-threshold polymodal nociceptors are C-fibers and stimulating them will only make the pain worse.

e: Many of these C-fibers ascend in the spinoreticular tract, and stimulating it will only make the pain worse.

65. **Answer d:**

Penicillin's action on gram-positive organisms is inhibited by tetracyclines.

a: Penicillin is the least toxic of the antimicrobial antibiotics.

b: Some people are allergic to penicillin and may have anaphylatic reactions.

c: Penicillin is a potent bactericide.

e: Penicillin is secreted by the renal tubules.

66. **Answer e:**

Virtually all carcinomas of the pancreas are of ductal origin and account for about 99% of tumors. Acinar cell carcinomas account for no more than 1% of pancreatic adenocarcinomas.

a: The ascinar cells account for only 1% of pancreatic adenocarcinomas.

b: Carcinoma of the pancreas is not associated with islet beta cells.

c: Carcinoma of the pancreas is not associated with islet alpha cells.

d: Carcinoma of the pancreas is not associated with interstitial fibroblasts.

67. **Answer e:**

A lumbar puncture to obtain CFS is typically performed by inserting the needle between L3 and L4 or L4 and L5. The spinal cord typically ends between L1 and L2.

a, b, c, d: Cord injury is a risk here, as the spinal cord has not yet terminated at this level.

68. **Answer d:**

The bulbourethral glands of the male are located within the deep perineal space.

a: Fibers of the ischiocavernosus muscle cover the crura of the penis and clitoris and are located within the superficial perineal space.

b: The bulb of the penis lies superficial to the perineal membrane and is thus located within the superficial perineal space.

c: The superficial transverse perinei muscles are quite small and are located within the superficial perineal space along the posterior margin of the urogenital diaphragm.

e: The crura of the penis lie superficial to the perineal membrane and as such lie within the superficial perineal space.

69. **Answer b:**

Patients commonly respond to physicians as if they were significant figures from the patient's past, such as a parent. The phenomena, termed transference, can interfere with the physician-patient relationship, if not addressed.

a: In projection, a defense mechanism is used in which unacceptable impulses are attributed to others.

c: The defense mechanism of regression involves an individual reverting to an earlier stage of development.

d: Reflection is an interviewing technique in which the physician reflects or mirrors patient-provided information.

e: Tangentiality is an example of a patient's inability to demonstrate goal-directed thought.

70. **Answer b:**

Some of the smooth muscle cells of the afferent arteriole, the granular cells, are the major site of renin synthesis.

a: The granular cells are located in the afferent arteriole.

c: The nucleus tractus solitarius is not a site of renin synthesis. This nucleus is important in neural regulation of cardiovascular function.

d: The paraventricular nucleus is the major site of oxytocin synthesis.

e: The posterior pituitary gland primarily secretes anti-diuretic hormone and oxytocin.

71. **Answer a:**

The base change mutation that gives rise to sickle cell anemia occurs in a cleavage site for the Mst I restriction enzyme. By preventing digestion with this enzyme, a larger than normal restriction fragment is produced and detected upon electrophoresis.

b: The deoxygenated form of sickle hemoglobin exposes the new valine residue, which then associates with the new valines on other molecules to initiate sickling.

c: The change of a glutamic acid (-1 charge) to the uncharged amino acid, valine, changes the electrophoretic mobility.

d: The mutation causes an amino acid change, not a deletion.

e: Oxygenated sickle hemoglobin has normal solubility.

72. **Answer b:**

The decidua basalis is not part of the placental barrier. Instead, it represents transformed endometrial tissue.

a: The endothelium of fetal capillaries is a component of the placental barrier.

c: The mesenchyme in fetal villi is a component of the placental barrier.

d: The basal lamina of fetal capillaries is a component of the placental barrier.

e: Syncytiotrophoblasts are a component of the placental barrier. The basal lamina of the trophoblast and the cytotrophoblast layer (present during the first few months of pregnancy only) were not included in the choices.

73. **Answer a:**

Compliance indicates the extent to which vessels distend as pressure increases.

b: Flow = pressure/resistance.

c: Pressure = flow $\times$ resistance.

d: Stroke volume/end-diastolic ventricular volume is an ejection fraction.

e: CO $\times$ MAP is a meaningless calculation.

74. **Answer b:**

Alzheimer's disease is a cortical dementia. The other diseases mentioned are subcortical dementias.

a: AIDS patients can have subcortical dementias.

c: Patients with Huntington's disease can have subcortical dementias.

d: Patients with Parkinson's disease can have subcortical dementias.

e: Patients with Wilson's disease can have subcortical dementias.

75. **Answer b:**

$t_{1/2} = 0.693 \cdot V/CL$

$C_{SS} = F \cdot Dose/CL \cdot T$

$C_{SS} = F \cdot Dose \cdot t_{1/2}/0.693 \cdot V \cdot T$

$C_{SS} = 0.6 \cdot 50 \text{ mg} \cdot 6 \text{ hr}/0.693 \cdot 70 \text{ L} \cdot 24 = 150$ ng/ml

76. **Answer e:**

The vestibular ganglia are sensory ganglia and do not receive autonomic input.

a: The ciliary ganglion receives autonomic input from the parasympathetic Edinger-Westphal nucleus.

b: The otic ganglion receives autonomic input from the parasympathetic inferior salivatory nucleus.

c: The pterygopalatine ganglion receives autonomic input from the parasympathetic superior salivatory nucleus.

d: The submandibular ganglion receives parasympathetic autonomic input.

77. **Answer d:**

The light microscope is not very helpful in determining whether a cell has undergone a reversible injury or a lethal one. Answer "D" is an electron microscopic change that does define a lethal cellular injury.

a: Cytoplasmic vacuolation is a common event in both reversible and lethal cellular injury. It is caused by loss of ATP synthesis, which in turn causes the sodium pump to fail.

b: Nuclear pyknosis is a cellular change seen in dead cells.

c: Fatty change is also a change that may be seen in either reversible or lethal cell injury and is due to the accumulation of new fat in the cell. The mechanism for the accumulation of fat may have multiple components.

e: Karyorrhexis, like nuclear pyknosis, is a nuclear change associated with dead cells.

78. **Answer b:**
    Specifically, puromycin mimics tyrosinyl-tRNA.

    a: When a peptide is esterified to the tRNA, it no longer shares a structural analogy with puromycin.
    c: Peptidyl transferase enzymatically joins puromycin to the nascent polypeptide chain, causing its premature release from the ribosome.
    d: The release factors cause an appropriate release of the completed peptide by recognizing the termination codon.
    e: Formulation of the alpha amino group on methionine limits its binding to the peptidyl site. Puromycin can only bind to the aminoacyl site.

79. **Answer a:**
    Because of the potential toxicity and availability of other effective drugs, chloramphenicol is recommended only for symptomatic *Salmonella* infections.

    b: Chloramphenicol is used to treat *H. influenzae* meningitis.
    c: Chlormaphenicol is used to treat meningococcal meningitis in patients allergic to penicillin.
    d: Chloramphenicol is used to treat brain abscesses.
    e: Because of the potential toxicity and availability of other effective drugs, chloramphenicol is recommended only for symptomatic *Salmonella* infections such as typhoid fever.

80. **Answer b:**
    Tardive dyskinesia occurs following chronic phenothiazine treatment.

    a: The tremor in Parkinson's disease is not choreoathetoid movement.
    c: Acute dystonic reactions are not choreoathetoid movements.
    d: The inability to remain in a sitting posture is not related.
    e: A perioral tremor is not a choreoathetoid movement.

81. **Answer a:**
    The dorsal longitudinal fasciculus contains descending autonomic output that originates in the hypothalamus.

    b: The fornix connects the hippocampus with the mammillary bodies.
    c: The medial lemniscus is an ascending tract carrying touch and proprioceptive information.
    d: The medial longitudinal fasciculus does not contain autonomic axons from the hypothalamus.
    e: The tectospinal tract is a descending tract originating in the superior colliculus.

82. **Answer e:**
    It is the drug of choice in *Corynebacterium, Chlamydia, Mycoplasma,* and *Legionella* infections.

    a: Erythromycin estolate is effective mainly against gram-positive organisms.
    b: Erythromycin estolate is the drug of choice for replacing penicillin in cases of penicillin allergy.
    c: Only 5% is excreted in the urine.
    d: Erythromycin estolate inhibits protein synthesis (50S unit).

83. **Answer b:**
    Rifampin is well absorbed orally and generally administered that way.

    a: Adverse reactions to rifampin include an orangish-pink coloration of body fluids.
    c: Rifampin does decrease the effectiveness of oral contraceptives.
    d: Para-aminosalicylic acid delays the absorption of rifampin.
    e: Rifampin is primarily excreted in the biliary and urinary tracts.

84. **Answer c:**
    Cholera infections are found exclusively within the lumen of the gut. The vibrios attach to the gut epithelium by means of their flagellae but never invade the cells.

    a: True. Cholera causes severe watery diarrhea, which may be life threatening.
    b: True. *V. cholerae* releases a potent endotoxin which causes an increase in cAMP.
    d: True. The diarrhea fluid produced by *V. cholerae* infection is unusual because it contains few acute inflammatory cells.
    e: True. *V. cholerae* infection may be successfully treated by oral replacement of the massive fluid loss from the gut.

85. **Answer d:**
    Nystagmus will not result from a lesion of the III nerve.

    a: External strabismus will occur because of the unopposed action of the lateral rectus and superior oblique muscles.
    b: Loss of accommodation will occur because parasympathetic fibers have been interrupted.

c: Mydriasis will occur because of the interruption of parasympathetic fibers and the unopposed activity of the sympathetic fibers of the iris diaphragm.

e: Ptosis will occur because of the unopposed action of the orbicularis oculi muscle, which is innervated by nerve VII.

86. **Answer a:**

The dorsal and ventral cochlear nuclei receive direct input from the axons of the spiral ganglion.

b: The inferior colliculus is a relay nucleus of auditory information but does not get direct input from the spiral ganglion.

c: The medial geniculate nucleus is also a relay nucleus of auditory information.

d: The superior colliculus has an auditory map and probably receives most of its input from the inferior colliculus.

e: The superior temporal gyrus receives auditory information after it has been processed at multiple brain stem sites.

87. **Answer c:**

Diffusion of K^+ down its electochemical potential from cell to extracellular potential is primarily responsible for the intracellular negative resting membrane potential.

a: The Na^+, K^+ ATPase is electrogenic, but it directly contributes only about 15% of the membrane potential.

b: The Na^+, K^+ ATPase contributes directly only about 15% of the resting membrane potential; its main effect is to establish ion concentration gradients.

d: The electrochemical gradient in a resting cell favors diffusion of Na^+ into the cell, which would tend to make the cell interior positive.

e: Na^+, glucose cotransport in epithelial cells will bring a net positive charge from Na^+ into the cell, which tends to depolarize the cell membrane.

88. **Answer e:**

The lateral vestibulospinal tract is found in the ventral funiculus of the spinal cord.

a: The lateral vestibulospinal tract is found in tegmentum of the pons not in the basilar region.

b: The lateral vestibulospinal tract is not found in the lateral funiculus of the spinal cord.

c: The lateral vestibulospinal tract originates from the lateral vestibular nucleus in the pons not from the rectum of the mesencephalon.

d: The lateral vestibulospinal tract originates from the lateral vestibular nucleus in the pons not from the tegmentum of the mesencephalon.

89. **Answer b:**

The capsule of *Klebsiella pneumoniae* is most closely associated with the pathogenesis of the organism.

a: Although produced by *Klebsiella,* urease is not considered a virulence factor for the organism.

c: Fimbriae are not associated with the pathogenesis of *Klebsiella.*

d: Hemolysins are not produced by *Klebsiella.*

e: Flagella play no role in the pathogenesis of *Klebsiella.*

90. **Answer b:**

GALT is an acronym for "gut-associated lymphoid tissue." Therefore students are asked to identify lymphoid tissue that is not associated with the gastrointestinal (GI) system. Tracheal lymphoid nodules are associated with the respiratory rather than the GI system.

a: Palatine tonsils are associated with the oral cavity (GI system).

c: Peyer's patches are associated with the ileum (GI system).

d: Mucosal lymphoid nodules are associated with the esophagus, a component of the GI system.

e: Mucosal lymphoid nodules are associated with the appendix, a component of the GI system.

91. **Answer d:**

Omeprazole irreversibly inhibits the gastric parietal cell proton pump, thus totally stopping gastric acid secretion.

a: Sucralfate is a mucosal protective agent.

b: Famotidine is an H_2 receptor antagonist.

c: Misoprostol is a prostaglandin antagonist.

e: 5-aminosalicylic acid stimulates acid secretion.

92. **Answer d:**

K^+ reabsorption normally occurs primarily in the proximal tubule, and is a passive process, driven by the urine, to plasma K^+ concentration gradient.

a: Angiotenin II is a peripheral vasoconstrictor.

b: Angiotensin II in the hypothalamus stimulates drinking.

c: Angiotensin II and plasma [K$^+$] are the two major regulators of aldosterone secretion.

e: Angiotensin II stimulates the proximal Na$^+$, H$^+$ antiport, increasing Na$^+$ reabsorption.

93. **Answer b:**

By definition, autoregulation means little or no change in flow when pressure changes.

a: Proportional increases in flow, with an increase in pressure, would be characteristic of a rigid vascular system.

c: Both GFR and RBF are autoregulated.

d: Both GFR and RBF are auotregulated.

e: In response to an increase in pressure, vasodilation would increase flow proportionately more than pressure, characteristic of passive relaxation of the vasculature.

94. **Answer c:**

The most common adverse effects are GI related: nausea, vomiting, heartburn.

a: Cardiovascular-related effects are not adverse effects of valproate.

b: Renal-related effects are not adverse effects of valproate.

d: Visual disturbances are not adverse effects of valproate.

e: Mental confusion is not an adverse effect of valproate.

95. **Answer d:**

Ciprofloxacin, as a member of the fluoroquinolone group, acts by inhibiting DNA synthesis.

a: Ciprofloxacin does not act by interfering with cell wall synthesis.

b: Ciprofloxacin does not act by competitive antagonism of folic acid synthesis.

c: Ciprofloxacin does not act by altering the function of plasma membrane.

e: Ciprofloxacin does not act by inhibiting protein synthesis.

96. **Answer c:**

Calmodulin binds four molecules of calcium causing its activation through a conformational change. The calcium calmodulin complex, in turn, activates various enzymes including kinases, cyclases, and phosphodiesterase.

a: GTP binds to the alpha-subunit of Gs-protein when the Gs-protein interacts with a stimulated hormone receptor. The Gs-protein-GTP complex then activates adenylate cyclase, which increases the intracellular concentration of cyclic AMP.

b: Inositol 1,4,5-triphosphate (IP$_3$) is produced when hormones stimulate the action of phospholipase C to break down phosphatidylinositol 1,4,5-triphosphate. The IP$_3$ causes rapid release of calcium from intracellular stores allowing its second messenger function both by combination with calmodulin and by direct stimulation of protein kinase C.

d: Diacylglycerol (DAG) is also produced by the action of phospholipase C on phosphatidylinositol 1,4,5-triphosphate. DAG acts to increase the activity of membrane-bound protein kinase C, which, in turn, regulates other proteins through a phosphorylation mechanism.

e: Cyclic adenosine monophosphate (cAMP) acts as a second messenger by activating protein kinase A by binding to its regulatory subunits. The further action of protein kinase A can regulate enzymes, ion channels, and DNA binding proteins.

97. **Answer a:**

Astrocytes proliferate to repair damaged tissue in the CNS.

b: Microglia phagocytize material in the CNS.

c: Oliogodendroglia myelinate axons in the CNS.

d: Ependymal cells line spaces such as ventricles and the central spinal canal in the CNS.

e: Significant numbers of meningeal neutrophils do not exist under normal circumstances.

98. **Answer c:**

The splenium of the corpus callosum connects the right and left occipital lobes.

a: The anterior commissure connects portions of the two temporal lobes.

b: Arcuate (U) fibers connect adjacent gyri in the same hemisphere.

d: The cingulum is the fiber tract connecting portion of the cingulate gyrus.

e: The posterior commissure, although important in visual reflexes, does not connect the two occipital lobes.

99. **Answer e:**

As it exits the greater sciatic foramen and enters the gluteal region, fibers of the piriformis muscle lie superiorly to the tendon of the obturator internus muscle. The sciatic nerve also enters the gluteal region inferiorly to the piriformis muscle.

a: Fibers of the piriformis muscle give rise to a tendon that passes posterior to the femoral neck to insert upon the greater trochanter of the femur.

b: Contraction of the fibers of the piriformis muscle results in lateral or external rotation of the thigh.

c: The fibers of the piriformis muscle take their origin from the pelvic aspect of the middle three sacral segments. The sacral plexus of nerves lies on the anterior surface of the muscle.

d: The piriformis muscle receives its innervation via branches of the sacral plexus of nerves.

100. **Answer d:**

Liver damage caused by hepatitis A virus is most likely mediated by an immunopathologic response and not virus-induced cytopathology. Hemorrhagic fever is not a common clinical manifestation of infection by hepatitis A.

a: Hantaan virus infection is often associated with hemorrhagic fever with renal syndrome.

b: Ebola virus causes severe or fatal hemorrhagic fevers.

c: Of the Arenaviruses, Lassa fever is most commonly associated with hemorrhagic fever.

e: Marburg virus causes severe or fatal hemorrhagic fever.

101. **Answer d:**

The plantar calcaneonavicular ligament is often termed the "spring ligament" and provides the primary support for the medial longitudinal arch of the foot.

a: The long plantar ligament lies superficially to the "spring ligament" and provides the primary support for the lateral longitudinal arch of the foot.

b: The plantar calcaneocuboid ligament lies deep to the long plantar ligament and is often referred to as the short plantar ligament. It assists in supporting the longitudinal arch of the foot.

c: The deltoid ligament is also known as the medial ligament of the ankle joint.

e: As one of the lateral ligaments of the ankle joint, the calcaneofibular ligament connects the lateral malleolus with the calcaneus.

102. **Answer e:**

In operant conditioning a negative reinforcer is defined as anything that maintains or increases the likelihood of a response by removing an unpleasant stimulus. Thus, the electric shock is a negative reinforcer because it increases the probability that the rat will press the bar to avoid pain.

a: A conditioned stimulus, a term associated with classical conditioning, refers to a previously neutral stimulus that gains the capacity to evoke a response because of repeated pairings with an unconditioned stimulus.

b: A response that initially was evoked by a naturally occurring stimulus becomes known as a conditioned response in classical conditioning when it follows a conditioned stimulus.

c: Punishment is a term associated with operant conditioning. It refers to anything that decreases the probability a behavior will occur.

d: A positive reinforcer is defined as anything that maintains or increases the likelihood of a response by adding a stimulus to the environment and is also a term associated with operant conditioning.

103. **Answer a:**

The suicide rate for male physicians is equal to the rate for the general male population.

b: In contrast to males, female physicians are 4 times more likely to commit suicide than their counterparts.

c: Medical students seek psychiatric services readily, with estimates suggesting up to 20% may obtain psychiatric care, primarily in the outpatient setting.

d: The stress upon physicians and their families likely influences why most presenting problems center around issues of adjustment, depression, and marital conflict.

e: Estimates suggest that as many as 34% of physicians obtain 10 or more outpatient therapy visits a year.

104. **Answer b:**

Viruses having negative sense RNA genomes contain an RNA polymerase.

a: Only DNA viruses have early genes that encode DNA-binding proteins and enzymes.

c: No DNA intermediate is required for replication of negative sense RNA genomes.

d: Viruses having negative sense RNA genomes do not undergo recombination.

e: Amantadine has clinical efficacy against *Influenza A,* but not against *Influenza B* or other viruses.

105. **Answer b:**

Many supersecondary structure motifs are combinations of alpha helices and beta structure.

a: The zinc finger motif chelates zinc through a combination of histidine and cysteine side chains.

c: The arrangement of secondary structure into characteristic patterns, or motifs, permits the formation of independently folding functional units within the same molecule, which are called domains.

d: Although the supersecondary structure is three dimensional, it does not describe the *complete* native conformation, as required for tertiary structure.

e: Although the amino acid composition may not be identical, there is enough sequence homology within the same motif to endow the same function in different proteins, e.g., the helix-turn-helix motif appears in many different DNA binding proteins.

106. **Answer e:**

The site of injection of insulin does not influence significantly the onset and duration of action.

a: True. Dietary control is needed for type II diabetes.

b: True. The subcutaneous injection of insulin may cause lipodystrophies.

c: True. Insulin requirements are often increased by infection.

d: True. Regular exercise reduces insulin requirement.

107. **Answer d:**

CSF is formed at the rate of 0.35 cc/min or 500 to 700 ml/day.

a: CSF formation is decreased when there is local arteriolar vasoconstriction.

b: CSF formation is decreased when the patient is hypotensive.

c: Hyperventilation (low P_{CO_2}) causes vasoconstriction and decreased CSF formation.

e: Vasodilation increases CSF formation.

108. **Answer e:**

Amphitrichously flagellated bacteria have one or more flagella at each end.

a: Peritrichously flagellated bacteria have flagella surrounding the entire cell.

b: Bacteria with no flagella are called atrichous.

c: Monotrichously flagellated bacteria have one flagellum at one end.

d: Lophotrichously flagellated bacteria have two or more flagella at one or both ends.

109. **Answer e:**

This mutation is a termination (nonsense) codon (91) and appears two codons earlier than the existing termination codon (93). The effect is to shorten the protein by two amino acids.

a: The wobble position is in the third base of the codon, but the mutation only affected the first base. Mutations occurring at the wobble position can leave the protein unchanged.

b: A frameshift results from insertion or deletion of one or more bases, whereas the mutation in question is a substitution.

c: Mutation is DNA damage that has gone unrepaired. Mutations, because they are permanent, cannot be repaired.

d: The new codon is a termination codon, another term for a nonsense codon, therefore, it does not code for any amino acid.

110. **Answer d:**

Adult polycystic kidney disease is an autosomal dominant disease.

a: Hemophilia A is an X-linked recessive disease.

b: Hemophilia B is an X-linked recessive disease. In this disease, heterozygous women do not express the disease but are carriers. Males with a defective X chromosome will express the disease.

c: Duchenne-Becker muscular dystrophy is an X-linked recessive disease. In this disease heterozygous women do not express the disease but are carriers. Males with a defective X chromosome will express the disease.

e: Chronic granulomatous disease is an X-linked recessive disease. In this disease heterozygous women do not express the disease but are carriers. Males with a defective X chromosome will express the disease.

111. **Answer b:**

The tensor tympani muscle receives its innervation via the nerve to the medial pterygoid muscle, which is a branch of the mandibular division of the trigeminal nerve.

a: The stylohyoid muscle receives its innervation via a branch of the facial nerve.

c: A branch of the facial nerve innervates the stapedius muscle.

d: Branches of the facial nerve are responsible for innervating the buccinator muscle.

e: The posterior belly of the digastric muscle is innervated by the facial nerve, i.e., the 7th cranial nerve.

112. **Answer b:**

Hydralazine dilates arterioles but not veins, effectively decreases blood pressure, and elicits reflex tachycardia and sympathetic stimulation, which in turn may provoke angina and ischemic arrhythmias.

a: Methyldopa decreases blood pressure but does not trigger myocardial ischemia.

c: Guanethidine decreases blood pressure but does not trigger myocardial ischemia.

d: Hydrochlorothiazide decreases blood pressure but does not trigger myocardial ischemia.

e: Reserpine decreases blood pressure but does not trigger myocardial ischemia.

113. Answer a:

The conversion of 11-cis retinal to all-trans retinal is caused by absorption of a photon by a rhodopsin molecule.

b: Light activated rhodopsin activates transducin.

c: Transducin activates the phosphodiesterase enzyme.

d: The cascade of events, which begins with the absorption of a photon by a rhodopsin molecule, ultimately culminates in a resulting fall of sodium levels, which causes the cell to hyperpolarize.

e: See D above.

114. Answer c:

L-forms are stable-cell wall-less bacteria.

a: Protoplasts are unstable-cell wall-less forms from gram-positive bacteria.

b: Mycoplasmas are bacteria that have no cell wall.

d: Spheroplasts are unstable-cell wall-less forms from gram-negative bacteria.

e: Prions are small proteinaceous, infectious particles thought to be associated with some of the slow virus diseases.

115. Answer a:

The sensitivity of a test addresses the proportion of individuals with a disorder that will be correctly identified by the test (true positives divided by the sum of true positives and false negatives).

b: Validity denotes whether a test measures what it is intended to measure.

c: Reliability refers to the consistency and accuracy of a measurement over conditions or time.

d: In contrast to sensitivity, specificity is a related term that refers to the ability of the test to correctly identify individuals who do not have the disorder being measured (true negatives divided by the sum of false positives and true negatives).

e: Variability is the degree of difference between test scores, expressed through measures such as the range, variance, or standard deviation.

116. Answer d:

Injury to the radial nerve may occur subsequent to the improper use of crutches. Such injury may result in a condition known clinically as "wrist-drop."

a: The thoracodorsal nerve is most at risk in surgical procedures involving the contents of the axilla.

b: The long thoracic nerve is not usually at risk when crutches are used improperly.

c: Injury to the suprascapular nerve is not typical of improper use of crutches.

e: The ulnar nerve in the axilla arises from the medial cord of the brachial plexus and is not at risk during improper crutch use.

117. Answer b:

The damage from UV radiation consists of either a thymine dimer or a thymine-cytosine dimer ("6-4" photoproduct).

a: The damaged area is first detected by an excision endonuclease. DNA ligase participates as the last step in repair of UV damage.

c: The endonuclease only cleaves the damaged strand.

d: UV radiation does not cause transversion mutations (purine ↔ pyrimidine).

e: Stronger (ionizing) radiation (e.g., x-radiation or gamma radiation), is required to break the covalent structure of the DNA backbone.

118. Answer b:

Lymphocytes do not leave the blood vascular system and enter the PALS by passing through the walls of central arterioles/arteries. Rather, lymphocytes depart the blood vascular system via capillary beds of follicular arterioles, red pulp arterioles, and penicillar arterioles.

a: Lymphocyte stem cells leave the bone marrow and enter the blood vascular system by passing through the sinusoidal walls in bone marrow.

c: Lymphocyte stem cells leave the blood vascular system and enter thymic parenchyma by passing through the walls of capillary loops in the thymus.

d: Lymphocytes leave the splenic parenchyma (e.g., cords of Billroth) and enter the blood vascular system by passing through the walls of splenic sinusoids.

e: Lymphocytes leave the blood vascular system and enter the lymph node parenchyma by passing through the walls of postcapillary venules in the cortex of the lymph node.

119. Answer c:

Type III reactions are mediated by the formation of circulating immune complexes. Such complexes may be deposited in various sites such as the renal glomeruli. The immune complex fixes complement and thereby induces an inflammatory response by releasing C5a. The C5a will chemotactically attract neutrophils and macrophages to the site of deposition of the immune complex. The inflammatory response causes tissue damage.

a: Type I reactions are typical anaphylactic reactions that are mediated by IgE. These reactions occur in response to reexposure to an antigen to which the patient has been previously sensitized.

b: Type II reactions are cytotoxic reactions in which IgG and/or IgM antibodies are directed against antigens on cell surfaces or in connective tissue. These reactions often fix complement and develop the membrane attack complex, which causes cellular lysis. This type of reaction is also responsible for opsonization of bacteria.

d: Type IV reactions are cellular reactions mediated by T-lymphocytes and macrophages. This is the typical delayed hypersensitivity reaction, similar to that seen in a positive tuberculin test.

120. **Answer b:**

Sulfonamides interfere with the dihydrofolate synthesis in bacteria, therefore they are effective against those bacteria that synthesize their own folate.

a: Sulfonamides interfere with the dihydrofolate synthesis in bacteria. They do not affect dihydrofolate reductase.

c: Sulfonamides are synergistic with trimethoprim.

d: Sulfonamides are not effective against *Pseudomonas aeruginosa.*

e: There are resistant strains in sulfonamides.

121. **Answer a:**

Increased acidity decreases percent saturation of hemoglobin at any level of PO_2, i.e., acidity causes hemoglobin to release O_2 more readily for any given PO_2.

b: Increased acidity decreases percent saturation of hemoglobin at any level of PO_2, i.e., acidity causes hemoglobin to release O_2 more readily for any given PO_2.

c: Acidity is not an important factor in binding of carbon monoxide.

d: Increased acidity will increase oxygen release in metabolizing tissues.

e: Increased acidity shifts the curve to the right, i.e., more oxygen is released per mm Hg PO_2.

122. **Answer c:**

The axillary nerve is at risk in fractures involving the surgical neck of the humerus. The radial nerve is at risk when fractures involve the humeral shaft.

a: Although the axillary nerve may be injured in fractures of the surgical neck, the musculocutaneous nerve is not directly related to the humerus and is protected by soft tissue structures.

b: Although the axillary nerve may be injured in fractures of the surgical neck, the median nerve is not directly related to the humerus and is protected by soft tissue structures.

d: The ulnar nerve may be injured in fractures involving the medial epicondyle of the humerus. The musculocutaneous nerve is not usually at risk in fractures involving the humerus.

e: Although the radial nerve is at risk in humeral shaft fractures, the median nerve is not usually at risk in humeral fractures.

123. **Answer a:**

A physician is often requested to distinguish dementia from delirium. One important differentiating factor is the onset of the disorders. In contrast to the insidious onset of dementia, delirium often occurs suddenly.

b: Delirious patients show alterations in consciousness, whereas, patients with dementia tend to be alert.

c: Depending on the time of day, delirious patients will often show varying degrees of cognitive impairment. Although cognitive impairment can range from mild to severe dementia, daily fluctuations rarely occur unless the patient also has an overlapping delirium.

d: Ten to twenty percent of demented patients may meet the full criteria for a depressive disorder, and up to 50% of demented patients will have some symptoms of depression. At times, patients with a substantial level of cognitive impairment from depression, referred to as pseudodementia, may also be difficult to distinguish from patients with dementia.

e: In dementia, an underlying medical cause is almost always presumed, and a major task for the physician is to determine whether an intervention will lead to a reversal of the condition.

124. **Answer a:**

Neostigmine is a reversible cholinesterase inhibitor with sufficiently long action.

b: Succinylcholine is a nicotinic stimulant.

c: The action of ACh is too short.

d: DFP is an irreversible cholinesterase inhibitor.

e: Ephedrine has direct and indirect stimulating properties.

125. **Answer c:**

Dexamethasone is a long-acting glucocorticoid with low sodium-retaining activity.

a: Prednisone is short-acting.

b: Cortisone is short-acting.

d: Fludrocortisone is a mineralocorticoid with high sodium-retaining activity.

e: Desoxycorticosterone is a mineralocorticoid with high sodium-retaining activity.

126. **Answer c:**

The section of the brain stem at the intercollicular level leads to decerebrate rigidity since all descending inhibitory input to the vestibular nuclei and reticular activating system has been abolished.

a: Ataxia is not a manifestation of this lesion.

b: Ballism results from damage to the subthalamic nuclei.

d: Epilepsy is not a manifestation of this lesion.

e: Insomnia is not a manifestation of this lesion.

127. **Answer a:**

Synthesis of ATP can occur through substrate level phosphorylation of ADP by pyruvate kinase.

b: Phosphocreatine is important in muscle as a storage of high-energy phosphate, but it does not substitute for ATP. Instead, it regenerates ATP from ADP.

c: Energetically unfavorable reactions can be coupled through a common intermediate with an energetically favorable reaction, as long as the free energy change for both is negative.

d: The second terminal phosphate bond does not release more energy than the first, but the subsequent hydrolysis of pyrophosphate to inorganic phosphate (to be recycled back into ADP) creates a favorable free energy change that drives the synthetic process.

e: ATP is produced in the cytoplasm by pyruvate kinase (substrate level phosphorylation), and GTP is produced in the mitochondrion by succinate thiokinase.

128. **Answer b:**

While *ras* normally goes back and forth from an active to inactive state, when active, it excites downstream regulators of mitosis such as MAP kinases. When *ras* has been mutated, it becomes stuck in the "on" position and sends a constant barrage of mitogenic signals.

a: Apoptosis is prevented by *bcl*-2 through a mechanism that is still not clear. When it is overexpressed, as in the t(14:18)(q32:q21) translocation that is commonly found in Burkitt's lymphoma, it prevents normal programmed cell death. In this case, the gene is abnormally activated by being translocated to a site where the control sequences for immunoglobulin synthesis cause activation.

c: Examples of oncogenes that function as growth factor receptors are *erb* and *fms*. If they are mutant, they may be in a constant state of activation. In some cases, they are structurally normal but are present in extreme numbers.

d: Nuclear regulatory genes include *myc, myb, jun,* and *fos*. Their mode of function is not completely understood, but they function in starting and stopping transcription of DNA within the nucleus.

129. **Answer d:**

The right suprarenal gland lies in contact with the inferior vena cava (IVC). A portion of its venous drainage is also directly into this vessel. As such, the IVC is at risk during removal of the organ.

a: The portal vein lies within the hepatoduodenal ligament and is not at risk.

b: The abdominal aorta is separated from the right suprarenal gland by the IVC.

c: The right renal artery is located too far inferiorly to be at risk.

e: The hepatic portal vein is formed by the union of the superior mesenteric and splenic veins deep to the pancreas and is not at risk.

130. **Answer b:**

Confabulation refers to the creation of false details to compensate for memory loss. This phenomenon is often associated with Korsakoff's syndrome as the patient has a chronic amnestic syndrome with a prominent loss of recent memory.

a: Perseveration occurs when an individual continues to respond to previous stimulus although a new stimulus has been presented. In perseveration, a patient will often repeat previous statements in response to new questions.

c: Flight of ideas, a phenomenon often seen in mania, refers to the rapid shifting from one idea to another partially related idea.

d: Malingering occurs when an individual consciously provides false information in order to obtain secondary gain. Although patients with Korsakoff's syndrome often present false information, the false details are presented to compensate for a memory loss.

e: Neologisms refer to the creation of nonexistent words for idiosyncratic reasons.

131. **Answer b:**

Fertilization typically occurs in the ampulla of the oviduct.

a: It is not typical for fertilization to occur in the uterus.

c: Fertilization never occurs in the vagina because capacitation does not take place until the sperm reaches the uterus.

d: Fertilization never occurs in the cervix because capacitation does not take place until the sperm reaches the uterus.

e: It is not typical for fertilization to occur in the intramural portion of the oviduct.

132. **Answer c:**

There is a direct sigmoidal relationship between the arterial blood pressure and the frequency of firing of baroreceptors.

a: Increasing pressure causes the vascular walls to stretch and increases firing of baroreceptors.

b, d, e: Firing increases to a maximum at a mean pressure of about 200 mm Hg.

133. **Answer b:**

No stem cells are present in nerve fascicles. Nerve fascicles are composed of nerve processes and connective tissue elements.

a: Erythrocyte and leukocyte stem cells are injured and killed, which results in a decreased hematocrit and white blood cell count differential.

c: Injury and death of stem cells in the gastric mucosa (in the neck region of the glands) results in sloughing of the gastric epithelium followed by nausea. Stem cells are located in the neck of the gastric glands.

d: Damage to stem cells in hair follicles results in partial to complete hair loss in areas where radiation damage is specifically incurred and nonspecific hair loss due to chemotherapy.

e: Damage to stem cells in crypts of Lieberkühn results in sloughing of the intestinal epithelium and subsequent diarrhea.

134. **Answer e:**

Suppression of the immune response may be accomplished by elimination, not stimulation, of antigen levels.

a: Feedback inhibition by antibodies may suppress the immune response.

b: Immunologic intolerance may suppress the immune response.

c: Feedback inhibition by cytokines may suppress the immune response.

d: Regulation of networks of idiotypes and anti-idiotypes may suppress the immune response.

135. **Answer d:**

In some instances, the white cell response to an acute infection may be so pronounced that it may be mistaken for an acute leukemia. Leukemoid reaction may be diagnosed by a high leukocyte alkaline phosphatase, toxic granulation, Döhle's bodies, and significant maturation of the neutrophils, such that the majority of the cells present are more mature than myelocytes. Promyelocytes may certainly be present in small numbers.

a: Toxic granulation of neutrophils is a diagnostic indicator of leukemoid reaction.

b: Döhle's bodies in neutrophils are a diagnostic indicator of leukemoid reaction.

c: High neutrophil leukocyte alkaline phosphatase is associated with leukemoid reaction.

e: Promyelocytes may be present in small numbers in leukemoid reaction.

136. **Answer e:**

In the nonhabituated individual, an ethyl alcohol blood level of 300 mg/dl would result in coma and possible respiratory arrest.

a: At 50 mg/dl there is some loss in cognitive function, but not coma.

b: At 100 mg/dl there is impairment of motor function and judgement, but not coma.

c: At 150 mg/dl there is significant impairment of motor function, but not coma.

d: At 200 mg/dl a person will "pass out" (narcosis), but will not fall to a coma until 300 mg/dl.

137. **Answer e:**

Despite the unequivocal presence of acute renal failure in these patients, there is no morphologic hallmark that suggests a cause. That no permanent structural damage is present is suggested by the fact that these kidneys regain function, if the hepatic cirrhosis is reversed, and in the same token, they function normally when transplanted.

138. **Answer a:**

Cryptorchidism is clinically significant because of two factors; first the testis will become sterile if it remains cryptorchid. Boys who are bilaterally cryptorchid may be sterile if the condition persists beyond the second year of life. Second, there is about a 35 fold increase in risk of developing a germ cell malignancy in a testis that has been cryptorchid beyond the tenth year of life.

b: Boys who are bilaterally cryptorchid may be sterile if the condition persists beyond the second year of life.

c, d: There is a 35 fold increase in the risk of developing a germ cell malignancy in a testis that has been cryptorchid beyond the tenth year of life.

e: Orchiopexy should be performed before the second birthday to prevent sterility and development of germ cell malignancies.

139. **Answer b:**

Periosteum refers to a specialized layer of connective tissue that covers the outer surface of osseous tissue. The periosteum is not used to classify bone embryologically, histologically, or grossly.

a: Bone is classified embryologically as either intramembranous or endochondral, depending on what type of tissue it replaces.

c: Bone is classified as woven or lamellar, depending on its histologic appearance.

d: Bone is classified grossly as either compact or spongy depending on its gross morphology.

e: Bone is classified as lamellar or woven, depending on its histologic appearance.

140. **Answer e:**

Creatine kinase is an enzyme that is not associated with liver function or hepatic damage. Creatine kinase is elevated in injury to muscle (both skeletal and cardiac), and to the CNS, and is sometimes secreted by tumors.

a: An increase in conjugated bilirubin is associated with cholestasis.

b: An increase in blood cholesterol is associated with cholestasis.

c: An increase in circulating bile acids is associated with cholestasis.

d: An increase in serum alkaline phosphatase is associated with cholestasis.

141. **Answer b:**

Urea will diffuse into the cell along its concentration gradient. Water will also diffuse into the cell, because of the osmotic effect of intracellular proteins. Because the urea readily penetrates the cell, it does not exert any extracellular osmotic effect to oppose the effect of the intracellular proteins.

a: Although the osmolality of the urea solution is about equal to normal plasma osmolality, the fact that the membranes are permeable to urea means that urea does not exert any osmotic effect to oppose the effect of intracellular proteins. The proteins will draw water into the cell until it lyses.

c: The osmolality of the urea solution is about equal to normal plasma osmolality.

d: As urea diffuses into the cell, water also diffuses in, due to the osmotic effect of the intracellular proteins.

e: The cells will swell as urea and water diffuse in, and continue to swell until they lyse, due to the osmotic effect of the intracellular proteins.

142. **Answer e:**

Mumps infection may cause a transient acute pancreatitis. It is usually of little significance.

a: Alcoholism is strongly associated with chronic pancreatitis.

b: Biliary tract disease is associated with chronic pancreatitis.

c: Hypercalcemia disease is associated with chronic pancreatitis.

d: Hyperlipidemia disease is associated with chronic pancreatitis.

143. **Answer a:**

Delusions are false beliefs, maintained rigidly by an individual, despite objective data. Challenging a psychotic patient's delusions often results in the patient becoming increasingly suspicious, agitated, or angry and decreases rapport.

b: As a psychotic patient is rarely a reliable historian, secondary sources of information tend to be critical in diagnostic formulation and treatment planning.

c: A directive interviewing style tends to assist a psychotic patient in providing necessary information and ensures that all areas are appropriately assessed.

d: Maintaining formality and respect for a psychotic patient tends to set the patient at ease.

e: By focusing on concrete skills, especially activities of daily living, a psychotic patient will be less threatened and the interviewer will obtain critical information necessary for treatment planning.

144. **Answer c:**

Cardiac output is the limiting factor in whole body exercise.

a: There is little or no change in arterial P_{O_2} in maximal exercise, indicating that pulmonary uptake of oxygen is not limiting oxygen consumption.

b: Caloric intake is not the limiting factor.

d: Sensitivity of the baroreceptors is not the limiting factor.

e: The increase in cardiac output that occurs with exercise is primarily due to an increase in heart rate, with only a small change in stroke volume. Therefore it is the maximal heart rate that is limiting, not stroke volume.

145. **Answer b:**

The definition of Km is the substrate concentration that produces one-half the maximal velocity. Remember that Km is a substrate concentration and not a velocity.

a: The velocity becomes independent of the substrate concentration when the enzyme becomes saturated with substrate.

c: The velocity will begin to fall when the temperature begins to denature the protein.

d: Enzymes have an optimum pH that is determined by the overall stability of the molecule and by any ionizable side chains located at the active site.

e: Enzyme initial rates are higher at first and then slow down as substrate is depleted and product inhibition occurs.

146. **Answer b:**

In almost every other human autosomal dominant disease, heterozygotes are less affected than homozygotes. In Huntington's syndrome this is not true. Having a single HD gene will produce the full-fledged syndrome within the usual time course of the disease. Huntington's syndrome may be the only human genetic disease to show complete dominance.

a: Huntington's syndrome is caused by the dominant gene 4pl6.3.

c: Symmetric atrophy of the caudate nuclei is a morphologic finding of Huntington's disease.

d: The small neurons of the caudate and putamen are depleted in Huntington's disease.

e: The age of onset for Huntington's disease is usually about 40.

147. **Answer c:**

Lactose intolerance is a common condition in which absence of lactase (a disaccharidase) from the brush border of enterocytes results in accumulation of lactose in the bowel, and causing osmotic diarrhea.

a: Pancreatic amylase does not digest a disaccharide like lactose.

b: Osmotic diarrhea due to accumulation of sucrose in the bowel does not cause lactose intolerance.

d: An excess of lactose or any other non-reabsorbed solute will result in osmotic diarrhea.

e: Dissacharidases are located in the brush border membrane of enterocytes.

148. **Answer e:**

Cytokinesis and endocytosis are functions attributable to microfilaments.

a: Microtubules function in cell migration.

b: Microtubules function in intracellular transport of secretory granules.

c: Microtubules function in movement of chromosomes during mitosis.

d: Microtubules function in maintenance of asymmetric shapes.

149. **Answer a:**

This vessel is a branch of the subscapular artery and normally supplies muscle on the dorsal aspect of the scapula. In this instance, however, blood flow is reversed in the circumflex scapular and subscapular arteries forming a collateral circulation around the scapula.

b: Directional flow in the transverse cervical artery, a branch of the thyrocervical trunk, remains normal and feeds into the collateral circulation.

c: Directional flow in the posterior intercostal arteries remains normal.

d: Directional flow in the suprascapular artery, a branch of the thyrocervical trunk, remains normal and feeds into the collateral circulation.

e: The profunda brachii artery is not involved in this collateral circulation, since it arises from the brachial artery distal to the origin of the subscapular artery from the axillary artery.

150. **Answer c:**

Enuresis (bedwetting) is not associated with narcolepsy.

a: Cataplexy is a symptom associated with narcolepsy.

b: Daytime drowsiness is a symptom associated with narcolepsy.
d: Hypnogogic hallucinations are a symptom associated with narcolepsy.
e: Sleep paralysis is a symptom associated with narcolepsy.

151. **Answer a:**

The area postrema is a circumventricular organ that lacks a blood-brain-barrier. It thus is sensitive to circulating bacterial endotoxins, chemicals, and some drugs and can induce the vomiting reflex.

b: The hypothalamus is not the trigger for the vomiting reflex.
c: The organum vasculosum lacks a blood-brain-barrier but is not the trigger for the vomiting reflex.
d: The pineal gland lacks a blood-brain-barrier but is not the trigger for the vomiting reflex.
e: The subfornical organ lacks a blood-brain-barrier but is not the trigger for the vomiting reflex.

152. **Answer b:**

In atropine poisoning the skin is hot, dry and red, and there is no sweating.

a: Hyperthermia is a characteristic symptom of atropine poisoning.
c: Mydriasis is a characteristic symptom of atropine poisoning.
d: Tachycardia is a characteristic symptom of atropine poisoning.
e: Hallucinations are a characteristic symptom of atropine poisoning.

153. **Answer b:**

Cones rather than rods are present exclusively in the fovea centralis.

a: Rods possess rhodopsin.
c: Rod disks are replaced on a regular basis.
d: Rods are more numerous than cones.
e: Rods function during periods of low-light intensity.

154. **Answer c:**

The presence of numerous profiles of rER is not consistent with other morphologic features observed in the typical PCT cell. These cells do not synthesize large amounts of protein for export.

a: Cells of the PCT function mainly in reabsorption. Hence, proteins and large peptides are reabsorbed by endocytosis, which is why there are so many vesicles in the apical cytoplasm.

b: Cells of the PCT function mainly in reabsorption. Hence, one would expect to see eosinophilic cytoplasm that is caused by mitochondria.
d: Cells of the PCT function mainly in reabsorption. Hence, one would expect to see striations near the basal cell surface that are caused by longitudinally-oriented mitochondria and intervening infoldings of basal plasma membrane.
e: Cells of the PCT function mainly in reabsorption. Hence, one would expect to see numerous microvilli on the apical cell surface.

155. **Answer e:**

Repeated stimulation of polymodal nociceptors lowers their threshold and sensitizes them to fire with a lesser stimulus than previously.

a: Cold receptors do not lower their threshold after repeated stimulation.
b: Golgi tendon organs cannot be sensitized.
c: Meissner's corpuscles cannot be sensitized.
d: Pacinian corpuscles cannot be sensitized.

156. **Answer b:**

Secretin is produced by enteroendocrine cells. These are not present in the islets of Langerhans.

a: B cells in the pancreatic islets of Langerhans secrete insulin.
c: D-1 cells in the pancreatic islets of Langerhans secrete VIP.
d: A cells in the pancreatic islets of Langerhans secrete glucagon.
e: D cells in the pancreatic islets of Langerhans secrete somatostatin.

157. **Answer a:**

Transitional epithelial cells protect underlying tissue from urine, which in many cases can be acidic and thus toxic. If protection from abrasion is the primary function of transitional epithelium, it is much more likely that the urinary system would be lined with stratified squamous epithelium (nonkeratinized or parakeratinized).

b: Transitional epithelium lines the urinary bladder.
c: Transitional epithelium contains cells that prevent movement of water from the underlying tissues into urine.
d: Transitional epithelium lines the renal pelvis.
e: Transitional epithelium possesses binucleate cells in the most superficial layer.

158. **Answer b:**

Influenza virus A is the only virus in which mutation-derived changes in the hemagglutinins can cause "antigenic shifts."

a: Adenoviruses are nonenvelope viruses that have fibers that may act as a hemagglutinin, but there is no evidence that these hemagglutinins mutate to cause "antigenic shifts" in the virus.

c: Respiratory syncytial virus does not have hemagglutinins.

d: Poliovirus has no hemagglutinins.

e: Rhinoviruses have no hemagglutinins.

159. **Answer d:**

Sodium nitrite administered intravenously produces methemoglobin that binds cyanide ions.

a: Glyceryl trinitrate is not administered intravenously.

b: Amyl nitrate is not administered intravenously.

c: Papaverine is a smooth muscle relaxant and not useful in treating cyanide poisoning.

e: Erythrityl tetranitrate is not administered intravenously.

160. **Answer a:**

Haemophilus influenzae has not been shown to cause osteomyelitis in children.

b: *Haemophilus influenzae* causes cellulitis in very young children.

c: *Haemophilus influenzae* is one of the most common causes of otitis media in children.

d: *Haemophilus influenzae* is the most common cause of pediatric meningitis in nonimmunized children.

e: *Haemophilus influenzae* can cause life-threatening epiglottitis in nonimmunized children primarily in the 2- to 4-year age group.

161. **Answer d:**

The cells of the *Mycoplasma pneumoniae* bacterium are wall-less and would not be revealed on the Gram's stain. Infections by this organism often result in a positive cold agglutinins titer.

a: *Streptococcus pneumoniae* probably would have been seen on the Gram's stain. This organism does not cause a rise in cold agglutinins.

b: *Klebsiella pneumoniae* would likely have appeared on a Gram's stain. It, also, does not produce cold agglutinins.

c, e: Neither *Chlamydia pneumoniae* nor *C. psittaci* would appear in the Gram's stain, but they do not produce cold agglutinins.

162. **Answer a:**

Because metoprolol is the only beta blocker in the group, it is the only one that may inhibit reflex tachycardia.

b: Minoxidil is a vasodilator.

c: Spironolactone is a mineralocorticoid antagonist.

d: Sodium nitroprusside is a vasodilator via the release of nitric oxide.

e: Enalapril is an ACE inhibitor, which does not evoke reflex tachycardia.

163. **Answer d:**

The A portion of pertussis toxin has ADP-ribosylating activity and interferes with the transfer of signals from cell-surface receptors to intracellular mediator systems.

a: Pertussis toxin can block immune effector cells and can cause lymphocytosis and hypoglycemia.

b: Pertussis toxin is composed of six protein subunits.

c: Pertussis toxin is an important component in newly developed vaccines.

e: Pertussis toxin aids in the adherence of *Bordetella pertussis* to respiratory epithelial cells.

164. **Answer b:**

Halothane may cause liver damage, however, there is no clear explanation for the mechanism.

a: Methoxyflurane exerts nephrotoxicity.

c: Diazepam causes adverse effects related to CNS depression and muscle relaxation.

d: Nitrous oxide causes practically no toxicity.

e: Thiopental depresses the cardiovascular system and the medullary respiratory center.

165. **Answer d:**

Nitrogen equilibrium, or the excretion of nitrogen equaling nitrogen intake, occurs in normal adults when dietary intake of protein is adequate. Tyrosine is a nonessential amino acid, since it can be synthesized from phenylalanine provided in the balanced diet. Therefore, the protein intake would be considered adequate and of high quality.

a: Negative nitrogen balance, or the excretion of more nitrogen than is ingested, will occur when protein intake is insufficient or of low quality (i.e., lacking a balance of essential amino acids).

b: Nitrogen balance generally will not have transient periods in the positive or negative direction, since the conditions that lead to nitrogen imbalance are more of a chronic nature. For example, negative nitrogen balance is brought on following surgery, in advanced stages of cancer, or in starvation syndromes, such as kwashiorkor.

c: Phenylalanine is an essential amino acid and is not synthesized by the body.

e: An increase in urea excretion would indicate a possible negative nitrogen balance due to the inability of the body to use an incomplete protein. Since the protein intake is a complete protein, this would not occur.

166. **Answer d:**

Meckel's diverticulum is a true diverticum. It has all three layers of the normal bowel wall, mucosa, submucosa, and muscularis propria.

a: True. Meckel's diverticulum may cause appendicitis-like symptoms.

b: True. Meckel's diverticulum may contain ectopic foci of gastric mucosa.

c: True. Meckel's diverticulum may contain ectopic foci of pancreatic tissue.

d: True. Meckel's diverticulum arises from persistence of the vitelline duct.

167. **Answer c:**

Most pulmonary emboli are silent and cause no clinical symptoms. The reason for this is that they are small and tend to lodge in the periphery of the lung. In most cases, the dual circulation of the lung plus collateral circulation is sufficient to provide oxygen to the compromised tissue.

a: True. Most pulmonary emboli arise in the lower extremities.

b: True. Deep vein thrombosis is associated with venous stasis.

d: True. Deep vein thrombosis is associated with oral contraceptives.

e: True. Large pulmonary emboli may be quickly fatal.

168. **Answer e:**

Lymphogranuloma venereum, a chlamydial disease transmitted by *C. trachomatis,* typically causes a small, painless vesicle at the point of innoculation. After the vesicle heals, the inguinal lymph nodes develop a combination of suppurative and granulomatous inflammation. The nodes may rupture and form fistula tracts. In some patients, the scarring will result in blockage of the pelvic lymphatics, resulting in lymphedema of the genitals and stricture of the rectum.

a: Gonorrhea is not associated with genital elephantiasis and rectal strictures.

b: Syphillis is not associated with genital elephantiasis and rectal strictures.

c: Chancroid is not associated with genital elephantiasis and rectal strictures.

d: Mycoplasma is not associated with genital elephantiasis and rectal strictures.

169. **Answer c:**

Hantaan virus is not an arbovirus and is not transmitted by an arthropod vector.

a: Dengue virus is transmitted by the Aedes mosquito.

b: St. Louis encephalitis virus is transmitted by the Culex mosquito.

d: Eastern equine encephalitis virus is transmitted by the bite of either Aedes or Culiseta mosquitos.

e: Powassan is transmitted to humans by Ixodes ticks.

170. **Answer c:**

The pontine nuclei give rise to axons of the pontocerebellar tract. These axons decussate in the basilar pons and form the entire middle cerebellar peduncle.

a: The external (lateral, accessory) cuneate nucleus gives rise to the cuneocerebellar track, which enters the cerebellum through the inferior cerebellar peduncle.

b: The inferior olive gives rise to the olivocerebellar tract. These axons decussate in the medulla and enter the cerebellum through the inferior cerebellar peduncle.

d: The nucleus dorsalis of Clark gives rise to axons in the posterior spinocerebellar tract. These axons enter through the inferior cerebellar peduncle.

e: The reticular formation gives rise to reticulocerebellar axons, which enter through the inferior cerebellar peduncle.

171. **Answer b:**

Facilitated diffusion is passive and does not have a direct requirement for hydrolysis of ATP.

a: The protein carrier molecules that mediate facilitated diffusion allow water soluble substrates to cross the lipid barrier of the cell membrane.

c: The limited number of carrier sites in a membrane results in saturation kinetics at high substrate concentration.

d: Carriers distinguish between different classes of substrates.

e: Similar substrates (e.g., different types of sugars), compete for diffusion with carriers, resulting in competitive inhibition of transport.

172.   **Answer a:**
Parathyroid hormone has a role in restoring extracellular fluid calcium by mobilization of bone
calcium, reducing renal clearance of calcium. It
also stimulates the synthesis in the kidney of
$1,25\text{-}(OH)_2$ cholecalciferol, which increases calcium absorption from the gut. Excesses of PTH
will exaggerate both of these processes.

b: The formation of $24,25\text{-}(OH)$ cholecalciferol
from $25\text{-}(OH)$ calciferol is stimulated at *low* PTH
levels.
c: Formation of $1,25\text{-}(OH)$ cholecalciferol from
$25\text{-}(OH)$ cholecalciferol is stimulated by PTH, as
well as low serum phosphate levels.
d: 7-dehydrocholesterol is formed photochemically
as a direct result of exposure to sunlight, and as
such, is not regulated.
e: PTH indirectly stimulates the uptake of calcium
by stimulating $1,25\text{-}(OH)$ cholecalciferol synthesis in the kidney.

173.   **Answer d:**
C fibers are the smallest fibers and are unmyeli-
nated. They are the axons of the polymodal nociceptors, which transmit slow, burning pain.

a: Axons carrying discriminative touch information
belong to the A-beta fiber group.
b: Axons carrying flutter information belong to the
A-beta group.
c: Axons carrying information about limb proprioception are the most heavily myelinated and belong to the A-alpha group.
e: Axons carrying information about vibration sense
belong to the A-beta group.

174.   **Answer c:**
The lenticulostriate arteries are small arteries that
exit from the large middle cerebral artery and provide part of the blood supply to the internal capsule.

a: The central (rolandic) branch of the middle cerebral artery usually supplies the precentral and
postcentral gyrus and thus could cause both motor and sensory deficits. However, it is not one of
the first arteries that come off the middle cerebral
artery, nor does it supply the posterior limb of the
internal capsule.
b: The callosomarginal artery is a branch of the anterior cerebral artery.
d: The pericallosal artery is a branch of the anterior
cerebral artery.
e: The recurrent artery of Heubner is one of the first
branches of the anterior cerebral artery.

175.   **Answer c:**
Supersensitivity occurs when the hormone for a
receptor is absent for a long period; in this case,
the vascular smooth muscle cells will synthesize
an increased number of alpha-adrenergic receptors for norepinephrine.

a: Specificity refers to the affinity of a receptor for a
particular ligand.
b: Ligand gating refers to ion channels that open or
close in response to binding of ligands to receptors on the cells containing the channels.
d: Down regulation is a decrease in the number of
receptors on a cell; it will result in a decrease in
sensitivity to the ligand (norepinephrine in this
case).
e: Saturation occurs when all receptors of a particular type are occupied by ligand.

176.   **Answer c:**
The interfascicular oligodendroglia are the predominant glial cells found in the white matter.

a: Ependymal cells are found lining ventricular cav-
ities.
b: Fibrous astrocytes do not predominate.
d: Perineuronal oligodendroglia are found in gray
matter.
e: Tanycytes are not found in white matter.

177.   **Answer c:**
The enzyme can not hydrolyze paraoxon, because
the complex can not dissociate, thus the enzyme
is inactivated.

a: Alkylphosphates do not influence the synthesis of
acetylcholinesterase.
b: There is no natural cholinesterase inhibitor.
d: Parathion is converted to paraoxon by oxidative
desulfuration.
e: Alkylphosphates do not influence the catabolism
of acetylcholinesterase.

178.   **Answer c:**
Pralidoxime binds to both the enzymes and the
inhibitor and is capable of reactivating the enzyme.

a: Alkylphosphates do not influence the synthesis of
acetylcholinesterase.
b: Neostigmine is a cholinesterase inhibitor.
d: Decreased catabolism would enhance the effect.
e: Atropine does not influence the activity of the enzyme.

179. **Answer c:**
Thickening (not thinning) of the skin on the palms and soles (increased keratin formation) is characteristic of arsenic poisoning along with all the symptoms mentioned in A, B, D, and E.

a: Nausea, anorexia, and diarrhea are all symptoms of arsenic poisoning.
b: Dermatitis and thickening of the palms and soles due to increased keratin formation are characteristics of arsenic poisoning.
d: Arsenic poisoning can cause capillary damage.
e: Personality changes result from arsenic poisoning.

180. **Answer e:**
Vibrio cholerae produces its effect exclusively by the action of its exotoxin on the gut mucosa, causing the cells to secrete isosmotic fluid in massive quantities. It is not tissue invasive and causes no acute inflammation and, hence, no fecal leukocytosis.

Matching answers 181 through 185

181. **Answer f:**
Actinomyces israelii produces multiple abscesses connected by sinus tracts and sulfur granules associated with these abscesses.

182. **Answer c:**
Clostridium perfringens produces a lecithinase (demonstrated on egg yolk agar) and is a cause of bacterial food poisoning.

183. **Answer a:**
Clostridium difficile is associated with pseudomembranous colitis, and in the hospital setting can be a major source of outbreaks.

184. **Answer d:**
Clostridium botulinum is a gram-positive bacillus that produces a neurotoxin that blocks the release of acetylcholine.

185. **Answer b:**
Clostridium tetani produces a neurotoxin that blocks release of neurotransmitters of inhibitory synapses.

Matching answers 186 and 187

186. **Answer c:**
Histrionic personality disorder refers to a pattern of excessive emotionality and attention seeking. These patients often present in a seductive or dramatic fashion.

187. **Answer e:**
A pattern of preoccupation with orderliness, perfectionism, and control suggests a diagnosis of obsessive-compulsive personality disorder is most applicable. This personality disorder is separate from an obsessive-compulsive disorder, which is diagnosed when obsessions and compulsions are present.

a: The hallmark characteristic of a paranoid personality disorder is a pattern of mistrust and suspiciousness.
b: Antisocial personality disorder refers to a pattern of social disregard, in which the rights of others are violated.
d: Avoidant personality disorder is characterized by a pattern of social inhibition, sense of inadequacy, and fear of negative evaluation.

Matching answers 188 and 189

188. **Answer c:**
Also known as an endodermal sinus tumor, this neoplasm is among the most common germ cell tumors in children. The characteristic microscopic structure of this tumor is the Schiller-Duval body, which is a microcyst containing a glumerulus-like structure. The tumor cells stain positively for alpha$_1$-fetoprotein, which also forms a tumor marker in the serum. Embryonal carcinomas frequently contain a yolk sac component, even in adults.

189. **Answer a:**
Seminoma is the most common germ cell tumor found in males. It constitutes about 30% to 50% of germ cell tumors. Seminoma occurs in several histological variants: classic, anaplastic, and spermatocytic.

Matching answers 190 and 191

190. **Answer a:**
The Tarasoff I ruling stated that a physician or psychotherapist who believes a patient may injure or kill another individual must warn the potential victim, the potential victim's relatives, or the authorities.

191. **Answer c:**
The Wyatt v. Stickney case was a class action suit leading to a ruling that persons committed to a mental institution have a constitutional right to treatment that affords them a reasonable opportunity for cure or improvement.

b: Tarasoff II, an extension of the Tarasoff I case, broadened the duty to warn to a duty to protect.

d: The M'Naghten rule was originally established in 1843 through British courts. It asserts that individuals are not guilty of a crime by reason of insanity if they had a mental disease that led them to be unaware of the nature, quality, and consequences of their actions or if they were not capable of distinguishing between right and wrong.

e: The Durham rule was an attempt to qualify the M'Naghten rule by requiring demonstration that criminal behavior was a product of mental disease for a "not guilty by reason of insanity" plea to be valid. This rule was disregarded because it was believed to be open to subjective interpretation.

Matching answers 192 and 193

192. **Answer h:**
Coronaviruses are the second most prevalent cause of the common cold.

193. **Answer i:**
The polyprotein of HIV-1, gp160, is cleaved into the glycoproteins gp41 and gp120.

Matching answers 194 through 197

194. **Answer e:**
Carboxypeptidases split amino acids from the carboxyl end of a peptide; they are exopeptidases because they cleave the last link in a peptide chain.

195. **Answer a:**
Amylase is a starch-digesting enzyme secreted by the salivary glands and the pancreas.

196, 197. **Answer b:**
Trypsin is an endopeptidase that cleaves peptides at the carboxyl group of arginine or lysine.

c: Elastase was not referred to in this set of questions.

d: Chymotrypsin was not referred to in this set of questions.

Matching answers 198 through 200

198, 199. **Answer c:**
Proliferation of the endometrium occurs during the first half of the cycle and overlaps the time that the follicles are developed (late follicular phase, Question 198), and during the period of increasing plasma estradiol (Question 199).

200. **Answer e:**
The secretory phase occurs during the second half of the cycle under the influence of progesterone, which is increasing at this time.

a: The ischemic phase occurs in the second half of the cycle; this choice was not used in this question set.

b: The peak plasma level of LH occurs at midcycle; this choice was not used in this question set.

d: Menstruation occurring at the end of the cycle does not correspond to any of the three lettered items; this choice was not used in this question set.

Categories and Answers for Exam 3

Question Number	Answer	Check Here If Correct	Category 1	Category 2	Category 3
1	B	☐	Physiology	Endocrine System	Main Effects
2	B	☐	Anatomy	Lower Limb	Clinical Anatomy
3	C	☐	Pathology	Female Reproductive System	Neoplasia
4	D	☐	Physiology	Cells & Tissues	General Properties
5	E	☐	Pharmacology	Central Nervous System	Clinical Uses
6	C	☐	Neuroscience	Central Nervous System	Normal Anatomy
7	E	☐	Microbiology	Virology	Diseases
8	C	☐	Microbiology	Mycology	Epidemiology
9	D	☐	Physiology	Cells & Tissues	General Properties
10	B	☐	Histology	Female Reproductive System	Normal Function
11	B	☐	Physiology	Cardiovascular System	Microcirculation
12	B	☐	Physiology	Urinary System	Regulation
13	D	☐	Physiology	Gastrointestinal System	General Properties
14	D	☐	Pharmacology	General Principles	Pharmacokinetics
15	B	☐	Microbiology	Bacteriology	Epidemiology
16	A	☐	Neuroscience	Head & Neck	Normal Anatomy
17	B	☐	Physiology	Cardiovascular System	The Heart as a Pump
18	A	☐	Microbiology	Bacteriology	Diseases
19	B	☐	Neuroscience	Back & Spinal Cord	Lesions
20	E	☐	Pathology	Gastrointestinal System	Diseases
21	C	☐	Microbiology	Virology	Pathogenesis
22	B	☐	Microbiology	Mycology	Diseases
23	E	☐	Physiology	Gastrointestinal System	Secretion
24	A	☐	Neuroscience	Motor Systems & Reflexes	Lesions
25	A	☐	Biochemistry	Endocrine System	Diseases
26	B	☐	Anatomy	Thorax	Normal Anatomy
27	C	☐	Physiology	Cardiovascular System	Regulation
28	E	☐	Pathology	Blood & Lymph	Diseases
29	E	☐	Microbiology	Bacteriology	Epidemiology
30	C	☐	Histology	Gastrointestinal System	Secretion
31	A	☐	Physiology	Respiratory System	Mechanics of Breathing
32	D	☐	Physiology	Endocrine System	Normal Function
33	A	☐	Anatomy	Pelvis & Perineum	Normal Anatomy
34	B	☐	Pharmacology	Autonomic Nervous System	Main Effects
35	A	☐	Physiology	Endocrine System	Secretion
36	A	☐	Pathology	Cardiovascular System	Diseases
37	D	☐	Anatomy	Upper Limb	Normal Anatomy
38	D	☐	Physiology	Urinary System	Normal Function
39	D	☐	Neuroscience	Central Nervous System	Normal Anatomy
40	D	☐	Pathology	Immune System	Immune Response
41	D	☐	Pharmacology	Chemotherapy	Treatment
42	C	☐	Neuroscience	Central Nervous System	Lesions
43	D	☐	Pathology	Immune System	Immune Response
44	D	☐	Biochemistry	Enzymes	Inhibition
45	E	☐	Neuroscience	Motor Systems & Reflexes	Normal Anatomy
46	E	☐	Physiology	Respiratory System	Transport
47	C	☐	Physiology	Gastrointestinal System	Regulation
48	B	☐	Neuroscience	Back & Spinal Cord	Normal Anatomy
49	E	☐	Anatomy	Upper Limb	Normal Anatomy
50	E	☐	Pathology	Endocrine System	Diseases

Categories and Answers for Exam 3

Question Number	Answer	Check Here if Correct	Category 1	Category 2	Category 3
51	C	☐	Pharmacology	Blood & Lymph	General Properties
52	C	☐	Pharmacology	Chemotherapy	Metabolism
53	D	☐	Pharmacology	Endocrine System	Main Effects
54	A	☐	Pharmacology	General Principles	Pharmacodynamics
55	D	☐	Pharmacology	General Principles	Pharmacodynamics
56	C	☐	Biochemistry	Molecular Genetics	Genetics
57	B	☐	Neuroscience	Central Nervous System	Lesions
58	C	☐	Microbiology	Bacteriology	Epidemiology
59	C	☐	Microbiology	Bacteriology	Diseases
60	D	☐	Pathology	Central Nervous System	Clinical Anatomy
61	E	☐	Pathology	Female Reproductive System	Lesions
62	D	☐	Neuroscience	Central Nervous System	Normal Function
63	D	☐	Pharmacology	Autonomic Nervous System	Main Effects
64	D	☐	Microbiology	Bacteriology	Pathogenesis
65	C	☐	Biochemistry	Amino Acids & Proteins	Structure
66	C	☐	Physiology	Gastrointestinal System	Secretion
67	E	☐	Histology	Cells & Tissues	Structure
68	A	☐	Pharmacology	Toxicology	Main Effects
69	C	☐	Physiology	Cardiovascular System	General Properties
70	D	☐	Neuroscience	Central Nervous System	Normal Anatomy
71	C	☐	Pathology	Cells & Tissues	Neoplasia
72	D	☐	Biochemistry	Molecular Genetics	Regulation
73	E	☐	Neuroscience	Central Nervous System	Normal Anatomy
74	C	☐	Physiology	Cardiovascular System	General Properties
75	C	☐	Physiology	Endocrine System	Main Effects
76	A	☐	Pharmacology	Autonomic Nervous System	Main Effects
77	D	☐	Microbiology	Bacteriology	Structure
78	C	☐	Anatomy	Lower Limb	Normal Anatomy
79	D	☐	Physiology	Respiratory System	General Properties
80	E	☐	Pharmacology	General Principles	Pharmacokinetics
81	B	☐	Pharmacology	Cardiovascular System	Treatment
82	B	☐	Histology	Cells & Tissues	Normal Tissues
83	B	☐	Pharmacology	Autocoids & Diuretics	Main Effects
84	D	☐	Microbiology	Parasitology	Pathogenesis
85	C	☐	Histology	Endocrine System	Normal Function
86	E	☐	Histology	Respiratory System	Normal Tissues
87	A	☐	Histology	Male Reproductive System	Clinical Anatomy
88	A	☐	Microbiology	Bacteriology	Epidemiology
89	B	☐	Anatomy	Back & Spinal Cord	Normal Anatomy
90	B	☐	Anatomy	Pelvis & Perineum	Normal Anatomy
91	E	☐	Neuroscience	Central Nervous System	Lesions
92	E	☐	Pharmacology	Chemotherapy	Clinical Uses
93	C	☐	Microbiology	Mycology	Diseases
94	C	☐	Pharmacology	General Principles	Pharmacokinetics
95	B	☐	Pharmacology	Central Nervous System	Side Effects
96	E	☐	Anatomy	Thorax	Normal Anatomy
97	E	☐	Biochemistry	Purine & Pyrimidine Metabolism	Synthesis
98	E	☐	Microbiology	Virology	Epidemiology
99	E	☐	Pharmacology	Autonomic Nervous System	Main Effects
100	A	☐	Neuroscience	Head & Neck	Lesions

Categories and Answers for Exam 3

Question Number	Answer	Check Here if Correct	Category 1	Category 2	Category 3
101	D	☐	Microbiology	Bacteriology	Diseases
102	C	☐	Physiology	Respiratory System	Mechanics of Breathing
103	C	☐	Pharmacology	Cardiovascular System	General Properties
104	B	☐	Neuroscience	Head & Neck	Normal Anatomy
105	A	☐	Physiology	Respiratory System	Regulation
106	D	☐	Pathology	Cardiovascular System	Immune Response
107	C	☐	Anatomy	Pelvis & Perineum	Normal Anatomy
108	A	☐	Histology	Immune System	Immune System Cells
109	D	☐	Biochemistry	Amino Acids & Proteins	General Properties
110	C	☐	Pathology	Musculoskeletal System	Diseases
111	D	☐	Anatomy	Thorax	Clinical Anatomy
112	A	☐	Biochemistry	Molecular Genetics	Synthesis
113	A	☐	Pharmacology	Blood & Lymph	Diseases
114	A	☐	Neuroscience	Central Nervous System	Lesions
115	D	☐	Physiology	Cells & Tissues	General Properties
116	C	☐	Microbiology	Virology	General Properties
117	B	☐	Neuroscience	Head & Neck	Lesions
118	C	☐	Anatomy	Back & Spinal Cord	Normal Anatomy
119	D	☐	Pharmacology	Endocrine System	Side Effects
120	D	☐	Microbiology	Bacteriology	Epidemiology
121	A	☐	Histology	Blood & Lymph	Structure
122	C	☐	Histology	Immune System	Normal Anatomy
123	E	☐	Histology	Urinary System	Structure
124	D	☐	Histology	Cells & Tissues	Structure
125	A	☐	Pharmacology	Central Nervous System	Clinical Uses
126	B	☐	Anatomy	Upper Limb	Normal Anatomy
127	D	☐	Pathology	Female Reproductive Tract	Neoplasia
128	E	☐	Neuroscience	Central Nervous System	Normal Anatomy
129	A	☐	Pharmacology	Chemotherapy	Clinical Uses
130	A	☐	Neuroscience	Central Nervous System	Normal Anatomy
131	E	☐	Pharmacology	Cardiovascular System	Main Effects
132	E	☐	Pathology	Gastrointestinal System	Diseases
133	E	☐	Neuroscience	Neurotransmitters	Synthesis
134	D	☐	Microbiology	Bacteriology	General Properties
135	C	☐	Histology	Gastrointestinal System	Diseases
136	A	☐	Microbiology	Immune System	Immune System Cells
137	D	☐	Neuroscience	Neurotransmitters	Synthesis
138	E	☐	Pathology	Bacteriology	Immune System Cells
139	B	☐	Histology	Immune System	Structure
140	D	☐	Neuroscience	Central Nervous System	Normal Anatomy
141	B	☐	Pathology	Forensic Medicine	Clinical Anatomy
142	A	☐	Pathology	Blood & Lymph	Diseases
143	B	☐	Pathology	Gastrointestinal System	Diseases
144	B	☐	Biochemistry	Amino Acids & Proteins	General Properties
145	B	☐	Physiology	Cells & Tissues	Regulation
146	D	☐	Biochemistry	Molecular Genetics	Structure
147	A	☐	Pathology	Cardiovascular System	Cell Injury & Cell Death
148	A	☐	Pathology	Blood & Lymph	Diseases
149	A	☐	Pathology	Urinary System	Lesions
150	C	☐	Biochemistry	Liver & Pancreas	Diseases

Categories and Answers for Exam 3

Question Number	Answer	Check Here if Correct	Category 1	Category 2	Category 3
151	A	☐	Physiology	Endocrine System	Main Effects
152	A	☐	Histology	Gastrointestinal System	Secretion
153	B	☐	Microbiology	Bacteriology	Structure
154	C	☐	Histology	Endocrine System	General Properties
155	D	☐	Histology	Ear	Normal Anatomy
156	D	☐	Anatomy	Thorax	Normal Anatomy
157	C	☐	Biochemistry	Molecular Genetics	Recombinant DNA
158	C	☐	Pathology	Musculoskeletal System	Immune System Cells
159	C	☐	Physiology	General Principles	Transport
160	C	☐	Neuroscience	Central Nervous System	Normal Anatomy
161	A	☐	Anatomy	Head & Neck	Normal Anatomy
162	E	☐	Microbiology	Parasitology	Epidemiology
163	B	☐	Anatomy	Head & Neck	Normal Anatomy
164	A	☐	Neuroscience	Cells & Tissues	Normal Function
165	D	☐	Microbiology	Virology	Pathogenesis
166	D	☐	Pathology	Head & Neck	Neoplasia
167	D	☐	Pharmacology	Central Nervous System	Interactions
168	D	☐	Biochemistry	Membranes	Transport
169	D	☐	Histology	Endocrine System	Normal Function
170	C	☐	Physiology	Urinary System	Regulation
171	D	☐	Pharmacology	Autocoids & Diuretics	Main Effects
172	B	☐	Neuroscience	Head & Neck	Lesions
173	E	☐	Pathology	General Principles	Diseases
174	B	☐	Biochemistry	Intermediary Metabolism	Metabolism
175	D	☐	Histology	Gastrointestinal System	Normal Function
176	D	☐	Pathology	Cardiovascular System	Diseases
177	E	☐	Pathology	Musculoskeletal System	Neoplasia
178	C	☐	Anatomy	Back & Spinal Cord	Normal Anatomy
179	E	☐	Biochemistry	Intermediary Metabolism	Glycolysis & Gluconeogenesis
180	C	☐	Pharmacology	Autonomic Nervous System	Side Effects
181	C	☐	Neuroscience	Motor Systems & Reflexes	Normal Anatomy
182	D	☐	Physiology	Musculoskeletal System	Signaling
183	E	☐	Microbiology	Immune System	General Properties
184	A	☐	Microbiology	Immune System	Immune System Cells
185	E	☐	Biochemistry	Lipids & Steroids	Diseases
186	D	☐	Biochemistry	Lipids & Steroids	Diseases
187	H	☐	Pathology	General Principles	Neoplasia
188	B	☐	Pathology	General Principles	Neoplasia
189	C	☐	Microbiology	Virology	Diseases
190	B	☐	Microbiology	Virology	Diseases
191	D	☐	Microbiology	Virology	Laboratory Diagnosis
192	A	☐	Physiology	Endocrine System	Metabolism
193	C	☐	Physiology	Endocrine System	Metabolism
194	A	☐	Physiology	Endocrine System	Metabolism
195	B	☐	Physiology	Endocrine System	Metabolism
196	B	☐	Physiology	Endocrine System	Metabolism
197	L	☐	Neuroscience	Central Nervous System	Normal Anatomy
198	I	☐	Neuroscience	Central Nervous System	Lesions
199	B	☐	Biochemistry	Nitrogen Metabolism	Diseases
200	E	☐	Biochemistry	Nitrogen Metabolism	General Properties

1. **Answer b:**

    Amino acid concentrations decrease; insulin stimulates uptake of amino acids by muscle.

    a: Insulin decreases release of glucose from liver and stimulates glucose uptake by muscle, lowering the plasma level.

    c: Insulin lowers the FFA concentration in plasma by lowering release from adipose tissue.

    d: Insulin lowers release of FFA from adipose tissue, which results in less ketone body production.

    e: Insulin stimulates K^+ uptake by muscle and liver, thus decreasing the plasma level.

2. **Answer b:**

    The superior gluteal nerve innervates the gluteus medius, gluteus minimus, and tensor fasciae latae muscles.

    a: The gluteus maximus muscle receives its innervation via the inferior gluteal nerve.

    c: The nerve to the obturator internus innervates the muscle of the same name.

    d: The piriformis is innervated by branches of the sacral plexus.

    e: The nerve to the quadratus femoris innervates the muscle of the same name.

3. **Answer c:**

    Various studies have quoted survival statistics of 70% to 90% in women with stage I breast cancer. Eighty percent is a reasonable average. This situation of progressive disease in women with no obvious spread of tumor from the primary site is a dilemma that still lacks a solution. Currently there is no satisfactory prognostic tool to predict if a woman is in the cured group or the group that will have progressive disease.

4. **Answer d:**

    This equation is valid because P_{CO_2} of inspired air $= 0$, and arterial P_{CO_2} (Pa_{CO_2}) equals alveolar P_{CO_2}. Therefore the volume of CO_2 expired/min is:

    $$V_{ECO2} = (V_A \times Pa_{CO_2})/K$$

    K is a constant to correct for differences in units. This equation may be readily solved for V_A. V_A is calculated from the volume of expired CO_2 per minute, V_{ECO2}, assuming (1) P_{CO_2} of inspired air $= 0$, and (2) arterial P_{CO_2} (Pa_{CO_2}) equals alveolar P_{CO_2}.

5. **Answer e:**

    Trihexyphenidyl is an anticholinergic antiparkinson drug.

    a: Carbidopa inhibits DOPA decarboxylase.

    b: Bromocriptine is a dopamine agonist.

    c: Amantadine is an antiviral agent with effects on the dopaminergic system.

    d: L-DOPA is a precursor of dopamine.

6. **Answer c:**

    Brainwave activity does *not* include gamma activity.

    a: Brainwave activity does include alpha activity.

    b: Brainwave activity does include beta activity.

d: Brainwave activity does include delta activity.
e: Brainwave activity does include theta activity.

7. **Answer e:**
   Renal failure is not a common occurrence in coxsackie virus infection.

   a: Viral or aseptic meningitis is commonly associated with picornaviruses such as coxsackie and echovirus.
   b: Herpangina is a common clinical manifestation of coxsackie A virus.
   c: Pleurodynia, also known as Bornholm disease, is a manifestation of infection by coxsackie B virus.
   d: Vesicular lesions are commonly associated with hand-foot-and-mouth disease, caused by coxsackie A16.

8. **Answer c:**
   Coccidioidomycosis most frequently occurs in the San Joaquin Valley in California, in Arizona, and in the southwestern counties of Texas.

   a: North American blastomycosis is endemic primarily in the Ohio and Mississippi Valley region.
   b: Histoplasmosis is found primarily in the Ohio and Mississippi Valley region.
   d: Candidiasis is an opportunistic pathogen that occurs worldwide.
   e: Cryptococcosis occurs throughout the world.

9. **Answer d:**
   $RV = TLC - VC = 6 - 4.8 = 1.2$ L
   $FRC = ERV + RV$, so $ERV = FRC - RV = 2.4 - 1.2 = 1.2$ L
   $VC = IRV + VT + ERV$
   $4.8 = IRV + 0.5 + 1.2$ so $IRV = 3.1$.

10. **Answer b:**
    Inhibin is a hormone that regulates the *male* (not the female) reproductive system. It is secreted by Sertoli cells in the seminiferous tubules and inhibits adenohypophysial activity.

    a: Estrogen regulates changes in the endometrium of the uterus.
    c: Progesterone regulates changes in the endometrium of the uterus.
    d: Luteinizing hormone regulates follicular development in the ovary.
    e: Follicular-stimulating hormone regulates follicular development in the ovary.

11. **Answer b:**
    Decreasing cellular utilization of glucose will decrease the concentration gradient for glucose between plasma and cell, and therefore decrease glucose transport (diffusion) from plasma to cell.

    a: Glucose transport depends on diffusion, and concentration gradient is one determinant of the rate of diffusion.
    c: An increase in blood flow will maintain plasma glucose concentration locally in the muscle, maintaining the rate of glucose diffusion.
    d: Opening capillaries will increase glucose delivery to the muscle and allow more transport (diffusion) of glucose to occur.
    e: Glucose diffuses through these vesicles; increasing their number will increase glucose transport (diffusion).

12. **Answer b:**
    A decrease in blood volume stimulates ADH secretion via cardiopulmonary mechanoreceptors (vagal afferents).

    a: An increase in blood pressure will suppress ADH secretion via the baroreceptors.
    c: A decrease in plasma osmolality will inhibit ADH secretion via the osmoreceptors.
    d: An increase in extracellular fluid volume will inhibit ADH secretion via cardiopulmonary mechanoreceptors (vagal afferents).
    e: A decrease in plasma K^+ concentration will have little or no effect on ADH secretion.

13. **Answer d:**
    Stimulation of the myenteric plexus increases velocity of the peristaltic waves.

    a: Stimulation of the myenteric plexus increases tone of the intestinal wall and increases the velocity of peristaltic waves.
    b: Stimulation of the myenteric plexus increases the strength of rhythmic contractions of the intestinal wall and increases the velocity of peristaltic waves.
    c: Stimulation of the myenteric plexus increases the rate of rhythmic contractions of the gut wall and increases the velocity of peristaltic waves.
    e: Stimulation of the myenteric plexus inhibits contraction of sphincters and increases velocity of peristaltic waves.

14. **Answer d:**

    Phenytoin induces the enzymes metabolizing dig-itoxin, thus increases its metabolism.

    a: Chloramphenicol inhibits the metabolism of tol-butamide.
    b: Disulfram inhibits the metabolism of ethanol.
    c: Isoniazid inhibits the metabolism of coumarin.
    e: Cimetidine inhibits the metabolism of diazepam.

15. **Answer b:**

    Mycoplasma pneumoniae is usually acquired by in-halation of aerosolized droplets.

    a: There is no evidence that *Mycoplasma pneumoniae* is transmitted by an arthropod vector.
    c: *Mycoplasma pneumoniae* is not acquired by aspira-tion of contaminated food.
    d: *Mycoplasma pneumoniae* infection is not acquired by inoculation through a break in the skin.
    e: There is no evidence to suggest that *Mycoplasma pneumoniae* infection occurs as a result of im-munocompromising an individual by drug ther-apy.

16. **Answer a:**

    The abducens nucleus is a nucleus of the general somatic efferent type.

    b: The abducens nucleus is not a general visceral af-ferent nucleus.
    c: The abducens nucleus is not a special somatic af-ferent nucleus.
    d: The abducens nucleus is not a special visceral ef-ferent nucleus.
    e: The abducens nucleus is not a general visceral ef-ferent nucleus.

17. **Answer b:**

    When the ventricle begins to contract, increasing ventricular pressure causes the atrioventricular valves to close.

    a: The second heart sound is caused by the closing of the aortic and pulmonic valves at the end of ventricular ejection.
    c: The second heart sound is caused by the closing of the aortic and pulmonic valves at the end of ventricular ejection.
    d: The first heart sound occurs at the beginning of systole.
    e: The first heart sound occurs at the beginning of systole.

18. **Answer a:**

    Pseudomonas cepacia is a common respiratory pathogen in individuals with cystic fibrosis.

    b: *Pseudomonas maltophilia* is not commonly found in patients with cystic fibrosis.
    c: *Pseudomonas pseudomallei* is not commonly found in patients with cystic fibrosis.
    d: *Moraxella catarrhalis* is a common cause of bron-chitis, sinusitis, and otitis.
    e: *Acinetobacter calcoaceticus* is an opportunistic pathogen most commonly associated with noso-comial respiratory infections.

19. **Answer b:**

    This patient probably has had a hemisection of the spinal cord at T12 on the left side (Brown-Séquard's syndrome). This would interrupt the first order axons in the dorsal columns on the left side leading to loss of fine tactile discrimination, vibration sense, and conscious proprioception. The lesion would also interrupt the ascending crossed fibers of the spinothalamic system leading to loss of pain and temperature on the right side. The motor tracts would also be affected leading to the spastic hemiparesis, hyperreflexia, and Babinski sign on the left side. Other symptoms, which could have been mentioned in the stem, include: (1) total loss of all sensation of T12 due to destruction of the dorsal root at its entrance at the level of the lesion and (2) hypotonic paralysis and muscle atrophy at the level of the lesion due to loss of alpha motor neurons and their exiting axons.

    a: An anterior spinal artery infarct might destroy both lateral corticospinal tracts and both spinothalamic tracts leading to bilateral symp-toms. However, the dorsal columns would be spared with no loss of fine tactile discrimination, vibration sense, and conscious proprioception.
    c: A left posterior inferior cerebellar artery infarct may interrupt fiber tracts in the inferior cerebellar peduncle and may get the pain and temperature fibers. However, it would fail to interrupt the fine touch and conscious proprioceptive fibers, which would now have decussated and be in the right medial lemniscus. Similarly, this lesion would not interrupt the as yet undecussated motor axons in the pyramids.
    d: A right posterior artery infarct would interrupt the fine touch and conscious proprioceptive fibers in the right fasciculus gracilis and cuneatus. How-ever, the motor tracts in the right lateral and ven-tral funiculi would be spared as well as the axons in the anterolateral system below the level of the lesion.
    e: A right vertebral artery lesion would interrupt ax-ons in the right pyramid and medial lemniscus but would spare the pain and temperature fibers in the anterolateral system.

20. **Answer e:**

Barrett's esophagus is metaplasia of the normal squamous epithelium of the esophagus in which it is replaced by columnar epithelium. It commonly becomes dysplastic. When the dysplasia is severe (high-grade), there is significant danger of malignant transformation.

    a: Esophageal strictures are not the most serious sequelae of developing Barrett's esophagus.

    b: Esophageal varices are not the most serious sequelae of developing Barrett's esophagus.

    c: Mallory-Weiss syndrome is not the most serious sequelae of developing Barrett's esophagus.

    d: Hematemesis is not the most serious sequelae of developing Barrett's esophagus.

21. **Answer c:**

Rotavirus causes a syndrome that varies from severe gastroenteritis to mild diarrhea with no CNS involvement.

    a: The temporal lobe of the brain is targeted in herpes simplex encephalitis.

    b: The anterior horn of the spinal cord and motor neurons are affected by Enterovirus infections such as poliomyelitis.

    d: The hippocampus, brain stem, ganglionic cells of pontine nuclei, and Purkinje's cells of the cerebellum are affected in rabies virus infection.

    e: Measles virus is a potential cause of viral encephalitis.

22. **Answer b:**

The yeast phase of *Histoplasma capsulatum,* a dimorphic fungus, is found predominantly in macrophages.

    a: *Coccidioides immitis* is also a dimorphic fungus, but its tissue phase is the spherule, which is not found in macrophages.

    c: *Cryptococcus neoformans* is not dimorphic; it grows only in a budding yeast in infected tissue.

    d: Mucor species have only a filamentous phase.

    e: *Aspergillus* species also are *filamentous fungi* with no yeast phase.

23. **Answer e:**

A negative feedback loop exists that causes increases in portal venous bile salt concentration to inhibit bile salt synthesis.

    a: Parasympathetic stimulation may increase bile salt secretion but has greater effects to stimulate gallbladder contraction.

    b: Sympathetic stimulation will relax the gallbladder; it does not effect bile salt synthesis.

    c: Cholecystokinin, as the name implies, stimulates gallbladder contraction.

    d: Motilin is released from the intestinal mucosa; it stimulates gallbladder contraction.

24. **Answer a:**

Babinski's sign is a sign of an upper motor neuron (UMN) lesion. Diabetes mellitus is associated with lower motor neuron (LMN) neuropathy.

    b: Decreased deep tendon reflexes is one sign of LMN disease.

    c: Decreased muscle tone is one sign of LMN disease.

    d: Fasciculations in denervated muscles is one sign of LMN disease.

    e: Muscle atrophy is one sign of LMN disease.

25. **Answer a:**

Obesity is believed to contribute to the development of maturity onset diabetes by contributing to insulin resistance.

    b: Although juvenile diabetes (Type I) is characterized by low or absent insulin release, Type II diabetes is characterized by normal or even high levels of insulin, coupled with insulin resistance.

    c: Ketoacidosis is only present in Type I diabetes, where the absence of insulin permits fat mobilization and oxidation to continue unabated. The normal circulating insulin levels in Type II diabetes are sufficient to suppress the development of ketoacidosis.

    d: While glycosylation, or chemical modification by covalent attachment of glucose, contributes to microvascular damage, cataracts are due to increased production in the lens of sorbitol from glucose. Tissues, such as lens, retina, and kidney, which have low levels of the enzyme sorbitol dehydrogenase, are vulnerable to sorbitol accumulation. This causes damaging osmotic effects due to cell swelling.

    e: Patients with poorly controlled diabetes demonstrate a marked *increase* in blood levels of hemoglobin A_{1C}, which is produced by covalent attachment of glucose.

26. **Answer b:**

   The middle cardiac vein lies in the posterior interventricular groove with the posterior interventricular artery.

   a: The great cardiac vein accompanies the anterior interventricular or left anterior descending artery (LAD) in the anterior interventricular groove.
   c: The small cardiac vein accompanies the marginal branch of the right coronary artery within the atrioventricular groove.
   d: The anterior cardiac veins enter the right atrium directly and do not accompany any of the major branches of the coronary arteries.
   e: The coronary sinus lies in the atrioventricular groove on the diaphragmatic surface of the heart.

27. **Answer c:**

   By increasing the slope of the pacemaker potential, the time to reach threshold is decreased, thus increasing heart rate.

   a: Increased sympathetic activity increases heart rate and decreases the duration of systole.
   b: Increased sympathetic activity is a vasoconstrictor in most tissues.
   d: Increased sympathetic nervous activity increases ventricular contractility.
   e: Hyperpolarization of the pacemaker would decrease heart rate.

28. **Answer e:**

   Patients with pernicious anemia have the obvious characteristics of a macrocytic anemia (MCV 102). Because of the profound destruction of red cells within the marrow, the LDH may rise to spectacular values. With the history given, some degree of iron deficiency could be present but could not be verified from the information given. Folate deficiency would also be a possibility but was not one of the choices given.

29. **Answer e:**

   Bacteremia is uncommon in *Shigella* infections.

   a: *Shigella* infection is usually associated with fecal-oral transmission.
   b: *Shigella* has no lower animal reservoirs.
   c: *Shigella* does invade the intestinal mucosa.
   d: *Shigella* often causes a watery diarrhea without blood or mucus.

30. **Answer c:**

   Intrinsic factor, which avidly binds vitamin B_{12} so that it can be absorbed, is secreted by parietal cells.

   a: Enteroendocrine cells do secrete somatostatin.
   b: Enteroendocrine cells do secrete gastrin.
   d: Enteroendocrine cells do secrete secretin.
   e: Enteroendocrine cells do secrete cholecystokinin.

31. **Answer a:**

   Total lung capacity is not changed by obstructive disorders. Instead, obstruction of the airways decreases indicators of air flow.

   b: FVC is the maximal volume that can be forcibly exhaled after inhaling to total lung capacity. FVC and other measures of airway obstruction are reduced in emphysema.
   c: FEV_1 is the maximal volume of air exhaled in 1 second. FEF_1 and other measures of airway obstruction are reduced in emphysema.
   d: $FEV_1/FVC\%$ and other measures of airway obstruction are reduced in emphysema.
   e: $FEF_{25\text{-}75}$ is the maximal mid expiration flow rate. Forced vital capacity, $FEF_{25\text{-}75}$, and other measures of airway obstruction are reduced in emphysema:

32. **Answer d:**

   Insulin acts to increase or preserve storage forms of metabolic fuels.

   a: Injection of insulin causes hypoglycemia by stimulating insulin uptake by muscle and adipose tissue.
   b: Insulin increases synthesis of lipids, glycogen, and protein.
   c: Insulin directs metabolic pathways toward glycogenesis.
   e: Insulin directs metabolism toward lipid synthesis, not lipolysis.

33. **Answer a:**

   The ducts of the bulbourethral glands exit the deep perineal space and enter the initial portion of the spongy urethra.

   b: The bulbourethral glands are located within the deep perineal space.
   c: Fibers of the sphincter urethrae muscle surround the bulbourethral glands within the deep perineal space.

d: The bulbourethral glands of the male are homologous with the greater vestibular glands of the female.

e: The ducts of the bulbourethral glands pierce membrane as they exit the deep perineal space.

34. **Answer b:**

Alpha$_1$ agonists increase blood pressure, decrease heart rate (baroreflex), and produce mydriasis.

a: Systemic administration of an alpha$_1$ agonist would not produce hypotension.

c: Systemic administration of an alpha$_1$ agonist would not produce an increase in blood flow to the skeletal muscles.

d: Systemic administration of an alpha$_1$ agonist would not produce tachycardia.

e: Systemic administration of an alpha$_1$ agonist would not be expected to produce an increase in GI tone nor an increase in blood flow to the kidneys.

35. **Answer a:**

Insulin inhibits glucagon secretion.

b: Hypoglycemia stimulates glucagon secretion.

c: Arginine stimulates glucagon secretion.

d: Acetylcholine stimulates glucagon secretion.

e: Catecholamine stimulates glucagon secretion.

36. **Answer a:**

Unless a myocardial infarction was to injure a heart valve in some remote fashion, it would not be expected to increase the likelihood of developing bacterial endocarditis. The other factors mentioned either scar the valves, resulting in potential sites of infection, or introduce large numbers of pathogenic organisms into the blood.

b: Mitral valve prolapse can scar the valves, resulting in potential sites of infection.

c: Congenital heart disease can scar the valves, resulting in potential sites of infection.

d: Rheumatic valvulitis can scar the valves, resulting in potential sites of infection.

e: Intravenous drug use can introduce large numbers of pathogenic organisms into the blood.

37. **Answer d:**

Stability of the glenohumeral joint is largely the result of the arrangement of tendons of the "rotator cuff" muscles, i.e., supraspinatus, infraspinatus, subscapularis, and teres minor.

a: Although the cartilaginous glenoid labrum is attached to the margin of the glenoid fossa, it contributes little in terms of stability of the joint.

b: Although fibers of the deltoid lie anterior, superior, and posterior to the joint, they contribute little to the stability of the joint.

c: The size and shape of the articular surfaces are well suited for a large range of motion, however, they do not contribute to the stability of the joint.

e: The short head of the biceps brachii muscle is attached proximally to the coronoid process of the scapula and does not contribute to the stability of the glenohumeral joint.

38. **Answer d:**

An increase in tubular reabsorption of Ca^{2+} is a major renal effect of PTH.

a: PTH stimulates formation of 1,25 dihydroxyvitamin D3.

b: PTH inhibits proximal tubular reabsorption of phosphate.

c: Ca^{2+} is not secreted by the kidneys.

e: Phosphate is not secreted by the kidneys.

39. **Answer d:**

The fornix connects the hippocampus with the septal area.

a: The arcuate fasciculus is a major association bundle into the temporal lobe.

b: The dorsal longitudinal fasciculus is mylinated fibers reciprocally connecting the periventricular zone of the hypothalamus and the ventral part of periaqueductal gray.

c: The fasciculus retroflexus is fibers arising in the habenula and passing ventrally to the interpeduncular nucleus of the midbrain and the adjacent reticular formation.

e: The stria medulloris thalami is fibers connecting the septal region to the habenular nuclei.

40. **Answer d:**

T-cell mediated immunity is one of the two major causes of granulomatous inflammation and is the cause associated with infection by mycobacteria or fungi. Another cause is the presence of poorly digestible irritants such as foreign bodies or, on occasion, accumulation of abnormal cellular products.

a: IgM is usually formed in response to an initial exposure to an antigen and is more typical of viral or bacterial infections.

b: IgG is produced in response to acute infections or during an amnestic response.

c: A fall in complement is not associated with typical granulomatous infections. It is more typically seen in massive bacterial infections or inflammatory conditions.

e: An abscess is the hallmark of acute inflammation and is typically the result of the action of neutrophils rather than macrophages.

41. **Answer d:**

Praziquantel is the drug of choice in schistosomiasis.

a: True. Mebendazole is a broad spectrum anthelmintic and is the drug of choice for infections due to ascaris, enterobius (pinworm), or hookworms (necator and ancylostoma).

b: True. Praziquantel is the drug of choice for the treatment of tapeworm infections.

c: True. Pyrantel pamoate is used for the treatment of pinworm (enterobiasis).

e: True. Metronidazole is effective for the treatment of trichomonas and giardia infections.

42. **Answer c:**

Brain acetylcholine is not higher in brains from Alzheimer's patients compared to brains from healthy patients. Alzheimer's disease is correlated with a loss of cholinergic neurons, particularly in the nucleus basalis of Meynert.

a: True. There is generalized cortical neuronal loss.

b: True. Neuronal loss is prominent in the nucleus basilis of Meynert.

d: True. Neurofibrillary tangles are prominent.

e: True. Granulovacuolar degeneration occurs.

43. **Answer d:**

TXA_2, thromboxane A_2, is a product of arachidonic acid metabolism produced by platelets as well as monocytes and macrophages. It is a strong vasoconstrictor and also functions to cause the second wave of platelet aggregation.

a: PGL_2 is a strong vasodilator and bronchodilator. It also functions to inhibit inflammatory cell function.

b: PDG_2 is a strong vasodilator, which also can cause bronchodilitation and inhibition of inflammatory cell function.

c: PGF_2 is a vasodilator but causes bronchoconstriction.

e: LTB_4 is a chemotactic that attracts phagocytic cells. It also functions to stimulate adherence of phagocytic cells, as well as to increase vascular permeability.

44. **Answer d:**

A noncompetitive inhibitor will slow the enzyme due to competition for the active site, but sufficient concentrations of substrate will outcompete the inhibitor, allowing saturation with substrate that is by definition the V_{max}.

a: A change in pH has the potential to alter the charge distribution within the active site with dramatic effects on the catalytic properties of the enzyme.

b: An increase in temperature above the optimum will slow the reaction rate, due to denaturation of the enzyme.

c: A noncompetitive inhibitor will directly affect the V_{max} by reducing the number of active enzyme molecules available.

e: Increased ionic strength can affect the V_{max} by causing denaturation of the enzyme due to binding water in hydration shells and thus reducing the hydration of the enzyme.

45. **Answer e:**

The cornea only has free nerve endings, which transmit pain information. Thus, the spinal nucleus of nerve V would be the nucleus in which these axons would synapse.

a: The chief sensory nucleus of nerve V transmits information about fine tactile discrimination and vibratory sense.

b: The facial nucleus is involved in the corneal reflex, but it provides the motor component of this reflex.

c: The mesencephalic nucleus of nerve V transmits unconscious proprioceptive information. This type of information is not carried by these axons.

d: Nucleus solitarius is not involved in sensory information from the cornea.

46. **Answer e:**

90% of CO_2 is carried as HCO_3^- formed from CO_2 diffusing into the red blood cells, 5% is carried as carbamino compounds, and 5% as dissolved CO_2.

47. **Answer c:**

Spike potentials occur when slow waves depolarize below (become less negative than) -40 millivolts.

a: Slow Ca^{2+} channels are responsible for mediating intestinal smooth muscle action potentials, whereas fast Na^+ channels are responsible for neuronal action potentials.

   b: Ca^{2+} and calmodulin mediate the combination of actin and myosin for contraction in smooth muscle.

   d: Intestinal spike potentials last about 10 to 40 times longer than action potentials in nerve fibers.

   e: Spike potentials initiate contraction in intestinal smooth muscle.

48. **Answer b:**

Most of the axons from the nucleus gracilis will cross as internal arcuate fibers, travel in the medial lemniscus, and terminate in the contralateral VPL nucleus, which receives somatic sensation from the body.

   a: The VA nucleus receives motor information.

   c: The ipsilateral postcentral gyrus is the wrong answer for two reasons. The axons decussate after leaving the nucleus gracilis and terminate in the VPL nucleus. Axons originating in the VPL nucleus then terminate on neurons in the postcentral gyrus.

   d: Since the axons crossed in the medulla, they would not terminate on the ipsilateral side. Also, since the information carried by these axons related to information gathered in the legs and trunk, it would not be sent to VPM, which receives information regarding somatic sensation from the face.

   e: VL receives most of its information from the basal ganglia and cerebellum.

49. **Answer e:**

The tendon of the teres minor muscle attaches most inferiorly on the greater tubercle of the humerus.

   a: The tendon of the supraspinatus muscle attaches most superiorly on the greater tubercle of the humerus.

   b: The tendon of the infraspinatus muscle attaches between that of the supraspinatus and teres minor muscles on the greater tubercle of the humerus.

   c: The tendon of the subscapularis muscle attaches to the lesser tubercle of the humerus.

   d: The tendon of the teres major muscle attaches to the medial lip of the intertubercular groove of the humerus.

50. **Answer e:**

Chromophobe adenomas of the adenohypophysis generally secrete prolactin or are apparently hormonally inactive.

   a: Adrenal cortical adenoma is associated with Cushing's syndrome.

   b: Corticotrope hyperplasia of the adenohypophysis is associated with Cushing's syndrome.

   c: Diffuse adrenal hyperplasia is associated with Cushing's syndrome.

   d: Exogenous corticosteroids are associated with Cushing's syndrome.

51. **Answer c:**

Aspirin inhibits the cyclooxygenase enzyme, and thus interferes with thromboxane production.

   a: Ranitidine does not activate the fibrinolytic system.

   b: There is no such disease as late onset hemophilia.

   d: Ranitidine rarely shows any hematologic toxicity.

   e: Antacids do not induce vitamin K deficiency (vitamin K is rather lipophilic).

52. **Answer c:**

Cyclophosphamide has to be bioactivated; the cyclic phosphamide ring must be opened before the active group of molecules can ionize and alkylate.

   a: Doxorubicin is metabolized by the liver.

   b: Bleomycin is fully active.

   d: L-asparaginase is an enzyme.

   e: Methotrexate is not metabolized in the body.

53. **Answer d:**

Methyrapone inhibits 11-hydroxylation, interfering with cortisol and corticosterone synthesis, therefore it indirectly increases ACTH release.

   a: Cortisone inhibits ACTH release as a feedback mechanism.

   b: Reserpine inhibits the release of ACTH by interfering with the regulatory mechanisms of the release.

   c: Morphine inhibits the release of ACTH by interfering with the regulatory mechanisms of the release.

   e: Chlorpromazine inhibits the release of ACTH by interfering with the regulatory mechanisms of the release.

54. **Answer a:**
    The lower the dose that evokes an effect, the greater the potency. Drug X is the most potent.

    b: Drug Y is less potent than drug X.
    c: Drug Z is the least potent.
    d: The potency of drug X is definitely higher than that of drug Z.

55. **Answer d:**
    Efficacy reflects the limit of the dose-response relation on the response axis. Drugs X and Z are similar because they can elicit the same maximum response.

    a: The efficacy of drugs X and Z are similar.
    b: The efficacy of drugs X and Z are similar.
    c: The efficacy of drug Y is definitely less than that of drugs X and Z.

56. **Answer c:**
    The primase that initiates DNA synthesis by making a short (9-10bp) RNA primer is a DNA-directed RNA polymerase.

    a: Chain growth is continuous on the leading strand only. It is discontinuous during synthesis of the lagging strand.
    b: DNA synthesis proceeds bidirectionally from the point of origin.
    d: Chain growth always occurs at the 3′ end in the synthesis of DNA (and RNA).
    e: Nuclease activity is exhibited in proofreading by both DNA polymerases I and III, not DNA ligase.

57. **Answer b:**
    Thalamic pain is not related to activation of nociceptors.

    a: Excitation of nociceptors does not lead to thalamic pain.
    c: Thalamic pain is not an example of referred pain.
    d: There is no such thing as subliminal pain.
    e: Visceral pain originates in the viscera.

58. **Answer c:**
    Transient exposure to the tick vector is unlikely to result in transmission of *Borrelia burgdorferi*. Usually 24 to 48 hours of attachment by the tick is required.

    a: Isolation of the causative organism is sufficient to make a diagnosis of Lyme disease.
    b: Demonstration of diagnostic levels of either IgG or IgM are also sufficient tò make a diagnosis of Lyme disease.

    d: A significant rise in antibody titer between acute and convalescent sera is sufficient to confirm Lyme disease.
    e: Erythema migrans $\geq$ cm at the site of a tick bite from the known vector is sufficient to confirm Lyme borreliosis.

59. **Answer c:**
    Syphilis is not associated with a toxemia.

    a: Diphtheria is associated with a potent exotoxin.
    b: Whooping cough is associated with pertussis toxin.
    d: Scarlet fever is associated with an exotoxin.
    e: Plague is associated with both an exotoxin and an endotoxin.

60. **Answer d:**
    Arnold-Chiari malformation (Chiari type II malformation) is a malformation associated with a small posterior fossa. The vermis of the cerebellum is present and extends through the foramen magnum. These patients generally have hydrocephalus and a lumbar meningomyelocele, as well as the posterior fossa malformation. Other associated abnormalities include cerebral heterotopias, downward displacement of the medulla, and a malformed tectum.

    a: Arnold-Chiari malformation is associated with a large, not a small, posterior fossa.
    b: In Arnold-Chiari malformation the cerebellum is present and extends through the foramen magnum.
    c: A midline ependymal-lined cyst is not associated with Arnold-Chiari malformation.
    e: A cervical syrint is not associated with Arnold-Chiari malformation.

61. **Answer e:**
    Any of the smooth muscle tumors may be submucosal, intramural, or subserosal. The other characteristics mentioned provide clues to the nature of the lesion. The two most important criteria are the mitotic count and cellular atypia.

    a: The extent of the necrosis can be used to distinguish leiomyosarcoma from leiomyoma.
    b: Cellular atypia is one of the most important criteria for distinguishing leiomyosarcoma from leiomyoma.

c: Mitotic count is one of the most important criteria for distinguishing leiomyosarcoma from leiomyoma.

d: Extension into the surrounding myometrium can be used to distinguish leiomyosarcoma from leiomyoma.

62. **Answer d:**

The posterior hypothalamus is the heat generating center. Stimulation of this area leads to shivering, vasoconstriction, and an increased metabolic rate; it does not lead to sweating.

a: An increased basal metabolic rate would accompany stimulation of the heat generating center.

b: Stimulation of this area would cause shivering, and the person would seek out warm clothing.

c: Shivering occurs when the posterior hypothalamus is stimulated.

e: Vasoconstriction would occur as the person tries to conserve heat.

63. **Answer d:**

Labetalol blocks both alpha-1 and beta receptors.

a: Metoprolol is a beta$_1$ selective blocker.

b: Clonidine is an alpha$_2$ agonist.

c: Butoxamine is a beta$_2$ antagonist.

e: Pindolol is a nonselective beta antagonist with partial beta-agonist properties.

64. **Answer d:**

Blood is coagulated in the flea and the clot is dissolved in the human.

a: Blood is not coagulated in the human and the clot is not dissolved in the flea.

b: Blood is not coagulated in the rat nor is the clot dissolved in the flea.

c: Blood is not coagulated in the rat nor is the clot dissolved in the human.

e: Blood is not coagulated in the human nor is the clot dissolved in the rat.

65. **Answer c:**

Hydrophobic bonding is actually not true chemical bonding but is instead the result of hydrophobic side chains being "repelled away" from the aqueous environment toward the interior of the protein.

a: Electrostatic bonding is important in holding monomers together in forming quaternary structure.

b: Hydrogen bonding is important in maintaining the regular structure of alpha helices and beta structure.

d: Disulfide bonds help to stabilize tertiary structure in some proteins, but stable tertiary structure can be maintained without them.

e: Peptide bonds stabilize the primary structure (linear sequence of amino acids) of protcins.

66. **Answer c:**

As salivary flow increases, HCO_3^- concentration increases due to secretion of HCO_3^- into the saliva.

a: Secretion of HCO_3^- alkalinizes saliva.

b: Osmolality increases as saliva flow increases, although it always remains below plasma osmolality.

d: Amylase concentration remains constant or increases, as water is not added to saliva in the ducts.

e: K^+ concentration remains approximately constant during increased flow.

67. **Answer e:**

The anterior surface of the lens is lined with simple cuboidal or squamous epithelium.

a: The external auditory meatus is lined with stratified squamous keratinized epithelium.

b: Corneal epithelium is lined with stratified squamous, nonkeratinized epithelium.

c: The ventral surface of the tongue is lined with stratified squamous nonkeratinized or parakeratinized epithelium.

d: The lip is lined with stratified squamous, keratinized epithelium.

68. **Answer a:**

Sodium fluoride does not bind to BAL.

b: Mercury ions bind to BAL.

c: Arsenic ions bind to BAL.

d: Copper binds to BAL.

e: Antimony binds to BAL.

69. **Answer c:**

Opening of fast Na^+ channels allows the entry of Na^+, which is driven by electrical and concentration gradients, thereby depolarizing the membrane.

a: K^+ would leave the cell more rapidly along its concentration gradient, hyperpolarizing the membrane.

b: Cl^- would enter the cell, hyperpolarizing the membrane.

d: A decrease in Na^+ permeability will limit entry of a cation and have a hyperpolarizing effect.

e: Similar to the previous rationale, the concentration and electrical gradients favor diffusion of Ca^{2+} into the cell.

70. **Answer d:**

The globus pallidus cannot be seen looking at the cut surface of a midsagittal section of the brain.

a: The anterior commissure can be seen.
b: The corpus callosum can be seen.
c: The fornix can be seen.
e: The lamina terminalis can be seen.

71. **Answer c:**

The most important individual variable in malignant melanoma of the skin is the depth of invasion of the tumor. The potential for survival can be predicted from careful measurement of the thickness of the tumor.

<0.76 mm	93% 8-year survival
0.76-1.69 mm	86% 8-year survival
1.7-3.6 mm	60% 8-year survival
>3.6 mm	33% 8-year survival

The other factors mentioned are also predictors but not so in linear a fashion.

72. **Answer d:**

Depending on the gene involved, enhancers can be either upstream or downstream.

a: Enhancers can be effective when they are 1000 base pairs away from the promoter.
b: Actively regulated genes require an AT-rich sequence, known as the TATA box, presumably to facilitate local melting of the DNA for efficient binding of RNA polymerase.
c: In contrast to other locations in the genome, CG islands, which are repetitive sequences of several thousand (CG)n pairs, are unmethylated in the upstream region of housekeeping genes.
e: Enhancers act by stimulating the initiation of transcription in genes.

73. **Answer e:**

The fibers of the corona radiata converge to form the internal capsule.

a: The anterior commissure connects the two temporal lobes and some axons of one olfactory bulb with the contralateral bulb.
b: The corpus callosum connects the two cerebral hemispheres.

c: The external medullary lamina is in the thalamus.
d: The fornix is the tract connecting the hippocampus with the mammillary bodies.

74. **Answer c:**

Resistance = pressure/flow. Pulmonary resistance is least because the lungs receive the entire cardiac output, and peak systolic pulmonary pressure is about $\frac{1}{5}$ of peak aortic systolic pressure.

a: Resistance = pressure/flow. Pulmonary resistance is less: the lungs receive the entire cardiac output at a mean pulmonary arterial pressure of about 10 mm Hg, and the brain receives 15% of cardiac output at a mean arterial pressure of about 100 mm Hg.
b: Resistance = pressure/flow. Pulmonary resistance is less: the lungs receive the entire cardiac output at a mean pulmonary arterial pressure of about 10 mm Hg, and the heart receives 5% of cardiac output at a mean arterial pressure of 100 mm Hg.
d: Resistance = pressure/flow. Pulmonary resistance is less: the lungs receive the entire cardiac output at a mean pulmonary arterial pressure of about 10 mm Hg, and the liver receives 15% of cardiac output, about $\frac{1}{4}$ of which is delivered by the hepatic artery, at a mean arterial pressure of 100 mm Hg.
e: Resistance = pressure/flow. Pulmonary resistance is less: the lungs receive the entire cardiac output at a mean pulmonary arterial pressure of about 10 mm Hg, and the kidneys receive 25% of cardiac output at a mean arterial pressure of 100 mm Hg.

75. **Answer c:**

Coronary vasodilation is a beta-adrenergic effect.

a: Most vasoconstrictive responses are alpha-adrenergic.
b: Sweating is an alpha-adrenergic effect.
d: Contraction of the radial muscle leading to pupillary dilation is a sympathetic alpha-adrenergic effect.
e: Glycogenolysis in the heart is alpha-adrenergic, although in liver and muscle it may also be beta-adrenergic.

76. **Answer a:**

Fatty acid release from adipose tissues is mediated by beta-receptors; isoproterenol is a potent stimulant.

b: Methoxamine is an alpha$_1$ simulant.
c: Dopamine has agonistic effect on the beta receptor, however it is much weaker than isoproterenol.

d: Phenylephrine is an alpha receptor agonist.

e: Oxymetazoline is an alpha$_1$ stimulant.

77. **Answer d:**

Mesosomes act as attachment sites for the replicating bacterial chromosome.

a: Mesosomes are not attachment sites for flagella.

b: Mesosomes are not involved in endospore formation.

c: Mesosomes are not known to be receptors for chemotactic stimuli.

e: Mesosomes are not attachment sites for fimbriae.

78. **Answer c:**

Contraction of the right gluteus medius and minimum muscles permit the left lower limb to clear the ground during the swing phase of walking.

a: Gluteus maximus is a powerful extensor of the thigh but does not play a major role in hip stabilization during the swing phase of walking.

b: The semitendinosus is an extensor of the thigh and flexor of the left at the knee but does not stabilize the hip during walking.

d: The biceps femoris muscle flexes the leg and extends the thigh but does not stabilize the hip during walking.

e: Obturator externus helps maintain contact between the acetabulum and femoral head. It also rotates the thigh laterally. It does not play a major role in stabilization of the hip during the swing phase of walking.

79. **Answer d:**

As $\dot{V}_A/\dot{Q}$ increases, alveolar P_{CO_2} decreases and P_{O_2} increases, so that alveolar gas tends to resemble inspired air.

a: As $\dot{V}_A/\dot{Q}$ increases, the composition of alveolar gas becomes less like mixed venous blood and more like inspired air.

b: As $\dot{V}_A/\dot{Q}$ increases, the composition of alveolar gas becomes less like systemic capillary blood and more like inspired air.

c: As $\dot{V}_A/\dot{Q}$ increases, the composition of alveolar gas becomes less like systemic arterial blood and more like inspired air.

e: As $\dot{V}_A/\dot{Q}$ increases, the composition of alveolar gas becomes less like pulmonary arterial blood (which is equivalent to mixed venous blood) and more like inspired air.

80. **Answer e:**

G-6-PD introduces the pentose phosphate shunt and mediates the reduction of NADP, which plays an important role in the reduction of methemoglobin. Lack of methemoglobin reduction leads to hemolysis.

a: Pseudocholinesterase has no effect on the reduction of methemoglobin.

b: Cytochrome P-450 2B1 has no effect on the reduction of methemoglobin.

c: N-acetyltransferase has no effect on the reduction of methemoglobin.

d: Alcohol dehydrogenase has no effect on the reduction of methemoglobin.

81. **Answer b:**

Labetalol (the mixture of isomers of two optically active centers) has specific alpha-1 antagonist, nonspecific beta-antagonist, and partial beta-2 agonist activity. Therefore it may be used in hypertensive patients with obstructive pulmonary disease, but not to treat patients with second degree heart block.

a: Labetalol is used to treat patients with cardiac failure.

c: Labetalol is used to treat patients with peripheral vascular disease.

d: Labetalol is used to treat hypertensive patients with COPD.

e: Labetalol is used on young, physically active hypertensive patients.

82. **Answer b:**

The term macula occludens is derived from macula adherens and zonula occludens. However, there is no such structure called macula occludens.

a: Zonula occludens and tight junctions are synonymous terms that refer to a component of the junctional complex.

c: Desmosome and macula adherens are synonymous terms that refer to a component of the junctional complex.

d: Tight junctions and zonula occludens are synonymous terms that refer to a component of the junctional complex.

e: Macula adherens and desmosome are synonymous terms that refer to a component of the junctional complex.

83. **Answer b:**
Loop diuretics are the most effective, followed by the thiazide diuretics. The potassium-sparing diuretics are the weakest.

84. **Answer d:**
Leishmania species typically invade reticuloendothelial cells such as the macrophage where they are capable of replication and evading host immune responses.

 a: Macrophages are not involved in the life cycle of *Ascaris lumbricoides.*
 b: Schistosomes can evade the immune response by coating themselves with substances that the host recognizes as self.
 c: Trypanosomes do not invade cells of the reticuoloendothelial cell system.
 e: *Toxoplasma gondii* typically form cysts in chronic infections and do not invade macrophages.

85. **Answer c:**
The stimulation of calcium absorption by osseous tissue is a function of tyrocalcitonin secreted by the parathyroid gland. The effect is to decrease (rather than increase) blood-calcium levels.

 a: PTH enhances and stimulates bone resorption.
 b: PTH reduces calcium excretion by the kidneys.
 d: PTH stimulates osteoclast activity.
 e: PTH stimulates calcium absorption by the small intestine.

86. **Answer e:**
Sustentacular cells are a component of the olfactory epithelium but not the respiratory epithelium. Sustentacular cells are also located in other specialized epithelia such as the maculae of the utricle and saccule and the cristae ampullaris.

 a: Brush cells (short microvilli) are a component of the respiratory epithelium.
 b: Basal cells (stem cells) are a component of the respiratory epithelium.
 c: Goblet cells are a component of the respiratory epithelium.
 d: Ciliated cells are a component of the respiratory epithelium.

87. **Answer a:**
Of the five glands/tissues listed, the one farthest away from the prostatic urethra is least likely to be detected early and most likely to possess a malignant tumor. The main prostatic gland is the farthest away from the prostatic urethra and therefore is most likely to possess a malignant tumor.

 b: Submucosal glands are closer to the lumen of the prostatic urethra than the main prostatic gland.
 c: Mucosal glands are closer to the lumen of the prostatic urethra than either the submucosal or main glands.
 d: The epithelial lining of the prostatic urethra is obviously closer to the lumen of the prostatic urethra than is any other choice.
 e: The epithelial lining of the prostatic utricle is close to the lumen of the prostatic urethra.

88. **Answer a:**
Plague is usually transmitted by fleas.

 b: Mites are not known to be involved in the transmission of plague.
 c: Ticks are not known to be involved in the transmission of plague.
 d: Mosquitoes are not known to transmit plague.
 e: Lice are not involved in the transmission of plague.

89. **Answer b:**
The dens forms a synovial joint with the anterior arch of the atlas.

 a: The dens articulates with the posterior aspect of the anterior arch of the atlas and as such lies within the vertebral foramen of the latter.
 c: The dens, a characteristic feature of the axis, represents the developmental fusion of the body of the atlas with the second cervical vertebra.
 d: The dens and odontoid process are synonymous with one another.
 e: Vertical fibers of the cruciform ligament extend superiorly and connect the dens with the anterior margin of the foramen magnum of the occipital bone.

90. **Answer b:**
The pudendal (Alcock's) canal is located along the lateral wall of the ischioanal fossa at the inferior margin of the obturator internus muscle.

 a: The coccygeus forms part of the pelvic diaphragm and is not associated with the pudendal canal.
 c: The pubococcygeus forms part of the pelvic diaphragm and is not associated with the pudendal canal.
 d: The iliococcygeus forms part of the pelvic diaphragm and is not associated with the pudendal canal.
 e: The piriformis exits the pelvis via the greater sciatic foramen and is not associated with the pudendal canal, which lies in the ischioanal fossa.

91. **Answer e:**

Resting tremor is seen in patients with Parkinson's disease. The tremor observed in cerebellar lesions is an intention tremor.

a: Patients with neocerebellar lesions sometimes have poor articulation of speech, and their speech seems slurred and slow.

b: Patients with neocerebellar lesions often have trouble performing rapid alternating movements.

c: Patients with cerebellar lesions often exhibit past-pointing, since they cannot arrest the muscular movement at the desired point.

d: Patients with archicerebellar lesions often exhibit nystagmus.

92. **Answer e:**

Dapsone, a sulfonamide derivative, is recommended to treat lepromatous leprosy; a combination of dapsone and rifampin will decrease the development of resistance to the drug. It also may be used to treat Pneumocystis pneumonia in AIDS cases.

a: Dapsone is not used in tuberculosis.

b: Dapsone is not used to treat leishmaniasis.

c: Dapsone is not used to treat mycotic infections.

d: Dapsone is not used to treat superficial, mycotic infections.

93. **Answer c:**

Trichophyton schoenleinii is a dermatophytic fungus, which is a common cause of tinea or ringworm.

a: *Cryptococcus neoformans* usually has a pulmonary focus, but can cause meningitis and skin and bone lesions, but not tinea.

b: *Trichosporon beigelii* is a superficial fungus that causes white piedra of the hair shaft.

d: *Sporothrix schenckii* causes sporotrichosis, a disease usually acquired by traumatic implantation of the organism into deeper layers of the skin.

e: *Candida albicans* is an opportunistic fungus that can cause skin infections (not tinea) or more systemic manifestations.

94. **Answer c:**

$t\frac{1}{2}$ 0.693 . V/CL

CL 0.693 . V/t½

CL 0.693 . 70 L/6 hr = 0.693 . 7000 ml/360 min = 134.7 ml/min

95. **Answer b:**

Clozapine may cause agranulocytosis in up to 3% of patients.

a: Carbamazepine is a tricyclic compound marketed for trigeminal neuralgia, but it is useful in epilepsy as well.

c: Meperidine is a synthetic opioid.

d: Maprotiline is a heterocyclic antidepressant.

e: Trazodone is a heterocyclic antidepressant.

96. **Answer e:**

The phrenic nerves arise from spinal cord segments C3, C4, and C5.

a: Sensory innervation of the mediastinal pleura and central portion of the diaphragmatic pleura is provided by branches of the phrenic nerves.

b: The phrenic nerves are in contact with mediastinal pleura as they traverse the superior mediastinum.

c: The phrenic nerves provide motor innervation to the diaphragm and sensory innervation to the mediastinal and the central region of the diaphragmatic pleura.

d: The phrenic nerves lie on the anterior scalene muscles in the neck and pass through the thoracic inlet to enter the superior mediastinum.

97. **Answer e:**

Because ATP is used in GMP synthesis and GTP is used in AMP synthesis, if the amount of either is limiting, the synthesis of the other is correspondingly lowered. In addition, AMP and GMP directly regulate through feedback their own synthesis to maintain appropriate cellular levels.

a: Thymidine is never combined directly with PRPP. DeoxyUMP is first produced from UMP. This is followed by methylation with thymidylate synthetase using the folate cofactor, N^5, N^{10}-methylene tetrahydrofolate.

b: The *de novo* synthesis of purines is also inhibited by methotrexate at the two steps that use formyl-tetrahydrofolate.

c: The ring structures of purines are assembled attached to PRPP, such that each intermediate could be considered a PRPP derivative. The pyrimidine ring structure is assembled as the intermediate orotate, which then has the PRPP moiety added to it.

d: Orotate decarboxylase catalyzes the conversion of orotate monophosphate to UMP, an unlikely location in the synthetic pathway for a committed step. The committed step, which is also regulated, is catalyzed by carbamoyl phosphate synthetase II, the first enzyme in pyrimidine biosynthesis.

98. **Answer e:**

The Hantavirus group is not transmitted by an arthropod vector (mosquito).

a: Hantaviruses can be spread to humans by aerosol.

b: Rodents are the reservoir of Hantaviruses.

c: Hemorrhagic fever is sometimes associated with Hantavirus infection.

d: Nephritis and hemorrhagic necrosis of the kidney are manifestations of Hantavirus infection.

99. **Answer e:**

Methoxamine is an alpha$_1$ agonist; it increases blood pressure, which evokes a reflex bradycardia.

a: Isoprotenol lowers blood pressure and will not produce bradycardia.

b: Terbutaline lowers blood pressure and will not produce bradycardia.

c: Phentolamine lowers blood pressure and will not produce reflex bradycardia.

d: Clonidine is an alpha$_2$ agonist and lowers blood pressure by central mechanisms. It does not produce bradycardia.

100. **Answer a:**

Patients with a tumor invading only the optic chiasm would have total loss of vision in the temporal halves of both visual fields or a bitemporal hemianopsia.

b: A contralateral hemianopsia results from a lesion in the optic tract and causes complete loss of vision in the opposite half of the visual field.

c: Scotomas are very small lesions in the visual cortex.

d: Total blindness would not result unless the tumor became very large and invaded the area of both optic nerves or both optic tracts.

e: Quadrantic lesions occur when part of the optic tract is lesioned.

101. **Answer d:**

Haemophilus ducreyi (soft chancre) causes a painful lesion.

a: A painful lesion is not associated with infection caused by *Brucella abortus*.

b: A painful lesion is not associated with infection caused by *Borrelia burgdorferi* (Lyme disease).

c: Lesions associated with infections by *Mycobacterium leprae* (leprosy) are painless.

e: Lesions (chancres) produced as a result of infection with *Treponema pallidum* are not painful.

102. **Answer c:**

In obstructive diseases, lung compliance increases due to damage to elastic tissue. In restrictive lung disease, fibrosis decreases compliance.

103. **Answer c:**

The time to reach total body equilibrium following daily administration is proportional to the drugs half-life. The longer the half-life, the longer it takes to reach equilibrium. Digitoxin has a much longer half-life.

a: True. Digitoxin is eliminated primarily by metabolic transformation in the liver.

b: True. Digitoxin is more completely absorbed from the GI tract than digoxin.

d: True. Both digoxin and digitoxin have a narrow margin of safety.

e: True. Digitoxin binds to plasma proteins more than digoxin.

104. **Answer b:**

The hypoglossal nerve is derived from axons of the hypoglossal nucleus alone.

a: The glossopharyngeal nerve derives its motor axons from nucleus ambiguus.

c: The spinoaccessory nerve derives some of its axons from nucleus ambiguus. Its motor axons, which innervate the sternocleidomastoid and trapezius muscles, come from the spinoaccessory nucleus in the anterior horn of the upper spinal cord.

d: The vagus nerve derives some of its motor axons, which innervate the muscles of the larynx and pharynx from the nucleus ambiguus.

105. **Answer a:**

Chronic obstructive lung disease leads to respiratory acidosis. The compensatory increase in plasma HCO_3^- gradually buffers the acidosis in the CSF, removing the central chemoreceptor drive, leaving only the peripheral chemoreceptors driven primarily by changes in PaO_2.

  b: The aortic body is relatively insensitive to PCO_2; the primary drive is changes in PaO_2 sensed by the carotid body.

  c: Increased plasma HCO_3^- will decrease CSF H^+ and eliminate the central chemoreceptor drive.

  d: The primary drive is via peripheral chemoreceptors responding to changes in PaO_2.

  e: The medullary chemoreceptors respond primarily to changes in CSF H^+; the primary drive in chronic obstructive lung disease is via peripheral chemoreceptors responding to changes in PaO_2.

106. **Answer d:**

With the exception of the lung, in which the capillaries are also involved, the postcapillary venule is the major site of induction of adhesion molecules on the endothelium. Rolling neutrophils bind to this and then by diapedesis move through the endothelium and into the interstitial space.

  a: The artery is involved only in being the major supply of blood to the area. No active penetration of the vessel wall would occur.

  b: Precapillary arterioles are involved mainly in increasing the amount of blood in the area of inflammation. This is accomplished dilation. Movement of leukocytes through their walls is not a typical occurrence.

  c: Except for the lungs, the capillaries are not involved significantly with the adherence or penetration of leukocytes.

  e: The larger veins simply drain blood from the area of inflammation and usually are not involved in leukocytic adhesion or penetration.

107. **Answer c:**

The urethral crest is an elevated portion of the prostatic urethra located along its posterior wall.

  a: The prostatic urethra may become obstructed in the disease known as benign prostatic hypertrophy (BPH).

  b: The most dilatable portion of the male urethra is the prostatic urethra.

  d: The openings of the ejaculatory ducts are observed lateral to the prostatic utricle on the colliculus seminalis.

  e: Openings of the prostatic ductules are observed in the prostatic sinuses, which are shallow grooves on each side of the urethral crest.

108. **Answer a:**

The PALS is composed mostly of T lymphocytes.

  b: B lymphocytes predominate in lymphoid nodules within palatine tonsils.

  c: B lymphocytes predominate in lymphoid nodules within Peyer's patches.

  d: B lymphocytes predominate in lymphoid nodules within splenic white pulp.

  e: B lymphocytes predominate in lymphoid nodules in the outer cortex of lymph nodes.

109. **Answer d:**

A net 0 charge on a protein prevents it from migrating to either electrode during electrophoresis, hence the term isoelectric.

  a: It is physically impossible for simultaneous protonation of all carboxyl groups and unprotonation of all amino groups, since the pH required in each case is on opposite sides of neutrality.

  b: A protein does not have a pK, because the pK is a property of an individual ionizable group. The isoelectric point is a result of the additive effect of the pK values for all the ionizable groups in the protein.

  c: A pH that removes all of the protons from a protein would produce a net negative charge, whereas the isoelectric point produces a net 0 charge.

  e: If all groups have a positive charge, the protein would migrate toward the cathode during electrophoresis.

110. **Answer c:**

The usual histologic appearance of Paget's disease is a "crazy quilt" appearance of the lamellar bone. The pattern is caused by prominent cement lines between irregular segments of lamellar bone.

  a: Lack of bony remodeling with a woven appearance is not a histologic characteristic of Paget's disease.

  b: Heightened osteoelastic activity with enlarged Haversian canals is not a histologic characteristic of Paget's disease.

  d: Overgrowth of cartilage is not a histologic characteristic of Paget's disease.

111. **Answer d:**
     The long thoracic nerve is at risk in this region as it lies on the surface of the serratus anterior muscle.

     a: The thoracodorsal nerve, which innervates the latissimus dorsi muscle, lies too far laterally to be at risk during this procedure.
     b: The upper subscapular nerve supplies the subscapularis muscle and lies too far superolaterally to be at risk.
     c: The lower subscapular nerve innervates the subscapularis and teres major muscles and lies too far superolaterally to be at risk.
     e: The phrenic nerve is not at risk as it enters the superior mediastinum through the thoracic inlet and comes to lie within the thoracic cavity.

112. **Answer a:**
     Primer RNA is never found in the single-stranded form.

     b: Helicase opens up the DNA helix to allow primase to begin primer synthesis.
     c: Primer RNA is synthesized by primase.
     d: The 3′-group is always a hydroxyl that can esterify with the incoming phosphate.
     e: Primer RNA, like all other RNA, contain uracil in place of thymine, unless modified after transcription is completed.

113. **Answer a:**
     Higher doses of cyanocobalamin are used at the beginning of therapy to replenish body stores.

     b: True. In the absence of a neurologic disorder, the anemia should be treated with folic acid.
     c: True. The therapeutic goal is to support hemoglobin and red cell synthesis and replete liver stores of vitamin B_{12}.
     d: True. Treatment with cyanocobalamin or hydroxocobalamin will continue for life.
     e: True. The drug of choice is cyanocobalamin because hydroxocobalamin can give rise to allergic reactions.

114. **Answer a:**
     Hearing loss is a frequent manifestation of the use of aminoglycoside antibiotics. These drugs affect the outer hair cells, resulting in bilateral auditory ototoxicity. Patients may also exhibit vestibular problems, as well as nephrotoxicity.

     b: Insomnia is not a side effect.
     c: Resting tremors result from lesions to the substantia nigra as occurs in Parkinson's disease.

     d: Seizures are not a side effect.
     e: Tardive dyskinesias are not side effects of this drug treatment.

115. **Answer d:**
     Excess secretion of ADH will lead to inappropriate retention of water. Water will distribute throughout the body fluids, lowering the osmolality of compartments.

     a: Na^+ and its accompanying anions are the major determinants of extracellular fluid osmolality, so it is unlikely that osmolality would be increased when plasma $[Na^+]$ is decreased due to excessive ADH secretion.
     b: Plasma and interstitial fluids are separated by the capillary endothelium. This endothelium offers little barrier to the osmotic equilibration of water, so only very transient differences in osmolality could occur between plasma and interstitial fluid.
     c: Excess ADH will cause retention of water and an increase in total body water.
     e: An increase in body fluid osmolality is unlikely when plasma $[Na^+]$ is decreased and ADH is present in excess.

116. **Answer c:**
     Hepatitis D virus can replicate only in hepatitis B-infected cells and infects children and adults with underlying hepatitis B virus infection.

     a: Hepatitis D virus has a single-stranded, circular, RNA genome.
     b: Hepatitis D virus is a defective satellite virus and requires a helper virus for replication.
     d: Hepatitis D virus is spread in blood, semen, and vaginal secretions.
     e: Hepatitis D virus is responsible for about 40% of fulminant hepatitis infections.

117. **Answer b:**
     In an LMN lesion of the XII nerve, the tongue deviates to the same side as the lesioned nerve because of the unopposed action on the normal genioglossus muscles on the other side.

     a: Atrophy of muscles is typical in LMN lesions.
     c: Fasciculations are typical in LMN lesions.
     d: The tongue is furrowed because of the muscle atrophy.

118. **Answer c:**

This ligament helps prevent the dens from moving posteriorly into the spinal cord or medulla.

a: The alar ligaments interconnect the atlas and occipital bone.

b: Nodding of the head is achieved via motion at the atlanto-occipital joints.

d: The transverse ligament of the atlas interconnects the lateral masses of the atlas as it passes posterior to the dens.

e: The tectorial membrane is the superior extension of the posterior longitudinal ligament of the vertebral column and lies posterior to the transverse ligament of the atlas.

119. **Answer d:**

In insulin-induced hypoglycemia, the skin is cool and moist.

a: Dizziness is a sign of insulin-induced hypoglycemia.

b: Tachycardia is a symptom of insulin-induced hypoglycemia.

c: Weakness is a symptom of insulin-induced hypoglycemia.

e: Confusion is a symptom of insulin-induced hypoglycemia.

120. **Answer d:**

Clostridium botulinum is not associated with an animal reservoir.

a: *Vibrio parahemolyticus* is usually acquired by ingestion of improperly cooked seafood.

b: *Francisella tularensis* is often found in wild animals such as squirrels and rabbits.

c: *Salmonella enteritidis* is usually associated with poultry.

e: *Yersinia pestis* is usually associated with rodents, rabbits, or prairie dogs.

121. **Answer a:**

Ironically, plasma cells are not found in blood plasma and therefore would not appear in the buffy coat, a layer that, upon centrifugation, contains circulating white cells and platelets.

b: Lymphocytes are normally found in peripheral blood and therefore would appear in the buffy coat.

c: Neutrophils are all normally found in peripheral blood and therefore would appear in buffy coat.

d: Monocytes are all normally found in peripheral blood and therefore would appear in the buffy coat.

e: Eosinophils are all normally found in peripheral blood and therefore would appear in the buffy coat.

122. **Answer c:**

The thymus possesses a cortex and a medulla but no lymphoid nodules.

a: Primary or secondary lymphoid nodules are present in Peyer's patches.

b: Primary or secondary lymphoid nodules are present in splenic white pulp.

d: Primary or secondary lymphoid nodules are present in the outer cortex of lymph nodes.

e: Primary or secondary lymphoid nodules are present in the palatine tonsils.

123. **Answer e:**

Individual podocytes comprise the visceral layer of Bowman's capsule. These cells are not in any way a component of the JG apparatus.

a: Macula densa cells are a component of the JG apparatus, which is located adjacent to the vascular pole of Bowman's capsule.

b: Juxtaglomerular cells, as the name implies, are a component of the JG apparatus.

c: Modified smooth muscle cells in the wall of the afferent arteriole are a component of the JG apparatus.

d: Extraglomerular mesangeal cells are a component of the JG apparatus.

124. **Answer d:**

Cytokeratin is an intermediate filament found in many types of epithelial cells.

a: The extracellular matrix (ground substance) of hyaline cartilage is composed, in part, of hyaluronic acid.

b: The extracellular matrix (ground substance) of hyaline cartilage is composed, in part, of keratin sulfate.

c: The extracellular matrix (ground substance) of hyaline cartilage is composed, in part, of chondroitin sulfate.

e: Type II collagen is the major kind of collagen located in the extracellular matrix of hyaline cartilage.

125. **Answer a:**

Parkinson's disease is likely to respond well to treatment with antimuscarinic agents.

b: Tardive dyskinesia does not respond well to antimuscarinic agents.
c: Acute dystonic reactions do not respond well to antimuscarinic agents.
d: A sedative antihistamine is the drug of choice.
e: Perioral tremor is not a characteristic syndrome during treatment with antipsychotic drugs.

126. **Answer b:**

The radial nerve innervates the muscles of the extensor compartment of the arm, i.e., the three heads of the triceps brachii muscle.

a: The axillary nerve supplies the deltoid and teres minor muscles of the shoulder.
c: The musculocutaneous nerve supplies the muscles of the flexor compartment of the brachium.
d: The median nerve innervates muscles of the forearm and hand.
e: The ulnar nerve innervates muscles of the forearm and hand.

127. **Answer d:**

Gestational choriocarcinoma arises from an abnormal fertilization in which a sperm fertilizes an empty ovum (lacks functional DNA). The haploid number of chromosomes (23,X) duplicates into 46,XX, but all of the chromosomes are of paternal origin. Because of this, the embryo dies quickly, before placental circulation has developed. Fetal parts will always be absent. The usual result of this is the development of a complete hydatidiform mole, but in about 2% of cases the trophoblast becomes malignant. Since the trophoblast is derived from nonmaternal genetic material, it it nonself and hence can be considered an allograft.

128. **Answer e:**

Each of the two vertebral arteries supplies a branch that fuses in the midline to form a single anterior spinal artery.

a: Anterior inferior cerebellar artery branches do not form the anterior spinal artery.
b: Basilar artery branches do not form the anterior spinal artery.
c: Internal carotid artery branches do not form the anterior spinal artery.
d: Posterior inferior cerebellar artery branches do not form the anterior spinal artery.

129. **Answer a:**

Sulfonamides reversibly inhibit dihydrofolate synthesis.

b: Tetracycline inhibits protein synthesis.
c: Amphotericin B binds to ergosterol in the fungal cell membrane.
d: Methotrexate binds to the active catalytic site of dihydrofolate reductase.
e: Amantadine inhibits the uncoating of certain myxoviruses.

130. **Answer a:**

The lateral hypothalamus is the feeding center. Stimulation in this area causes an animal to eat, and it is activated by hunger.

b: Micturition (voiding reflex) is not initiated by the lateral hypothalamus.
c: The satiety center is the ventral medial nucleus of the hypothalamus.
d: The septal area is the pleasure center.
e: Thirst is not initiated by the lateral hypothalamus.

131. **Answer e:**

Clonidine decreases vascular resistance with maintained blood flow in the kidneys; it decreases renin secretion, decreases sympathetic nerve activity (central effect), and lowers blood pressure.

a: Clonidine decreases vascular resistance and lowers renin secretion.
b: Clonidine decreases blood pressure and lowers renin secretion.
c: Clonidine decreases blood pressure and sympathetic nerve activity.
d: Clonidine decreases vascular resistance and sympathetic nerve activity.

132. **Answer e:**

Carcinoma of the stomach is separated into two groups, based on the level of invasion. Tumors that are limited to the mucosa and submucosa are termed "early gastric carcinoma," and tumors that have invaded into the muscularis and beyond are termed "advanced gastric carcinoma." In early gastric carcinoma, a 5-year survival rate of greater than 90% can be achieved even with local lymph node metastases. Advanced gastric carcinoma has a dismal prognosis with a 5-year survival rate of less than 10%.

a: Depth of invasion, rather than histologic type, is a better predictor of outcome.

b: Depth of invasion rather than the region of the stomach involved, is a better predictor of outcome.

c: Depth of invasion rather than atrophic gastritis, is a better predictor of outcome.

d: Depth of invasion rather than achlorhydria, is a better predictor of outcome.

133. **Answer e:**

L-DOPA is an intermediate precursor in the synthesis of norepinephrine and dopamine.

a: 5-HIAA is not an intermediate precursor in the synthesis of norepinephrine and dopamine.

b: Choline is involved in acetylcholine synthesis.

c: Epinephrine is not an intermediate precursor in the synthesis of norepinephrine and dopamine.

d: GABA is not an intermediate precursor in the synthesis of norepinephrine and dopamine.

134. **Answer d:**

Mycoplasma lacks a typical bacterial cell wall with peptidoglycan, and therefore, is not susceptible to penicillin.

a: *Mycoplasma* requires sterols for growth.

b: *Mycoplasma* has no cell wall.

c: *Mycoplasma* is susceptible to tetracycline.

e: *Mycoplasma* replicates by binary fission.

135. **Answer c:**

This question tests knowledge of the anatomy of a typical tooth and the structures associated with it. In order for periodontal disease to occur, food particles must first become trapped in the gingival sulcus, a space (or potential space) between the enamel and the surrounding gingiva.

a: Food present in tonsilar crypts may cause bad breath but not periodontal disease.

b: Food is tasted when dissolved particles (of food) contact taste buds in papillary crypts.

d: Dental pulp is not normally accessible to food particles and bacterial debris.

e: The periodontal ligament is not associated with filiform papillae.

136. **Answer a:**

The final components of the immunoglobulin heavy chain variable region are assembled at the DNA level.

137. **Answer d:**

Proopiomelanocortin is the source of ACTH and beta-endorphin.

a: Proenkephalin is clipped to form one copy of leuenkephalin and six copies of metenkephalin.

b: Prodynorphin is clipped to form alpha-neoendorphin, beta-neoendorphin, and dynorphins A-C.

c: Prolactin is a hormone of the anterior pituitary gland.

e: Pancreatic polypeptide cannot be clipped to make beta-endorphin.

138. **Answer e:**

TNFa causes severe injury to the endothelium. It also induces the endothelium to produce other injurious cytokines.

a: C5a is the product of the activation of a complement and not a cytokine.

b: C3b is the product of the activation of a complement and not a cytokine.

c: IL-8 is a cytokine, but it is not the major factor involved in endothelial injury.

d: Nitric oxide is not a cytokine.

139. **Answer b:**

Alveolar macrophages are cuboidal to oval-shaped as contrasted to type I pneumocytes and endothelial cells, which are squamous-shaped. Since cuboidal/oval-shaped cells are thicker than squamous-shaped cells, air tends to pass more quickly through that part of the blood-air barrier, which is composed of squamous-shaped cells.

a: The cytoplasm of type I pneumocytes is one of four components that comprise a very thin blood-air barrier.

c: The cytoplasm of endothelial cells is one of four components that comprise a very thin blood-air barrier.

d: The basal lamina of type I pneumocytes is one of four components that comprise a very thin blood-air barrier.

e: The basal lamina of endothelial cells is one of four components that comprise a very thin blood-air barrier.

140. **Answer d:**

The mesencephalic nucleus of V contains first order cell bodies transmitting proprioceptive information from the face.

a: The chief sensory nucleus is a relay nucleus for fine touch and vibratory sensation. Its axons terminate on the third order VPM nucleus in the thalamus.
b: The nucleus cuneatus is a relay nucleus for fine touch and vibratory sensation from the body. Its axons terminate on the third order VPL nucleus in the thalamus.
c: The nucleus solitarius is a second order relay nucleus for taste sensation.
e: The spinal nucleus of V is a second order relay nucleus for pain and temperature sensation from the face. Its axons terminate on the third order VPM nucleus in the thalamus.

141. **Answer b:**

In gunshot wounds of the skull, the direction of the bullet can often be determined by examining the wounds in the skull. Typically, the defect in the skull will show increasing size in the direction of the bullet's travel. In this case, the travel of the bullet was from left to right such that the outer table of the skull on the left side would show a smaller defect than the inner table and similarly, the inner table on the right side would show a smaller defect than the outer table.

c: There is no indication that the assailant was in front of the victim.
d: There is no indication that the assailant was behind the victim.
e: From this information, you can determine that the assailant was to the left of the victim.

142. **Answer a:**

The Ann Arbor Staging System is based on the extent of disease, the Roman numeral component, and the presence or absence of symptoms, (the A or B component). Symptoms to be considered are fever, night sweats, or weight loss greater than 10% of the baseline weight.

Stage	Extent	Symptoms
I-A	Involves only a single lymph node region	Absent
I-B	Involves only a single lymph node region	Present
II-A	Involves two or more lymph node regions on the same side of the diaphragm	Absent
II-B	Involves two or more lymph node regions on the same side of the diaphragm	Present
III-A	Involves lymph node regions on both sides of the diaphragm	Absent
III-B	Involves lymph node regions on both sides of the diaphragm	Present
IV-A	Diffuse or disseminated involvement of one or more extralymphatic organs	Absent
IV-B	Diffuse or disseminated involvement of one or more extralymphatic organs	Present

This patient had involvement of only a single lymph node chain on one side of the diaphragm and had no symptoms. He therefore would be placed into stage I-A.

143. **Answer b:**

Crohn's disease has no curative treatment. Surgery is used for the treatment of complications such as fistulas and obstruction, rather than to affect a cure. Medical therapy has proven to be less than completely satisfactory, although the inflammation can be reduced by corticosteroids and cytotoxic agents.

a: Crohn's disease may affect any portion of the GI tract.
c: Fistula and intestinal obstruction are frequent complications of Crohn's disease.
d: The inflammation in Crohn's disease is typically transmural and skips from place to place.
e: Submucosal granulomas are prominent in Crohn's disease.

144. **Answer b:**

The best buffering occurs 1 pH unit above or below the pK (the half neutralization point).

a: The pK of a weak acid never changes. It is defined by the equilibrium between the conjugate acid and the conjugate base.
c: A weak acid loses its buffering capacity at titration points, which are more than 2 pH units above or below half neutralization (pK).
d: A pH of 7.0 is neutral only for purposes of definition of acids and bases. Half neutralization of a weak acid will occur at its pK, which will generally vary from pH 2 to pH 12.
e: At one half neutralization, by definition, the pH is equal to the pK.

145. **Answer b:**

Rapid equilibration of CO_2 between arterial blood and CSF allows the medullary chemoreceptors to play the major role in sensing CSF H^+ and therefore $PaCO_2$.

a: Exchange of CSF HCO_3^- for arterial Cl^- is not sufficiently rapid to account for ventilatory responses to changes in $PaCO_2$

c: Diffusion of H^+ into the CSF, which occurs in metabolic acidosis, stimulates medullary (not hypothalamic) chemoreceptors to increase ventilation, but this mechanism is not as important as the effect of PCO_2 on CSF pH.

d: An increase in $PaCO_2$ will not decrease CSF PO_2.

e: A decrease in PCO_2 will increase CSF pH and decrease ventilation.

146. **Answer d:**

Unlike spliceosomes, which process precursor mRNA in the nucleus, nucleosomes have no RNA as a part of their structure.

a: All nucleosomes have the same fundamental structure and are capable of associating in a cylindrical (solenoidal) geometry to form the higher order structure of chromatin.

b: There are five histoneproteins, each of which has a highly conserved structure.

c: There are 146 base pairs that wrap around the core, with the remainder (associated with histone H1) forming the linker between the cores.

e: Repetitive DNA can constitute up to 30% of the genome but does not serve a coding function.

147. **Answer a:**

Hypertrophy. Adult cardiac myocytes are incapable of mitosis. Any increase in mass must be due to an increase in the size of individual cells rather than an increase in the number of cells.

b: Hyperplasia by definition is an increase in the number of cells in an organ or tissue.

c: Metaplasia is when one adult type of cell changes into a different type of cell. For example, tall, columnar, cervical epithelial cells can change into squamous cells.

d: Atrophy is a diminution in size and function of a cell or organ.

e: Fatty change is the accumulation of fat in cells in an abnormal amount and would not be a process in this case.

148. **Answer a:**

Age is a major prognostic factor in acute lymphoblastic leukemia. Onset in a child under 1 year of age has a poor prognosis, as does onset in children over the age of 10 and in adults. Children in the window between 1 year and 7 years of age generally respond well to chemotherapy (except for the L3 subtype), and frequently have a permanent cure.

b: B-cell subtype is not a major factor affecting prognosis.

c: T-cell subtype is not a major factor affecting prognosis.

d: Null cell subtype is not a major factor affecting prognosis.

e: The presence of lymphadenopathy is not a major factor affecting prognosis.

149. **Answer a:**

This is a transitional cell papilloma, a benign lesion of the urothelium. For a long time, there was considerable controversy in the classification of these lesions, and many pathologists considered them to be low-grade malignancies. Current thinking is that they are not malignant but do represent an unstable urothelium. They recur in about 70% of cases, but the recurrence probably represents development of a new tumor rather than a true recurrence of the original lesion. About 7% of the lesions may develop into invasive transitional cell carcinoma.

150. **Answer c:**

A phosphorylase deficiency prevents the release of glucose from glycogen, but it leaves glucose production from gluconeogenesis unaffected. However, if glucose-6-phosphatase is absent, glucose from either source will be unable to enter the blood stream.

a: Phosphorylase deficiency only blocks the availability of glucose from glycogen for glycolytic metabolism. Glycolysis otherwise is unaffected.

b: Glucagon activates both phosphorylase and glucose-6-phosphatase. Phosphorylase is activated through a cascade of kinase enzyme, but glucose-6-phosphatase is activated by activating its gene to produce more enzyme.

d: Although liver phosphorylase is allosterically inhibited by glucose-6-phosphate, this does not explain the difference in severity of the hypoglycemia.

e: Glucose cannot be formed from fatty acids, but fatty acid oxidation can provide the energy needed for glyconeogenesis.

151. **Answer a:**

Glucocorticosteroids stimulate gastric acid secretion; all the other choices are correct descriptions of glucocorticoid actions.

152. **Answer a:**

Chief cells secrete pepsinogen, not lysozyme.

b: Serous cells in the parotid gland secrete lysozyme, which causes saliva to be bactericidal.

c: Serous cells in the lacrimal gland secrete lysozyme, which gives tears their bactericidal property.

d: Serous cells in the submandibular (submaxillary) gland secrete lysozyme, which causes saliva to be bactericidal.

e: Paneth cells in the crypts of Lieberkühn (primarily in the small intestine) secrete lysozyme which confers bactericidal properties on the intestinal lumina.

153. **Answer b:**

Vibrio cholerae is motile by means of conventional flagella.

a: *Leptospira interrogans* is motile by means of axial filaments.

c: *Borrelia burgdorferi* is motile by means of axial filaments.

d: *Treponema carateum* is motile by means of axial filaments.

e: *Treponema pallidum* is motile by means of axial filaments.

154. **Answer c:**

Melatonin is synthesized and secreted by the pineal gland.

a: Somatotropin is a trophic hormone secreted by the adenohypophysis.

b: Thyrotropin is a trophic hormone secreted by the adenohypophysis.

d: Luteinizing hormone is a trophic hormone secreted by the adenohypophysis.

e: Prolactin is a trophic hormone secreted by the adenohypophysis.

155. **Answer d:**

The stria vascularis is the only vascularized epithelial tissue in mammals. It secretes endolymph.

a: "Stria choroidalis" is a nonsense term that resembles the correct one.

b: The vestibular membrane is a bilaminar epithelioid membrane that separates endolymph in the scala media from perilymph in the scala vestibuli.

c: The endolymphatic sac is a component of the membranous labyrinth where endolymph is resorbed.

e: "Pia vascularis" is a nonsense term that resembles the correct one.

156. **Answer d:**

The conus arteriosus, or infundibulum, is the smooth-walled outflow tract of the right ventricle leading to the pulmonary trunk via the pulmonic valve.

a: Papillary muscles with attached chordae tendineae are characteristic features of both ventricles.

b: Trabeculae carneae are irregular muscular folds characteristic of both ventricles.

c: Chordae tendineae provide a connection between papillary muscles and cusps of the atrioventricular valve in both ventricles.

e: The venae cordis minimae open directly into all four chambers of the heart.

157. **Answer c:**

Heating is needed to dissociate the newly duplicated DNA sequences, and cooling is needed to allow primer annealing and chain polymerization.

a: A large excess of primers, rather than an equimolar quantity, is needed to provide enough primers to hybridize with the exponentially growing population of target DNA molecules.

b: Due to the use of thermostable DNA polymerase, which survives the heating cycle, additional polymerase enzyme is not needed.

d: Only the sequences (about 20 to 30 bases) at each end of the target DNA need to be known to direct primer annealing.

e: No other enzymes are needed in addition to DNA polymerase. Helicase and primase only act as a primosome during *cellular* DNA replication.

158. **Answer c:**

The majority of the lymphocytes present in the inflammatory infiltrate are CD4$^+$ T lymphocytes. The lymphoid infiltrate often takes the form of lymphoid follicles arranged in a perivascular orientation. Large numbers of B cells, plasma cells, and varying number of macrophages are also present. A number of neutrophils may be present in the synovium, but they rarely involve the articular surface itself.

159. **Answer c:**

Tm for glucose may be calculated as the difference between the filtered load and the amount excreted, when the reabsorptive mechanism is saturated. The calculation is as follows:

Tm = (GFR) (plasma [glucose]) − (urine flow) (urine [glucose])

Tm = (120 ml/min) (100 mg/100 ml) − (0.5 ml/min) (2 mg/ml) = 119 mg/min

(Note: plasma [glucose] is often expressed per 100 ml plasma.)

a: Incorrect units; the Tm is an amount per unit time, not volume/time.

b: 1.19 mg/ml is incorrect.

d: If glucose were completely reabsorbed there would be none in the urine.

e: 50 mg/ml is incorrect.

160. **Answer c:**

The precentral gyrus is immediately rostral to the central sulcus and dorsal to the lateral fissure.

a: The angular gyrus is posterior to the central sulcus.

b: The postcentral gyrus is posterior to the central sulcus.

d: The superior temporal gyrus is inferior to the lateral fissure.

e: The supramarginal gyrus is posterior to the central sulcus.

161. **Answer a:**

The pretracheal fascia is located deep in the infrahyoid muscles.

b: Pretracheal fascia is continuous laterally with the carotid sheath on each side.

c: The pretracheal fascia splits to enclose the thyroid gland.

d: The pretracheal fascia splits to enclose the esophagus.

e: The pretracheal fascia splits to enclose the trachea.

162. **Answer e:**

Diphyllobothrium latum is the fish tapeworm.

a: *Taenia solium* is the pork tapeworm.

b: *Taenia saginata* is the beef tapeworm.

c: *Hymenolepsis nana* is the dwarf tapeworm and does not involve fish in its life cycle.

d: *Echinococcus granulosus* causes hydatid cyst disease and does not involve fish.

163. **Answer b:**

The trochlear nerve emerges from the dorsal aspect of the brainstem and innervates the superior oblique muscle.

a: The medial rectus muscle is innervated by the oculomotor nerve, which arises from the ventral aspect of the brain.

c: The lateral rectus muscle is innervated by the abducent nerve, which arises from the ventral aspect of the brain.

d: The inferior oblique is innervated by the oculomotor nerve, which arises from the ventral aspect of the brain.

e: The levator palpebrae superioris muscle is innervated by the oculomotor nerve, which arises from the ventral aspect of the brain.

164. **Answer a:**

The burst cells are located in the PPRF and MPRF and initiate and fire during the saccade. Firing stops after completion of the saccade.

b: Burst-tonic cells fire like the motor neurons.

c: Oculomotor neurons continue firing after the saccade.

d: Pause cells fire at all times, except during a saccadic eye movement. They inhibit burst cells.

e: Tonic cells fire at a steady rate during fixation.

165. **Answer d:**

Falling levels of circulating CD4-positive and T-cells is a good indicator that HIV-1 infection is progressing toward AIDS.

a: The presence of anti-p24 IgM antibodies is an indicator of recent infection by HIV-1, but it is not a predictor of the progression toward AIDS.

b: Kaposi's sarcoma occurs in patients with AIDS.

c: Detecting reverse transcriptase in the patient's serum is no indicator of progression of the infection toward AIDS.

e: *Pneumocystis carinii* pneumonia occurs in AIDS patients with CD4-positive T-cell levels less than 500/mm^3.

166. **Answer d:**

One of the characteristic features of medullary carcinoma of the thyroid is the deposition of amyloid in the connective tissue stroma of the tumor. It is typically amyloid and shows positive apple-green birefringence when viewed with polarized light.

a: Papillary growth pattern is not a histologic feature of medullary carcinoma of the thyroid.

b: Well-developed follicular structure is not a histologic feature of medullary carcinoma of the thyroid.

c: The presence of lymphoid follicles is not a histologic feature of medullary carcinoma of the thyroid.

e: Undifferentiated and anaplastic tumor cells are not a histologic feature of medullary carcinoma of the thyroid.

167. **Answer d:**

Naltrexone is a potent opioid antagonist.

a: Fentanyl is a potent opioid agonist.

b: Sufentanyl is a potent opiate agonist used intravenously.

c: Dextromethorphan is essentially free of analgesic-additive effects and is used as an antitussive drug.

e: Pentazocine is a benzomorphane derivative analgesic.

168. **Answer d:**

Because a transporter molecule must bind the glucose and then change conformation to release it into the cell, a ligand-transporter complex exists for a finite period of time and can therefore be saturated.

a: Facilitated transport is always down a concentration gradient, just like simple diffusion.

b: There are five glucose transporters, the GLUT1-5 family, which mediate glucose transport in a tissue specific fashion.

c: Facilitated transport is not coupled to an energy source like ATP. It could be said to get its energy from the glucose concentration gradient.

e: GLUT-1 is abundant in the red blood cell, but not in skeletal muscle; whereas GLUT-4 is abundant in muscle and adipose tissue, showing a tissue-specific pattern of expression.

169. **Answer d:**

Since insulin promotes the uptake of glucose from peripheral blood it cannot also promote the release of glucose into the blood stream. That is the function of glucagon.

a: Insulin promotes the uptake of glucose from blood.

b: Insulin promotes the storage of glucose.

c: Insulin induces the phosphorylation of glucose.

e: Insulin promotes the synthesis of glycogen from glucose.

170. **Answer c:**

Increased renin secretion will result in increased angiotensin II and aldosterone levels, which will stimulate renal Na^+ reabsorption, maintaining blood volume.

a: A decrease in renal filtration fraction will decrease proximal tubular fluid reabsorption, tending to decrease blood volume.

b: Suppression of ADH secretion will cause water diuresis and a decrease in blood volume.

d: Increased glomerular filtration will tend to increase Na^+ and water excretion, decreasing blood volume.

e: Increased renal medullary blood flow will decrease solute concentration in the renal medulla, making the countercurrent mechanism less effective, thus increasing water excretion and decreasing blood volume.

171. **Answer d:**

H-1 antagonists block the effect of histamine at the receptor level.

a: H-1 antihistamines do not affect the release of histamine from mast cells.

b: H-1 antihistamines do not affect the metabolism of histamine.

c: H-1 antihistamines do not affect the methylation of histamine.

e: Gastric acid secretion by histamine is an H-2, not an H-1 effect.

172. **Answer b:**

A left internuclear ophthalmoplegia would interrupt the fibers of the left MLF that connect the right abducens nucleus with the left oculomotor nucleus. The patient would not be able to adduct the left eye (left medial rectus did not receive instructions to move eye to the right) on attempted gaze to the right.

a: This is the wrong MLF; it is the left MLF that is lesioned.

c: The left medial rectus should be abducting on attempted gaze to the right.

d: The right eye is fine in this patient. However, on attempted gaze to the right, the lateral rectus should abduct the eye.

e: On attempted gaze to the right, the left eye should be adducted.

173. **Answer e:**

The cause of essential hypertension is unknown, although a number of theories have been proposed. The other entities mentioned are known causes of hypertension in which the mechanism is well-defined and hypertension occurs as a secondary effect of a primary disease process.

a: Although renal disease leads to hypertension, the hypertension is a secondary effect of the primary disease process.

b: Although hyperaldosteronism leads to hypertension, the hypertension is a secondary effect of the primary disease process.

c: Use of oral contraceptive can lead to hypertension, but this is a secondary effect and is not considered essential hypertension.

d: Although increased intracranial pressure can lead to hypertension, the mechanism is known, and this is not considered essential hypertension.

174. **Answer b:**

Glucose-6-phosphate dehydrogenase catalyzes the first step in the pathway and is inhibited by high $NADPH/NADP^+$ ratios.

a: The pentose phosphate pathway is needed in red blood cells to maintain adequate levels of reduced glutathione.

c: One glucose carbon is lost as CO_2 from the action of 6-phosphogluconate dehydrogenase.

d: No NADH is produced in the pentose phosphate pathway, just NADPH.

e: The NADPH that is produced by the pentose phosphate pathway is used by glutathione reductase to regenerate reduced glutathione from the oxidized form. The oxidized form of glutathione is produced in the neutralization of hydrogen peroxide by the action of glutathione peroxidase.

175. **Answer d:**

It is generally agreed that taste buds associated with circumvallate papillae may detect bitter tastes.

a: Experts do not agree on this point, but it is believed by some that fungiform papillae throughout the tongue may detect acid tastes.

b: It is generally agreed that taste buds associated with fungiform papillae on the tip of the tongue may detect sweet tastes.

c: Experts do not agree on this point, but it is believed by some that fungiform papillae on the anterio-lateral-dorsal surface of the tongue may detect salty tastes.

e: It is generally agreed that taste buds associated with fungiform papillae on the posterio-laterol-dorsal aspect of the tongue may detect sour tastes.

176. **Answer d:**

Available statistics suggest that about 500,000 to 600,000 deaths per year occurring in the developed world are attributable to ischemic cardiac disease. That number would equate to about 80% of cardiac deaths. In the United States, ischemic heart disease is the leading cause of death and is responsible for 25% to 30% of all deaths.

a: Ischemic heart disease accounts for more than 50% of cardiac deaths.

b: Ischemic heart disease accounts for more than 60% of cardiac deaths.

c: Ischemic heart disease accounts for more than 70% of cardiac deaths.

e: Ischemic heart disease accounts for only about 80% of cardiac deaths.

177. **Answer e:**

This is a case of multiple myeloma. Although any of the carcinomas mentioned can and do metastasize to bone and produce bony destruction, they tend not to produce the typical round, punched-out lesions seen on x-ray film in multiple myeloma. The definitive factor is the finding of hyperproteinemia with a monoclonal spike. The diagnosis of multiple myeloma typically requires a number of findings including lytic bone lesions, a monoclonal spike of greater than 3 g/dl, or a urine M component, and sheets or nodules of plasma cells in the bone marrow.

178. **Answer c:**

The serratus posterior superior and serratus posterior inferior muscles constitute the intermediate layer of the extrinsic back muscles and are involved with respiration.

a: The trapezius muscle is a member of the superficial layer of extrinsic back muscles. This group of muscles unites the upper limb and trunk.

b: The latissimus dorsi muscle is a member of the superficial layer of extrinsic back muscles. This group of muscles unites the upper limb and trunk.

d: The rhomboid minor muscle is a member of the superficial layer of extrinsic back muscles. This group of muscles unites the upper limb and trunk.

e: The levator scapulae muscle is a member of the superficial layer of extrinsic back muscles. This group of muscles unites the upper limb and trunk.

179. **Answer e:**

If a preexisting glycogen chain of a few glucose monomers is not available, a primer must be initiated on the protein glycogenin.

a: The branching enzyme transfers short (5 to 8) unit chains from $alpha_{1,4}$ linkages to $alpha_{1,6}$ linkages to create branches. Glycogen synthase only adds glucose from UDP-glucose to make $alpha_{1,4}$ linkages.

b: The addition of glucose to the glycogen molecule is not reversible and can only be removed by the enzyme phosphorylase.

c: The phosphorylated form of glycogen synthetase is the inactive form.

d: Glucose 1-phosphate is converted to UDP-glucose by UDP-glucose pyrophosphorylase, and glucose is added to glycogen from UDP-glucose. There is no phosphate in glycogen.

180. **Answer c:**

Atropine dilates the pupils and may precipitate angle closure in patients with shallow anterior chambers.

a: Epinephrine increases aqueous outflow.

b: Propranolol reduces ocular pressure.

d: Diuretics are useful in reducing ocular pressure.

e: Captopril has no effect.

181. **Answer c:**

The axons from the dentate nucleus terminate in the VL nucleus.

a: The globus pallidus does not receive a direct projection from the dentate nucleus.

b: The subthalamic nucleus does not receive a direct projection from the dentate nucleus.

d: The VPM nucleus receives sensory input from the head.

e: The VPL nucleus receives sensory input from the body.

182. **Answer d:**

Arrival of the action potential at the presynaptic terminal results in quantal release of acetylcholine, which interacts with nicotinic postsynaptic receptors.

a: Acetylcholine is released from the nerve terminal, not the Schwann cell; the receptor is a nicotinic acetylcholine receptor.

b: CA^{2+} is released from the sarcoplasmic reticulum in response to the action potential.

c: The neuromuscular transmitter is acetylcholine, not norepinephrine.

e: Sequestration of Ca^{2+} ends the cross-bridge cycling and results in muscle relaxation.

Matching answers 183 and 184

183. **Answer e:**

Syngeneic mice are homozygous at every genetic locus and are genetically identical to all other mice in that strain.

184. **Answer a:**

The removal of introns from the primary nuclear RNA transcript in the formation of immunoglobulin mRNA is known as RNA splicing.

Matching answers 185 and 186

185. **Answer e:**

Familial hypertriglyceridemia is due to a genetic deficiency in lipoprotein lipase that impairs the ability to clear chylomicrons from the blood. This is not a risk factor for atherosclerosis, but pancreatitis is common.

186. **Answer d:**

Familial hypercholesterolemia results in elevated serum cholesterol by as much as 2 to 3 times normal, all due to increased LDL. The LDL elevation is due to an inherited deficiency in LDL receptors, resulting in delayed LDL clearance.

a: Mixed hypertriglyceridemia shows elevated chylomicron and triglyceride levels and modest increases in cholesterol. Lipoprotein lipase activity is normal.

b: Endogenous hypertriglyceridemia, as the term implies, is characterized by elevated serum triglycerides contained in VLDL. Elevated cholesterol is also seen with the increased VLDL levels, but LDL and HDL concentrations tend to be lowered.

c: Type III hyperlipoproteinemia is caused by a block in the conversion of triglyceride-rich VLDL to LDL. Like mixed hypertriglyceridemia, it is characterized by elevated triglyceride and cholesterol levels, but differs by having a much stronger increase in cholesterol and the appearance of a broad beta-migrating VLDL band on electrophoresis (hence the name broad beta disease).

Matching answers 187 and 188

187. **Answer h:**

Hepatic angiosarcomas are associated with previous exposure to the substances mentioned. The latent period is frequently lengthy and requires many years between exposure and development of the tumor. The tumors vary in malignant potential from rapidly fatal to relatively indolent.

188. **Answer b:**

The glomus tumor or glomangioma is a benign tumor derived from the glomus body. Glomus bodies are sensitive to temperature change and regulate arteriolar blood flow. A unique characteristic of these tumors is that they are painful.

Matching answers 189 through 191

189. **Answer c:**

The systemic spread of Varicella-zoster virus, as a result of viremia to the skin, causes lesions to develop in successive crops. Shingles is an adult clinical manifestation caused by this virus.

190. **Answer b:**

Herpes simplex virus II has been linked seroepidemiologically to human cervical cancer, possibly as a cofactor with human papilloma virus or other agent.

191. **Answer d:**

Infectious mononucleosis induced by the Epstein-Barr virus is usually documented by the demonstration of atypical lymphocytes, heterophile antibody, and positive serologic findings.

Matching answers 192 through 196

192. **Answer a:**

Insulin stimulates uptake of K^+, probably acting on the Na^+, K^+ ATPase, an effect important in the regulation of plasma K^+ concentration in response to a meal containing K^+.

193. **Answer c:**

Growth hormone inhibits glucose uptake by muscle.

194. **Answer a:**

Insulin increases transport of glucose into adipose and muscle cells via the glucose carriers in the cell membrane.

195. **Answer b:**

Glucagon belongs to this family of peptide hormones.

196. **Answer d:**

Glucagon acts on the liver and perhaps on the pancreatic beta cells.

e: Testosterone is not involved in any of the short-term metabolic effects listed. This choice was not used.

Matching answers 197 and 198

197. **Answer l:**

The internal medullary lamina separates the dorsal thalamus into a medial and lateral group of nuclei.

198. **Answer i:**

Damage to the genu of the internal capsule can cause a supranuclear facial palsy, since the UMN destined for the facial nucleus would be lost. The part of the facial nucleus that innervates the cheek area receives only crossed supranuclear innervation.

Matching answers 199 and 200

199. **Answer b:**

Urea cycle defects slow the disposal of free ammonia, causing it to build up. Ornithine transcarbamoylase deficiency in the mitochondrion blocks the entry of nitrogen into the urea cycle as carbamoyl phosphate. The buildup of mitochondrial carbamoyl phosphate eventually leaks into the cytoplasm, where it accelerates the synthesis of uracil, leading to its appearance in the urine.

200. **Answer e:**

Kinureninase converts kynurenine, an intermediate in the tryptophan degradation pathway, to 3-hydroxyanthranilate, a metabolite that can be subsequently converted to niacin or metabolized to acetyl CoA.

a: Carbamoyl phosphate synthetase II is the cytosolic form, which catalyzes one of the initial steps in pyrimidine synthesis. If this enzyme were deficient, any buildup of ammonia would be disposed of in the urea cycle, which would have a functional carbamoyl phosphate synthetase.

c: Serine hydroxymethyltransferase is an enzyme that reversibly transfers a single carbon unit from methylene tetrahydrofolate to glycine to synthesize serine.

d: Asparagine synthetase uses Mg-ATP to transfer the amide nitrogen from glutamine to aspartate. This differs from the glutamine synthetase reaction in that the latter uses free ammonia as the nitrogen source.

Categories and Answers for Exam 4

Question Number	Answer	Check Here If Correct	Category 1	Category 2	Category 3
1	E	☐	Neuroscience	Autonomic Nervous System	Normal Function
2	C	☐	Neuroscience	Neurotransmitters	Normal Anatomy
3	A	☐	Anatomy	Upper Limb	Clinical Anatomy
4	B	☐	Microbiology	Bacteriology	Structure
5	C	☐	Histology	Eye	General Properties
6	E	☐	Pathology	Liver & Pancreas	Neoplasia
7	C	☐	Behavioral Science	Professional Issues	Confidentiality
8	C	☐	Behavioral Science	Family Systems	General Properties
9	A	☐	Microbiology	Parasitology	Laboratory Diagnosis
10	C	☐	Physiology	Gastrointestinal System	Normal Function
11	D	☐	Microbiology	Virology	Pathogenesis
12	B	☐	Microbiology	Immune System	Immune System Cells
13	E	☐	Biochemistry	Molecular Genetics	Structure
14	B	☐	Pharmacology	Toxicology	General Properties
15	B	☐	Anatomy	Abdomen	Clinical Anatomy
16	C	☐	Biochemistry	Nitrogen Metabolism	Metabolism
17	C	☐	Anatomy	Thorax	Normal Anatomy
18	C	☐	Histology	Cells & Tissues	Normal Tissues
19	E	☐	Neuroscience	Head & Neck	Lesions
20	B	☐	Neuroscience	Head & Neck	Normal Anatomy
21	D	☐	Behavioral Science	Professional Issues	Physician-Patient Relationship
22	D	☐	Microbiology	Bacteriology	Diseases
23	B	☐	Pathology	Virology	Diseases
24	E	☐	Physiology	Cardiovascular System	General Properties
25	B	☐	Microbiology	Immune System	Immune System Cells
26	D	☐	Biochemistry	Lipids & Steroids	Metabolism
27	A	☐	Histology	Ear	Normal Anatomy
28	E	☐	Anatomy	Thorax	Normal Anatomy
29	D	☐	Behavioral Science	Psychopathology	Assessment
30	B	☐	Physiology	Respiratory System	General Properties
31	C	☐	Physiology	Cells & Tissues	General Properties
32	D	☐	Biochemistry	Intermediary Metabolism	Transport
33	E	☐	Neuroscience	Central Nervous System	Normal Anatomy
34	A	☐	Biochemistry	Nutrition	Diseases
35	A	☐	Pathology	Central Nervous System	Lesions
36	E	☐	Pharmacology	Cardiovascular System	Side Effects
37	B	☐	Pharmacology	Toxicology	Diseases
38	C	☐	Pharmacology	Cardiovascular System	Main Effects
39	C	☐	Microbiology	Mycology	Treatment
40	E	☐	Neuroscience	Back & Spinal Cord	Normal Anatomy
41	B	☐	Neuroscience	Central Nervous System	Normal Anatomy
42	D	☐	Behavioral Science	Molecular Genetics	Epidemiology
43	B	☐	Pharmacology	Urinary System	Main Effects
44	E	☐	Behavioral Science	Interviewing	Assessment
45	D	☐	Histology	Male Reproductive System	General Properties
46	A	☐	Pathology	Musculoskeletal System	Bones, Joints, & Soft Tissues
47	C	☐	Behavioral Science	Life Cycle	Psychosocial Development
48	A	☐	Physiology	Urinary System	Transport
49	D	☐	Histology	Cells & Tissues	Normal Tissues
50	E	☐	Physiology	Cardiovascular System	Regulation

Categories and Answers for Exam 4

Question Number	Answer	Check Here if Correct	Category 1	Category 2	Category 3
51	B	☐	Behavioral Science	Statistics	General Properties
52	B	☐	Anatomy	Head & Neck	Clinical Anatomy
53	D	☐	Microbiology	Immune System	Immune Response
54	C	☐	Neuroscience	Peripheral Nervous System	Normal Anatomy
55	C	☐	Neuroscience	Back & Spinal Cord	Normal Anatomy
56	B	☐	Microbiology	Bacteriology	Treatment
57	D	☐	Anatomy	Thorax	Clinical Anatomy
58	C	☐	Histology	Cardiovascular System	Circulation
59	B	☐	Pathology	Cardiovascular System	Diseases
60	A	☐	Physiology	Endocrine System	Signaling
61	E	☐	Histology	Blood & Lymph	Normal Tissues
62	C	☐	Neuroscience	Motor Systems & Reflexes	Normal Anatomy
63	D	☐	Neuroscience	Central Nervous System	Normal Function
64	C	☐	Pharmacology	Central Nervous System	General Properties
65	B	☐	Histology	Gastrointestinal System	Pathophysiology
66	B	☐	Pharmacology	Central Nervous System	Clinical Uses
67	E	☐	Behavioral Science	Life Cycle	Psychosocial Development
68	A	☐	Histology	Immune System	Immune System Cells
69	E	☐	Anatomy	Head & Neck	Normal Anatomy
70	B	☐	Neuroscience	Peripheral Nervous System	Normal Function
71	C	☐	Neuroscience	Motor Systems & Reflexes	Lesions
72	D	☐	Microbiology	Bacteriology	Structure
73	D	☐	Physiology	Musculoskeletal System	General Properties
74	D	☐	Physiology	Urinary System	Regulation
75	C	☐	Pharmacology	Autonomic Nervous System	Side Effects
76	D	☐	Pharmacology	Central Nervous System	Clinical Uses
77	B	☐	Pathology	Virology	Structure
78	A	☐	Neuroscience	Central Nervous System	Normal Anatomy
79	B	☐	Biochemistry	Intermediary Metabolism	Energy & Oxidation
80	C	☐	Pharmacology	Central Nervous System	General Properties
81	D	☐	Histology	Blood & Lymph	Genetics
82	B	☐	Microbiology	Bacteriology	General Properties
83	A	☐	Pathology	Cells & Tissues	Cell Injury & Cell Death
84	C	☐	Physiology	Endocrine System	Assessment
85	A	☐	Histology	Cardiovascular System	Normal Tissues
86	D	☐	Pathology	Musculoskeletal System	Bones, Joints, & Soft Tissues
87	B	☐	Neuroscience	Head & Neck	Normal Function
88	B	☐	Pharmacology	Cardiovascular System	Side Effects
89	D	☐	Physiology	Respiratory System	General Properties
90	C	☐	Pathology	Cells & Tissues	Cell Injury & Cell Death
91	B	☐	Histology	Cells & Tissues	Normal Tissues
92	B	☐	Physiology	Cardiovascular System	General Properties
93	E	☐	Histology	Cells & Tissues	Normal Tissues
94	E	☐	Pharmacology	Chemotherapy	Clinical Uses
95	A	☐	Pathology	General Principles	Diseases
96	E	☐	Pathology	Blood & Lymph	Neoplasia
97	E	☐	Physiology	Gastrointestinal System	Secretion
98	B	☐	Anatomy	Abdomen	Normal Anatomy
99	B	☐	Biochemistry	Molecular Genetics	Synthesis
100	D	☐	Biochemistry	Molecular Genetics	Structure

Categories and Answers for Exam 4

Question Number	Answer	Check Here If Correct	Category 1	Category 2	Category 3
101	D	☐	Biochemistry	Molecular Genetics	Synthesis
102	E	☐	Pharmacology	Blood & Lymph	Diseases
103	E	☐	Microbiology	Parasitology	Epidemiology
104	B	☐	Microbiology	Mycology	Epidemiology
105	B	☐	Pharmacology	Central Nervous System	Interactions
106	D	☐	Pharmacology	Toxicology	Pathogenesis
107	C	☐	Pathology	Cardiovascular System	Clinical Anatomy
108	B	☐	Pathology	Blood & Lymph	Synthesis
109	D	☐	Biochemistry	Intermediary Metabolism	Glycolysis & Gluconeogenesis
110	E	☐	Microbiology	Bacteriology	Pathogenesis
111	D	☐	Pharmacology	Chemotherapy	General Properties
112	A	☐	Pharmacology	Endocrine System	Main Effects
113	D	☐	Physiology	Urinary System	Regulation
114	B	☐	Neuroscience	Head & Neck	Normal Anatomy
115	B	☐	Microbiology	Bacteriology	Diseases
116	C	☐	Pharmacology	Central Nervous System	Side Effects
117	C	☐	Pharmacology	Central Nervous System	Side Effects
118	A	☐	Anatomy	Head & Neck	Normal Anatomy
119	A	☐	Neuroscience	Peripheral Nervous System	Normal Anatomy
120	D	☐	Neuroscience	Central Nervous System	Lesions
121	D	☐	Pharmacology	Toxicology	General Properties
122	C	☐	Physiology	Urinary System	Transport
123	D	☐	Physiology	Cardiovascular System	Circulation
124	E	☐	Pathology	Molecular Genetics	Diseases
125	C	☐	Histology	Male Reproductive System	Normal Function
126	B	☐	Histology	Musculoskeletal System	Normal Tissues
127	C	☐	Neuroscience	Motor Systems & Reflexes	Diseases
128	D	☐	Neuroscience	Central Nervous System	Normal Anatomy
129	E	☐	Anatomy	Pelvis & Perineum	Normal Anatomy
130	D	☐	Pathology	Bacteriology	Diseases
131	D	☐	Physiology	Cardiovascular System	The Heart as a Pump
132	C	☐	Anatomy	Abdomen	Normal Anatomy
133	E	☐	Microbiology	Immune System	Lesions
134	D	☐	Anatomy	Pelvis & Perineum	Normal Anatomy
135	A	☐	Physiology	Cardiovascular System	The Heart as a Pump
136	E	☐	Pathology	Liver & Pancreas	Diseases
137	E	☐	Pathology	Blood & Lymph	Diseases
138	B	☐	Microbiology	Bacteriology	Genetics
139	B	☐	Neuroscience	Central Nervous System	Normal Function
140	A	☐	Neuroscience	Back & Spinal Cord	Normal Anatomy
141	B	☐	Anatomy	Lower Limb	Normal Anatomy
142	C	☐	Behavioral Science	Statistics	Personality Disorders
143	D	☐	Pharmacology	Autonomic Nervous System	Main Effects
144	D	☐	Pathology	Male Reproductive System	Neoplasia
145	D	☐	Microbiology	Parasitology	Epidemiology
146	B	☐	Physiology	Cardiovascular System	The Heart as a Pump
147	C	☐	Physiology	Cardiovascular System	Regulation
148	D	☐	Pathology	Cells & Tissues	Neoplasia
149	B	☐	Physiology	Cardiovascular System	Regulation
150	A	☐	Pharmacology	Autonomic Nervous System	Interactions

Categories and Answers for Exam 4

Question Number	Answer	Check Here If Correct	Category 1	Category 2	Category 3
151	A	☐	Pharmacology	Autonomic Nervous System	Interactions
152	D	☐	Pharmacology	Autonomic Nervous System	Interactions
153	E	☐	Pharmacology	Autonomic Nervous System	Interactions
154	C	☐	Anatomy	Lower Limb	Normal Anatomy
155	B	☐	Histology	Cells & Tissues	Secretion
156	A	☐	Neuroscience	Central Nervous System	Normal Function
157	E	☐	Pathology	Cardiovascular System	Diseases
158	D	☐	Neuroscience	Head & Neck	Normal Anatomy
159	D	☐	Physiology	Cells & Tissues	General Properties
160	B	☐	Physiology	Urinary System	Transport
161	E	☐	Neuroscience	Central Nervous System	Lesions
162	A	☐	Anatomy	Pelvis & Perineum	Clinical Anatomy
163	B	☐	Physiology	Immune System	Immune System Cells
164	B	☐	Neuroscience	Peripheral Nervous System	General Properties
165	C	☐	Neuroscience	Central Nervous System	Normal Anatomy
166	D	☐	Anatomy	Abdomen	Normal Anatomy
167	E	☐	Pathology	Gastrointestinal System	Diseases
168	B	☐	Pathology	Gastrointestinal System	Diseases
169	A	☐	Pharmacology	Chemotherapy	General Properties
170	D	☐	Physiology	Gastrointestinal System	Secretion
171	C	☐	Pharmacology	Toxicology	Side Effects
172	D	☐	Microbiology	Immune System	Diseases
173	A	☐	Anatomy	Thorax	Normal Anatomy
174	D	☐	Microbiology	Immune System	Immune System Cells
175	C	☐	Neuroscience	Back & Spinal Cord	Normal Function
176	E	☐	Biochemistry	Molecular Genetics	Recombinant DNA
177	C	☐	Pharmacology	Autocoids & Diuretics	Main Effects
178	B	☐	Biochemistry	Enzymes	General Properties
179	E	☐	Biochemistry	General Principles	Diseases
180	D	☐	Biochemistry	General Principles	Diseases
181	F	☐	Microbiology	Immune System	Immune System Cells
182	G	☐	Microbiology	Immune System	Immune System Cells
183	D	☐	Biochemistry	Blood & Lymph	General Properties
184	E	☐	Biochemistry	Blood & Lymph	General Properties
185	A	☐	Behavioral Science	Life Cycle	Cognitive Development
186	C	☐	Behavioral Science	Life Cycle	Cognitive Development
187	D	☐	Microbiology	Bacteriology	Diseases
188	A	☐	Microbiology	Bacteriology	Diseases
189	E	☐	Microbiology	Bacteriology	Diseases
190	A	☐	Physiology	Endocrine System	General Properties
191	D	☐	Physiology	Endocrine System	Secretion
192	D	☐	Physiology	Endocrine System	Secretion
193	A	☐	Physiology	Endocrine System	General Properties
194	E	☐	Physiology	Endocrine System	General Properties
195	E	☐	Biochemistry	Lipids & Steroids	Synthesis
196	C	☐	Biochemistry	Lipids & Steroids	Synthesis
197	D	☐	Biochemistry	Purine & Pyrimidine Metabolism	Diseases
198	C	☐	Biochemistry	Purine & Pyrimidine Metabolism	Diseases
199	A	☐	Behavioral Science	Interviewing	Assessment
200	B	☐	Behavioral Science	Interviewing	Assessment

Answers and Explanations to Exam 4

1. **Answer e:**

   Parasympathetic stimulation causes a voluminous watery secretion. Sympathetic stimulation causes a very sparse viscous secretion.

   a: Arterial pressure is increased
   b: Blood glucose concentration is increased.
   c: Glycolysis in muscle is increased.
   d: Muscle strength is increased.

2. **Answer c:**

   The raphe nuclei release serotonin, and activity in some of these nuclei induces sleep. Destruction of these serotonergic neurons produces temporary insomnia.

   a: Cerebellar Purkinje cells release GABA.
   b: Locus ceruleus axons release norepinephrine.
   d: Substantia nigra pars compacta neurons release dopamine.
   e: Cerebellar granule cells release glutamate.

3. **Answer a:**

   The tendon of the supraspinatus muscle is the most frequently torn portion of the "rotator cuff." It may be weakened by trauma or disease.

   b: Although it forms part of the "rotator cuff," the infraspinatus tendon is not injured or torn that frequently.
   c: The tendon of the long head of the biceps brachii muscle does form part of the "rotator cuff" apparatus.

   d: Although it forms part of the "rotator cuff," the teres minor tendon is not injured or torn that frequently.
   e: Although it forms part of the "rotator cuff," the subscapularis tendon is not injured or torn that frequently.

4. **Answer b:**

   Capsules are one class of evasins that allow bacteria to resist phagocytosis.

   a: Capsules do not mimic host cell antigens in order to evade the immune response.
   c: Capsules are not capable of destroying secretory IgA molecules.
   d: Capsules are found on both gram-positive and gram-negative bacteria.
   e: The origin of flagella is within the cytoplasmic membrane.

5. **Answer c:**

   Light waves do not pass through the iris because its posterior margin (wall) is covered with two layers of pigmented epithelial cells and the stroma often contains numerous pigmented melanocytes.

   a: The vitreous humor is normally transparent, and this allows light to freely pass through it before striking the retina.
   b: The pupil is a space filled with aqueous humor and circumscribed by the iris. Therefore light passes freely through it before striking the retina.

    d: The cornea is normally transparent, and this allows light to freely pass through it before striking the retina.

    e: The lens is normally transparent, and this allows light to freely pass through it before striking the retina.

6. **Answer e:**

Hepatitis A is not a cause of cirrhosis, chronic infection, or hepatocellular carcinoma.

    a: Cirrhosis is associated with hepatocellular carcinoma.

    b: Aflatoxin has a strong association with the development of hepatocellular carcinoma, often in concert with hepatitis B infection.

    c: Hepatitis B is implicated as a major factor in the majority of hepatocellular carcinoma through mechanisms that are not entirely clear.

    d: Patients with hereditary tyrosinemia have a 40% incidence of developing hepatocellular carcinoma.

7. **Answer c:**

The patient's treatment team is considered an extension of, or a consultant to, the physician, and, therefore, a formal release of information is not required.

    a: Confidential information can only be released to a family member without the patient's consent if the family member is the legal guardian for the patient because the patient is a minor or deemed incompetent or in the event of an emergency. When an emergency occurs, the exchange of information should be limited to the details necessary for making immediate decisions.

    b: Information released to an attorney requires written consent by the patient or a *subpoena duces tecum.*

    d: Insurance carriers do not have a right to confidential information without a patient's signed release. However, insurance carriers can require that the patient provide written agreement to the exchange of information, at times including confidential details, prior to authorization of payment.

    e: Although communication between physicians providing inpatient care and primary care physicians facilitates treatment planning, written release is still required prior to the disclosure of confidential information.

8. **Answer c:**

Psychoanalytic theory hypothesizes that psychopathology arises when a fixation in psychosexual development occurs.

    a: Family systems theory states that the unit of psychological dysfunction is often the family, and the conflicts between family members often create the pathology seen in an individual.

    b: According to family systems theory each family member is viewed as serving a role in maintaining the family structure, and, at times, the identified patient is hypothesized as needing to develop pathology to continue to allow the family to maintain its formation.

    d: Dysfunctional family units are seen as the context for the development of pathology in many individuals according to family systems theory.

    e: Family systems therapists use family therapy to restructure the family in a healthy manner and alleviate the pathology seen within the identified patient.

9. **Answer a:**

The crescent-shaped gametocytes in a blood smear are diagnostic for *Plasmodium falciparum* (malignant tertian malaria).

    b: *Plasmodium ovale* causes enlargement of infected erythrocytes, but no gametocyte is seen.

    c: *Plasmodium malariae* produces no red cell enlargement and no gametocytes.

    d: *Plasmodium vivax* is similar to *Plasmodium ovale,* except that there are about twice as many merozoites in the schizont. No gametocyte is seen.

    e: *Plasmodium bergheii* causes rodent malariae and is not a human pathogen.

10. **Answer c:**

Colipase binds to pancreatic lipase to allow the lipase to bind to the oil-water interface of lipid droplets in the intestinal lumen.

    a: Pancreatic lipase hydrolyses triglycerides into monoglycerides and free fatty acids.

    b: Secretion of bicarbonate by the pancreas alkalinizes the intestinal contents, allowing lipase to act since the enzyme has an optimum of pH 7-8. The enzyme acts at the lipid-water interface of emulsified fat.

    d: Hydrolysis of phospholipids by phospholipose A_2 results in removal of one fatty acid molecule from the phospholipid.

    e: Absorption of cholesterol by enterocytes requires that the cholesterol be in the form of free sterol.

11. **Answer d:**
Opsonization of viruses by specific antibody has no role in their ability to evade the normal immune response.

a: Antigenic variation in the case of HIV results in genetic change after infection. It also causes annual genetic changes in influenza virus.
b: Hepatitis B virus inhibits interferon transcription.
c: Hepatitis B surface antigen is a blocking antigen to the humoral immune response.
e: HIV infection of CD4 T cells results in cytolysis of these cells.

12. **Answer b:**
The effect would be the prevention of expression of Class I MHC, since beta-2 microglobulin is an integral part of the immunoglobulin-like region of Class I MHC molecules.

a: TAP 1 and 2 proteins are encoded in the Class II MHC region.
c: Beta-2 microglobulin is part of Class I MHC and would not prevent expression of Class II MHC molecules.
d: Proteasomes are also a product of the Class II MHC genes.
e: Beta-2 microglobulin is encoded within Class I MHC genes.

13. **Answer e:**
Base stacking (hydrophobic) forces are comparable in magnitude with the forces produced by hydrogen bonding between the purine and pyrimidine bases.

a: Because the bases pair at an angle instead of directly across from each other, one groove (the major groove) is wider than the other (minor) groove.
b: Polynucleotides have a 5′ to 3′ polarity (direction), and in DNA each strand extends in opposite directions.
c: The classic Watson-Crick hydrogen bonding between AT and GC pairs is maintained in all three major forms of DNA: Z-DNA, and the B and A forms of DNA. These forms of DNA are different in the direction of coiling (left-handed for Z-DNA, right-handed for B- and A-DNA) and in the pitch of the helix (10 bases per turn for B-DNA, 11 and 12 for A-DNA and Z-DNA, respectively).

d: The B-form, which is most representative of that found in the cell, has 10 bases per turn and each turn is 34 angstroms in length. This is the form of DNA that is assumed, unless another form is specified.

14. **Answer b:**
The toxic properties of carbon monoxide are due to its binding to hemoglobin rendering hemoglobin incapable of normal oxygen transport; cyanide inhibits cytochrome oxydase.

a: Carbon monoxide is a chemical type of asphyxiation.
c: Carbon monoxide does combine with hemoglobin to form carboxyhemoglobin.
d: Carbon monoxide reacts with hemoglobin in a manner similar to oxygen.
e: Carbon monoxide produces cherry-colored blood.

15. **Answer b:**
Indirect inguinal hernias exit the abdominal cavity via the deep inguinal ring, which lies immediately lateral to the inferior epigastric vessels.

a: Indirect inguinal hernias exit the abdominal cavity via the deep inguinal ring, while direct inguinal hernias pass through the posterior wall of the inguinal canal.
c: Although indirect inguinal hernias occur in both sexes, they are much more common in males.
d: The indirect inguinal hernia occurs much more frequently in both sexes than do direct inguinal hernias.
e: Indirect inguinal hernias enter the deep inguinal ring, traverse the inguinal canal, and may exit the superficial inguinal ring to enter the scrotum or labia majora.

16. **Answer c:**
The amino groups of most amino acids are first transferred by a transaminase to alpha-ketoglutarate producing glutamate plus an alpha-keto acid, which corresponds to the original amino acid. The glutamate is then acted on by glutamate hydrogenase to produce free ammonia.

a: D-amino acids in the diet are metabolized by D-amino acid oxidase, but no such enzymes exist for the metabolism of L-amino acids, which are present in the tissues of humans (and other animals). Arginase is an enzyme whose activity is restricted to cleavage of urea from arginine in the urea cycle.

b: Glutaminase functions primarily in the kidneys and the intestine to remove free ammonia from glutamine. In the kidney, the ammonia is excreted, and in the intestine, it is transported directly to the liver, where it enters the urea cycle.

d: Argininosuccinate lyase is a part of the urea cycle where it catalyzes the cleavage of argininosuccinate into arginine and fumarate. Cytosolic carbamoyl phosphate synthetase is not part of the urea cycle. Rather, it is active in using free ammonia for pyrimidine synthesis.

e: Glutamine synthetase joins free ammonia to glutamate to provide glutamine needed for protein synthesis and to detoxify excess ammonia in the brain and the liver. Urease is a bacterial (and plant) enzyme that cleaves urea into carbon dioxide and ammonia. Excess urea, which makes its way to the gut (and therefore the gut flora) during kidney failure, can contribute to hyperammonemia.

17.   **Answer c:**
Fibers of the transversus thoracis muscle are located between the internal thoracic vessels and the parietal pleura on the deep surface of the anterior chest wall.

a: The internal intercostal muscles lie superficially to the parietal pleura and internal thoracic vessels.

b: The external intercostal muscles lie superficially to the parietal pleura and internal thoracic vessels.

d: The subcostalis muscles are located near the angles of the ribs and are too far laterally and posteriorly to be related to the internal thoracic vessels.

e: The costal cartilages are located superficially to the parietal pleura internal thoracic vessels.

18.   **Answer c:**
Figure 1 is a schematic cross section of a peripheral nerve showing eight nerve fascicles, each of which is bounded by a perineurium.

a: The epineurium refers to the connective tissue external to the perineurium.

b: A typical fascicle is composed of several myelinated nerve processes. Hence, numerous myelin sheaths are enclosed by each perineurium.

d: Schwann cell cytoplasm is closely associated with individual nerve axons.

e: The endoneurium refers to the connecting tissue elements within each fascicle.

19.   **Answer e:**
When the middle ear is filled with fluid, as occurs in otitis media, a conductive hearing loss of 30 dB can result.

a: Aging causes a sensorineural hearing loss.

b: Childhood rubella causes a sensorineural hearing loss.

c: Exposure to industrial noise causes a sensorineural hearing loss.

d: Exposure to ototoxic antibiotics causes a sensorineural hearing loss.

20.   **Answer b:**
The posterior belly of the digastric is supplied by the branchial motor component of the facial nerve.

a: The messeter is supplied by axons from the motor nucleus of nerve V.

c: The temporalis muscle is supplied by axons from the motor nucleus of nerve V.

d: The tensor tympani muscle is supplied by axons from the motor nucleus of nerve V.

e: The tensor veli palatini muscle is supplied by axons from the motor nucleus of nerve V.

21.   **Answer d:**
The described patient is making decisions while in a heightened emotional state. Providing counseling and education decreases the patient's anxiety and increases rational decision making. Postponing testing until emotional stability is regained provides the patient time to reconsider and strengthens the physician's ability to prevent suicidal behavior.

a: This patient is not in immediate danger of suicide unless testing is conducted, and, therefore, involuntary commitment is unlikely to be achievable. Even if commitment is feasible, this approach unnecessarily impinges on the patient's autonomy and represents an overreaction on the physician's part.

b: Providing false information is unethical and dangerous, disrespects patient autonomy, leads to mistrust, and interferes with treatment planning.

c: Fundamental duties of a physician include providing necessary health care, guiding rational decision making, and avoiding patient harm. Refusing testing without providing other services violates each of these duties.

35. **Answer a:**

    This is, of course, a meningioma. These are slow growing, indolent tumors that compress rather than invade the brain. They have a well-known propensity to erode the overlying skull, which can make complete removal difficult or impossible if they occur at the base of the brain.

36. **Answer e:**

    The set of symptoms associated with quinine toxicity is called cinchonism, referring to the cinchona tree, formerly the source of the drug.

    a: Lidocaine does not cause cinchonism.
    b: Verapamil does not cause cinchonism.
    c: Dopamine does not cause cinchonism.
    d: Nifedipine does not cause cinchonism.

37. **Answer b:**

    Lead encephalopathy develops in children only, probably because the blood-brain barrier is not yet fully functional.

    a: Arsenic produces only peripheral neuropathy.
    b: Mercury produces CNS symptoms in both adults and children.
    d: Chromium does not produce any neuropathy or encephalopathy.
    e: Beryllium does not produce any neuropathy or encephalopathy.

38. **Answer c:**

    Digitalis glycosides increase stroke volume, decrease heart rate, increase cardiac output, and decrease peripheral vascular resistance in patients with congestive heart failure.

    a: Increase in peripheral resistance is incorrect.
    b: Decrease in stroke volume and cardiac output is incorrect.
    d: Cardiac output is increased, peripheral vascular resistance is decreased.
    e: Stroke volume is increased.

39. **Answer c:**

    Griseofulvin is effective in the treatment of dermatophyte infections such as tinea capitis.

    a: Griseofulvin is not effective in the treatment of mucormycosis.
    b: Griseofulvin is not effective in the treatment of candidiasis or agents causing systemic mycoses.

d: Amphotericin B is the drug of choice for the treatment of coccidioidomycosis.
e: Sporotrichosis is effectively treated with oral potassium iodide (orally for subcutaneous lymphangitic sporotrichosis) or in systemic cases, amphotericin B.

40. **Answer e:**

    The cell bodies of the axons in the posterior spinocerebellar tract are in the ipsilateral nucleus dorsalis of Clark from T1-L2.

    a: The posterior spinocerebellar tract is uncrossed and the nucleus dorsalis of Clark is in lamina VII of Rexed.
    b: The posterior spinocerebellar tract is uncrossed. Nucleus proprius is laminae III and IV of Rexed.
    c: This tract originates from nucleus dorsalis of Clark, which extends from T1-L2 not C1-C8.
    d: The nucleus that gives rise to the tract is in lamina VII.

41. **Answer b:**

    The locus ceruleus has a blood-brain-barrier.

    a: Area postrema is a circumventricular organ and does not have a blood-brain-barrier.
    c: Median eminence is a circumventricular organ and does not have a blood-brain-barrier.
    d: The neurohypophysis is a circumventricular organ and does not have a blood-brain-barrier.
    e: The pineal is a circumventricular organ and does not have a blood-brain-barrier.

42. **Answer d:**

    Research studies have repeatedly suggested a genetic component exists regarding the inheritance of schizophrenia with monozygotic twins having the highest concordance rate, often estimated between 35% to 50%.

    a: Prevalence figures suggest that the rate of schizophrenia in the general population is about 1%, which is significantly lower than rates found in family members of schizophrenics.
    b: A prevalence rate of 0% would be even lower than that found in the general population (1%) and contradicts numerous studies supporting the presence of a genetic link for schizophrenia.

c: Although the probability that a schizophrenic's family member will have schizophrenia is strongly correlated with the closeness of the relationship, prevalence estimates for monozygotic twins rarely exceed 50%.

e: Although a single chromosome marker for schizophrenia has not been identified, numerous studies support a genetic link for the disorder.

43. **Answer b:**

Nicotinic acid (but not nicotinamide) inhibits VLDL secretion, thus lowering blood levels of cholesterol and lipoproteins.

a: Vitamin D has no effect on blood levels of lipoproteins.

c: Nicotinomide has no effect on blood levels of lipoproteins.

d: Thiamine has no effect on blood levels of lipoproteins.

e: Ascorbic acid has no effect on blood levels of lipoproteins.

44. **Answer e:**

The mental status examination represents the physician's attempt to systemically evaluate a patients' behavioral, emotional, and cognitive processes. Interpretation of a proverb requires the ability to engage in abstraction.

a: To assess memory, a patient will be asked to recall current and past historical details and may be given immediate and delayed recall tasks.

b: A patient's thought content is assessed throughout an interview with special emphasis placed on questions regarding the presence or absence of obsessions, compulsions, psychotic thought processes, and suicidal and homicidal ideation.

c: Attention is measured by tasks such as serial sevens, which require sustained focus.

d: Vocabulary is assessed based on the patient's usage and understanding of words.

45. **Answer d:**

Capacitation is the process by which spermatozoa are able to fertilize eggs after being in the female reproductive tract for a few days.

a: Spermiogenesis refers to a series of events in which spermatids, which are attached to Sertoli cells, are released to become free and independent cells.

b: Spermatogenesis refers to the process by which spermatogenia divide and differentiate into spermatids.

c: In females the process of luteinization (due to LH) regulates ovulation, the formation of the corpus luteum, and the final maturation of the ovarian follicles. Luteinizing hormone is also present in males, where it is referred to as interstitial cell-stimulating hormone (ICSH).

e: Differentiation refers to a process by which spermatozoa and many other rapidly dividing cell types transform from a primitive stage to a more mature stage.

46. **Answer a:**

Osteoarthritis, or degenerative joint disease, is the most common type of joint disease. It is the result of progressive erosion of the articular cartilage (wear and tear arthritis). It is thought to be primarily a disease of the articular cartilage in which chemical and metabolic changes cause its breakdown.

b: Rheumatoid arthritis is not the most common form of joint disease.

c: Pigmented villonodular synovitis is not the most common form of joint disease.

d: Gouty arthritis is not the most common form of joint disease.

e: Infectious arthritis is not the most common form of joint disease.

47. **Answer c:**

Freud labeled the period between 3 to 6 years of age the phallic stage as pleasure was connected with the genital area in this timeframe. During this phase boys were hypothesized to experience an Oedipal Complex, whereas, the term for the same phenomenon in girls was labeled the Electra Complex.

a: The oral phase of psychosexual development was hypothesized by Freud to encompass the first 18 months of life, and the source of gratification was oral contact, such as sucking and biting.

b: During the anal phase, age 18 months to 3 years, Freud proposed that pleasure was derived from the retention and expulsion of feces.

d: The latent phase in Freudian theory followed the phallic phase, lasting from ages 6 to 11, and represented a time period in which psychosexual development was temporarily curtailed within the developing child.

e: According to Freud, the genital phase represented the highest level of psychosexual development and began at the onset of puberty, corresponding with a focus on mature interpersonal relationships.

48. **Answer a:**

    Phosphate is one of many solutes cotransported with Na^+ in the proximal tubule.

    b: There is no such primary active transport.
    c: The electrical gradient in the last part of the proximal tubule is lumen positive and would oppose phosphate reabsorption.
    d: NH_4^+ and H^+ are secreted by antiport with Na^+.
    e: H^+ is secreted by antiport with Na^+.

49. **Answer d:**

    Hepatic bile ducts are primarily involved in the transportation, without significant modification, of secretory product. Therefore these ducts are not composed of epithelial cells characterized by longitudinally oriented mitochondria intermingled with numerous enfoldings of basal plasma membrane. These epithelial cells do not possess numerous microvilli.

    a: The renal PCT is composed of epithelial cells characterized by longitudinally oriented mitochondria intermingled with numerous enfoldings of the basal plasma membrane. These epithelial cells typically possess microvilli, and their lateral cell membranes are often tightly adhered to each other. These cells are characteristic of epithelial tissues that function in ion and fluid regulation.
    b: The inner sensory (nonpigmented) retinal epithelium of the ciliary body in the eye is composed of epithelial cells characterized by longitudinally oriented mitochondria intermingled with numerous enfoldings of the basal plasma membrane. These epithelial cells typically possess microvilli and their lateral cell membranes are often tightly adhered to one another. These cells are characteristic of epithelial tissues, which function in ion and fluid regulation.
    c: The striated duct in the submandibular gland is composed of epithelial cells characterized by longitudinally oriented mitochondria intermingled with numerous enfoldings of the basal plasma membrane. These epithelial cells typically possess microvilli, and their lateral cell membranes are often tightly adhered to one another. These cells are characteristic of epithelial tissues that function in ion and fluid regulation.
    d: The striated duct of the parotid gland is composed of epithelial cells characterized by longitudinally oriented mitochondria intermingled with numerous enfoldings of the basal plasma membrane. These epithelial cells typically possess microvilli, and their lateral cell membranes are often tightly adhered to one another. These cells are characteristic of epithelial tissues that function in ion and fluid regulation.

50. **Answer e:**

    There are no baroreceptors in muscular arterioles.

    a: The carotid sinuses are a major site of baroreceptors.
    b: The aortic arch is a major site of baroreceptors.
    c: Baroreceptors exist in the ventricles.
    d: The afferent arteriole contains a baroreceptor that mediates renin secretion.

51. **Answer b:**

    Skewed distributions occur when most scores are located at one end of a distribution. As the median represents the midpoint, it lies nearest the majority of scores for positively and negatively skewed distributions, and it is generally considered the best measure of central tendency when a skew occurs.

    a: The mean, the arithmetic average, which under normal circumstances is the most commonly used measure of central tendency, biasly estimates where the majority of scores are as it is pulled out toward the skew.
    c: The mode, the most frequently occurring score, will be misleading when a skewed distribution exists as it will not provide information regarding where the bulk of scores lie.
    d: The range, a measure of variance, is the highest score minus the lowest score, and is not a measure of central tendency.
    e: The variance is the average squared deviation from the mean and is not a measure of central tendency, rather it reflects variance.

52. **Answer b:**

    The facial nerve is at risk during a forceps delivery, since it exits the stylomastoid foramen medial to the mastoid process, which is underdeveloped at this stage.

    a: Branches of the trigeminal nerve are not at risk during a forceps delivery.
    c: The hypoglossal nerve is not at risk during a forceps delivery.

    d: The accessory nerve is not at risk during a forceps delivery.

    e: The greater occipital nerve is not at risk during a forceps delivery.

53. **Answer d:**

Immunoglobulins are antigen-specific, and therefore, are not classified as nonspecific defense mechanisms.

    a: Cytokines are not antigen specific, but do play an important role in modulating the immune response.

    b: Lactoferrin, from polymorphonuclear leukocytes, binds iron and competes with microorganisms for this metal.

    c: Mucus prevents colonization of bacteria to epithelial surfaces.

    e: Lysozyme from tears, saliva, and nasal secretions, catalyzes the hydrolysis of the peptidoglycan layer of bacteria.

54. **Answer c:**

Nuclear bag fibers are found in muscle and therefore do not belong to the group of cutaneous mechanoreceptors.

    a: Meissner's corpuscle is a cutaneous mechanoreceptor.

    b: Merkel's receptor is a cutaneous mechanoreceptor.

    d: Pacinian corpuscles are cutaneous mechanoreceptors.

    e: Ruffini's endings are cutaneous mechanoreceptors.

55. **Answer c:**

The oculomotor nerve is a pure motor nerve and does not contribute fibers to the spinal tract of nerve V.

    a: The facial nerve has some somatic afferent fibers from receptors in the skin of the external auditory meatus and a small patch of skin behind the auricle. The cell bodies are in the geniculate ganglion and the central processes enter the spinal trigeminal tract.

    b: The glossopharyngeal nerve supplies receptors in a small area of skin posterior to the auricle and the inner surface of the tympanic membrane. Central processes travel in the spinal tract of nerve V.

    d: Pain and temperature fibers from the face have their cell bodies in the trigeminal ganglion. Central processes enter the spinal tract of nerve V.

    e: The general sensory component of the vagus nerve supplies the skin of the external ear, external auditory canal, and surface of the tympanic membrane. Cell bodies are in the superior vagal ganglion. Central processes enter the spinal tract of nerve V.

56. **Answer b:**

BCG vaccination is not currently used in the United States.

    a: Therapy for all types of infections with mycobacteria is prolonged.

    c: Multiple antibiotics are administered simultaneously, because of the increasing problem of drug resistance.

    d: The usual isoniazid regimen for individuals exposed to *Mycobacterium tuberculosis* is 1 year.

    e: Control of *Mycobacterium bovis* infection in cattle herds does reduce human exposure.

57. **Answer d:**

The brachiocephalic veins lie most anteriorly within the superior mediastinum. There may also be some thymic remnants anterior to these veins.

    a: The trachea lies deep to the brachiocephalic trunk within the superior mediastinum.

    b: The brachiocephalic trunk is located between the left brachiocephalic vein anteriorly and the trachea posteriorly, within the superior mediastinum.

    c: The left common carotid artery arises from the aortic arch deep to the left brachiocephalic vein.

    e: The vagus nerves lie deep to the brachiocephalic veins, within the superior mediastinum.

58. **Answer c:**

Lymphatic capillaries selectively convey lipids away from the small intestine.

    a: Most proteins are carried away from the small intestine via capillaries.

    b: Most carbohydrates are carried away from the small intestine via capillaries.

    d: Steroids are not absorbed in significant amounts from the small intestine.

    e: Immunoglobulins are not absorbed in significant amounts from the small intestine.

59. **Answer b:**

The mitral valve is most often and severely affected by chronic rheumatic heart disease.

    a: The tricuspid valve is involved in only about 10% of cases, but usually only when the mitral valve and/or aortic valves are also involved.

c: The aortic valve is the *second* most commonly and severely affected valve in chronic rheumatic heart disease.

d: The pulmonic valve is rarely involved in chronic rheumatic heart disease.

e: Not all heart valves are affected equally. The mitral valve is the most often and severely affected valve. The aortic valve is the next most commonly involved valve. The tricuspid valve is involved in about 10% of cases but usually only when the mitral and/or aortic valves are also involved. The pulmonic valve is rarely involved.

60. **Answer a:**

The correct pairing is alpha$_1$ receptors with inositol triphosphate-diacylglycerol.

b: Alpha$_2$ receptors act via inhibiting adenylyl cyclase.

c: Beta-adrenergic receptors act via cAMP.

d: Beta-adrenergic receptors act via cAMP.

e: Beta-adrenergic receptors act via cAMP.

61. **Answer e:**

Figure 3 depicts a typical erythrocyte. Thus, the best response is the lumen of subcapsular sinus of lymph node, because it contains mostly mononuclear cells (lympohcytes and macro-phages). The four other choices all contain blood, the principal cell type of which is erythrocyte.

a: The right ventricle of the heart contains numerous erythrocytes and a relatively small number of white blood cells.

b: The lumen of a typical liver sinusoid contains many erythrocytes and a relatively small number of white blood cells.

c: The lumen of a typical splenic sinus contains many erythrocytes and a relatively small number of white blood cells.

d: The lumen of a typical renal arcuate artery contains many erythrocytes and a relatively small number of white blood cells.

62. **Answer c:**

The knee jerk is a simple reflex involving two neurons.

a, b, d, e: Chewing, coughing, locomotion, and swallowing are all complex movements, which have central pattern generators, which initiate the complex pattern of chained reflexes.

63. **Answer d:**

Penile tumescence is associated with REM sleep.

a: Bedwetting is associated with non-REM sleep.

b: A lowered arousal threshold is associated with non-REM sleep.

c: Night terrors are associated with non-REM sleep.

e: Sleep walking is associated with non-REM sleep.

64. **Answer c:**

Amatadine is an antiviral agent, which effects the dopaminergic system.

a: Carbidopa is not an antiviral agent; it inhibits DOPA decarboxylase.

b: Bromocriptine is a dopamine agonist with no antiviral effect.

d: L-DOPA is not antiviral; it is the precursor of dopamine.

e: Trihexyphenidyl is an anticholinergic antiparkinson drug with no antiviral effect.

65. **Answer b:**

Obstructive jaundice is caused by blockage in the bile drainage system. The smallest (terminal) components of that system is the bile canaliculus, which is created by adjacent hepatocytes that attach to one another via tight junctions. The obstruction eventually forces hepatocytes apart, rupturing their cell membranes and killing them.

a: Kupffer cells (liver macrophages) remain undamaged by obstructive jaundice.

c: Sinusoidal endothelial cells remain undamaged by obstructive jaundice.

d: Epithelial cells of Hering canals are not initially damaged when obstructive jaundice occurs. As obstructive jaundice worsens, larger components of the bile drainage system may be affected, which means that ducts of Hering and larger interlobular bile ducts may rupture, in turn, injuring or killing the epithelial cells that line them.

e: Fibroblasts in connective tissue of portal tracts remain undamaged by obstructive jaundice.

66. **Answer b:**

Diazepam administered intravenously is the drug of choice for immediate treatment of status epilepticus.

a: Triazolam has no particular anticonvulsive effect.

c: Clomipramine is a tricyclic antidepressant used for treatment of obsessive-compulsive disorder.

d: Naloxone is an opiate antagonist.

e: Fluphenazine is a potent antipsychotic.

67. **Answer e:**

Vulnerability theory hypothesizes that a combination of genetic and experiential factors must be present prior to the onset of a stressor for the stressor to result in a pathological reaction.

a: Double bind theory, an early concept regarding schizophrenia, associated the development of psychosis with a family environment in which the child received conflicting messages from a parent. Data supporting this theory has been limited.

b: The downward drift hypothesis refers to the theory that individuals with mental disorders slide down the socioeconomic scale as a result of their mental illness.

c: In contrast to the drift hypothesis, the social causation theory suggests that socioeconomic status is a significant contributor to the development of mental illness.

d: Attribution theory focuses on how individuals make internal and external attributions about the causes of behavior hypothesizing that individuals are likely to attribute their own behavior to situational causes but attribute others behavior to internal factors.

68. **Answer a:**

Macrophages synthesize and secrete a large variety of enzymes. However, they do not synthesize lipase, a lipid-degrading enzyme. An example of a cell type that does secrete lipase is the pancreatic acinar cell.

b: Macrophages secrete interleukin-1.

c: Macrophages secrete transforming growth factor (TGF).

d: Macrophages secrete acid phosphatase.

e: Macrophages secrete collagenase.

69. **Answer e:**

Taste fibers carried in the chorda tympani arise from neurons located in the geniculate ganglion of the facial nerve.

a: The superior cervical ganglion contains postganglionic sympathetic cell bodies.

b: The otic ganglion contains postganglionic parasympathetic cell bodies.

c: The pterygopalatine ganglion contains postganglionic parasympathetic cell bodies.

d: The ciliary ganglion contains postganglionic parasympathetic cell bodies.

70. **Answer b:**

A receptive field, by definition, is that area in which stimulation leads to activation of the receptor. Increasing stimulus intensity would not increase the receptive field of that receptor.

a: Increasing stimulation would cause a greater number of action potentials to be propagated.

c: Increasing stimulation would lead to a higher receptor potential amplitude.

d: Increasing stimulation would lead to a greater subjective sensation regarding the intensity of the stimulation.

71. **Answer c:**

A stroke affecting the left internal capsule is a lesion of the UMN so the signs will be opposite to the side of the lesion, because of the decussating pyramidal fibers. Signs of an UMN lesion include hyperactive deep tendon reflexes. These are the only signs that are on the correct side.

a: Babinski's reflex is an UMN sign, but this is on the wrong side.

b: Fasciculations are signs of an LMN lesion.

d: Increased tone is a UMN sign, but this is on the wrong side.

e: Telegraphic speech often accompanies a UMN lesion of the cortex, because of the involvement of Broca's area. However, this lesion did not involve Broca's area.

72. **Answer d:**

Lipopolysaccharides are heat stable.

a: Lipopolysaccharides contain lipid A.

b: Lipopolysaccharides contain a core polysaccharide.

c: Lipopolysaccharides are pyrogenic (cause fever production).

e: Lipopolysaccharides can activate complement cascade by the alternate pathway.

73. **Answer d:**

Ocular muscle is a fast muscle (twitch duration about $\frac{1}{10}$ of soleus), and fast muscles contain predominantly large fibers dependent on glycolysis for the immediate energy source for contraction.

a: Ocular muscle is a fast muscle that has large diameter fibers high in glycolytic capacity.

b: Ocular muscle is a fast muscle that contains relatively few mitochondria and is more dependent on glycolysis for energy than is slow muscle (soleus).

c: Ocular muscle is a fast muscle that has a relatively low capillary density and depends on glycolysis for energy.

e: Ocular muscle is a fast muscle that contains an extensive sarcoplasmic reticulum to support rapid provision of Ca^{2+} for fast contractile responses.

74. **Answer d:**

After a change in Na^+ in the diet, the kidney requires about 3 days to reestablish Na^+ balance; after an increase in Na^+ intake, there will be a positive Na^+ balance for 3 days and an increase in ECF volume.

a: An increase in plasma osmolality will stimulate thirst.

b: After an increase in Na^+ intake, aldosterone secretion decreases.

c: There is no reason under these conditions to expect a shift of K^+ into the intracellular fluid, and such a shift would, if anything, slightly decrease ECF volume.

e: Exchange of water between the interstitium and the plasma is determined by differences in oncotic pressure and hydrostatic pressure.

75. **Answer c:**

Systemic administration of a muscarinic stimulator produces relaxation of the trigone muscle, an increase in gastrointestinal activity, and an increase in blood flow to skeletal muscle.

a: Systemic administration of a muscarinic stimulator would not be expected to produce mydriasis, dry mouth, urinary retention, or hypotension.

b: Systemic administration of a muscarinic stimulator would not be expected to produce an increase in blood pressure, a decrease in heart rate, or mydriasis.

d: Systemic administration of a muscarinic stimulator would not be expected to produce salivation, sweating, or mydriasis.

e: Systemic administration of a muscarinic stimulator would not be expected to produce bronchodilation, increased bronchial secretion, or bradycardia.

76. **Answer d:**

Lithium is the first choice in the treatment of mild mania in maniac-depressive disorder.

a: Imipramine, a tricyclic antidepressant, might be used in the depressive phase.

b: Diazepam is a sedative/hypnotic.

c: Clomipramine, a tricyclic antidepressant, might be used in the depressive phase.

e: Doxepin, a tricyclic antidepressant, a might be used in the depressive phase.

77. **Answer b:**

Of the currently known hepatitis viruses, only hepatitis B has DNA as its genetic material. The other hepatitis viruses all have single-stranded RNA.

a: Hepatitis A has single-stranded RNA as its genetic material.

c: Hepatitis C has single-stranded RNA as its genetic material.

d: Hepatitis D has single-stranded RNA as its genetic material.

e: Hepatitis E has single-stranded RNA as its genetic material.

78. **Answer a:**

Cerebrospinal fluid flows directly from the 4th ventricle into the cisterna magna.

b: The cisterna magna is continuous with the cisterna pontis.

c: The interpeduncular cistern is found around the interpeduncular fossa.

d: The quadrigeminal cistern is found above the colliculi.

e: The suprasellar cistern is found above the sella turcica.

79. **Answer b:**

NADH dehydrogenase uses the cofactor flavin mononucleotide to transfer electrons from NADH to coenzyme Q.

a: The NAD/NADH pool serves a general oxidation function in the cell, and the NADP/NADPH pool provides reducing equivalents for biosynthetic synthetic reactions.

c: Only the terminal triphosphate for ATP is added during oxidative phosphorylation.

d: Electron transport uses several carriers: iron sulfur centers and flavin mononucleotide in NADH dehydrogenase, coenzyme Q, heme in each of the cytochromes, and copper in cytochrome oxidase.

e: Cyanide blocks the transfer of electrons from cytochrome oxidase to molecular oxygen.

80. **Answer c:**

Baclofen, a GABA derivative, stimulates the GABA$_B$ receptors, resulting in hyperpolarization.

a: Dantrolene interferes with excitation-contraction coupling in the muscle fibers.

b: Vecuronium is a steroid muscle relaxant.

d: Atracurium is an isoquinoline derivative.

e: Glycine is an amino acid with transmitter-modular function.

81. **Answer d:**

Reticulocytes do not possess nuclei and, therefore, are not capable of mitosis. The other four cell types possess nuclei. This is the only fact needed to answer the question correctly.

a: Proerythroblasts are relatively undifferentiated and mitotically active.

b: Basophilic erythroblasts are relatively undifferentiated and mitotically active.

c: Polychromatophilic erythroblasts are the last stage in erythrocyte development that is capable of mitosis.

e: Neutrophilic myelocytes are the last stage of neutrophil development that is capable of mitosis.

82. **Answer b:**

Diphtheria toxin does inactivate elongation factor 2.

a: Diphtheria toxin does not cause ADP-ribosylation of a membrane-bound G-protein leading to chloride secretion.

c: Diphtheria toxin is not an adenylate cyclase.

d: Diphtheria toxin plays no role in bacterial adhesion.

e: Diphtheria toxin is not an enterotoxin.

83. **Answer a:**

For reasons that are not well understood, the brain typically will undergo liquifaction necrosis rather than coagulation necrosis, when there is hypoxia severe enough to cause cell death.

b: Pancreas tissue undergoes coagulation necrosis under conditions of hypoxia.

c: Large intestine tissue undergoes coagulation necrosis under conditions of hypoxia.

d: Liver tissue undergoes coagulation necrosis under conditions of hypoxia.

e: Kidney tissue undergoes coagulation necrosis under conditions of hypoxia.

84. **Answer c:**

Addition of a known amount of radioactively labeled hormone to the unknown sample results in binding of the labeled hormone. The extent of binding of the labeled hormone depends on how much unlabeled hormone is present in the unknown to compete for binding with the labeled hormone.

a: The concentration is determined by measuring radioactivity, which is proportional to the amount of radioactive hormone added.

b: A standard curve is produced by adding varying amounts of unlabeled hormone to tubes containing labeled hormone and a limited amount of antibody.

d: Radioactive iodine is bound only by those hormones that are proteins or peptides; the iodine is bound to a sample of hormone used for the standard curve, not to the unknown. Other radioactive atoms are used for nonpeptide hormones.

e: If the antibody had a greater affinity for the unknown, the standard curve created with the known hormone would not give accurate results.

85. **Answer a:**

Multipolar neurons differentiate from neuroblasts rather than cardiac muscle cells.

b: Sinoatrial node cells are modified cardiac muscle cells that are smaller, have fewer myofibrils, and function to transmit nerve impulses (from the SA node to the arterioventricular (AV) node).

c: Purkinje fibers are modified cardiac muscle cells that are larger, have fewer myofibrils, and function to transmit nerve impulses throughout the ventricular myocardium.

d: AV node cells are modified cardiac muscle cells that are smaller, have fewer myofibrils, and function to transmit nerve impulses (from the SA node to the AV node).

e: Bundle of His cells are modified cardiac muscle cells that are larger, have fewer myofibrils, and function to transmit nerve impulses throughout the ventricular myocardium.

86. **Answer d:**

Osteoid osteoma is uncommonly painful for its small size (usually less than 2 cm in diameter). The pain is due to excess production of prostaglandin E2 and consequently is remarkably reduced by the administration of aspirin.

a: Osteoid carcinoma does frequently occur in the third and fourth decade of life.

b: Osteoid carcinoma is more frequent in males than females.

c: Osteoid carcinoma is usually found in the appendicular skeleton.

e: Osteoid carcinoma is readily cured by conservative surgery.

87. **Answer b:**

Axons from the pretectal area do not decussate in the anterior commissure. Instead, they decussate in the posterior commissure.

a: True. Axons in the brachium of the superior colliculus synapse in the pretectal area.

c: True. Axons from the nucleus of Edinger-Westphal terminate in the ciliary ganglion.

d: True. Ganglion cell axons terminate in the pretectal area.

e: True. Postganglionic parasympathetic axons originate from neurons in the ciliary ganglion.

88. **Answer b:**

Propranolol inhibits peripheral beta receptors, thus decreasing exercise tolerance, increasing airway resistance, and decreasing HDL levels.

89. **Answer d:**

Surfactant is synthesized by type II pneumocytes of the alveolar wall, not by capillary endothelium.

a: These are the main constituents of surfactant, although other lipids are present also.

b: This property of surfactant tends to prevent collapse of smaller alveoli.

c: Intermolecular repulsion between surfactant molecules in this lipid layer is responsible for decreasing surface tension.

e: Increasing pulmonary compliance reduces the work of breathing.

90. **Answer c:**

Chronic loss of blood supply to an organ may be a cause of atrophy. Sudden and virtually complete loss of blood supply will cause necrosis rather than atrophy.

a: Denervation of a skeletal muscle, as with injury to the brachial plexus, will cause a lack of tropic stimuli to the skeletal muscles that will, as a result, undergo atrophy.

b: Aging, for reasons that still are not well understood, is associated with multiple atrophic changes such as loss of muscle mass, brain weight, etc.

d: Casting of a limb causes atrophy of the skeletal muscle, since the tropic signals generated by work are absent.

e: Castration of either a male or female will result in the atrophy of the tissues that require specific hormonal support, for example the endometrium or the prostate.

91. **Answer b:**

Connective tissue has fewer cells and more intracellular substance than any of the other basic tissues.

92. **Answer b:**

The QRS complex corresponds to ventricular depolarization.

a: The P wave represents atrial depolarization.

c: The T wave represents ventricular repolarization.

d: The ST segment is the interval between ventricular depolarization and repolarization.

e: The P-P interval represents the interbeat interval.

93. **Answer e:**

Primitive mesenchymal cells are undifferentiated and thus functionally inactive. They do not synthesize significant amounts of protein for export, which is what occurs in cells that possess significant amounts of rER.

a: Plasma cells secrete a large amount of antibody, a protein that is exported.

b: Neurons secrete endorphins, enkephalins, gamma-aminobutyric acid, and glycine. These are peptide or protein neurotransmitters that are exported.

c: Osteoblasts secrete a large amount of tropocollagen, a precursor of type I collagen, a protein found in the extracellular matrix of all types of bone (e.g., spongy, compact, lamellar, woven, endochondral, intramembranous).

d: Young chondrocytes secrete a large amount of tropocollagen, a precursor of type II collagen, a protein present in the extracellular matrix of cartilage and especially hyaline cartilage.

94. **Answer e:**

Nystatin is not absorbed orally. It is given orally to suppress local *candida* infections; all nystatin taken orally is excreted in the feces.

a: True. Ketoconazole, an imidazole derivative, is clinically useful in a variety of systemic fungal diseases. It is given orally for systemic disease.

b: True. Amphotericin B is used for deep (systemic) mycotic infections. It is given intravenously when used for systemic disease.

c: True. Flucytosine is used for systemic mycotic infections. It is given orally when used for systemic disease.

d: True. Griseofulvin is used to treat mycoses of the skin, and it is given orally to treat skin and nail infections.

95.   **Answer a:**

Of the bullous diseases mentioned, only pemphigus vulgaris and its variants form vesicles by separation of the epidermis just above the basal layer.

b: In bullous pemphigoid, vessicles form between the epidermis and the dermis.

c: In junctional epidermolysis bullosa, vessicles form between the epidermis and the dermis.

d: In dermatitis herpetiformis, vessicles form between the epidermis and the dermis.

e: In dermolytic epidermolysis bullosa, vessicles form between the epidermis and the dermis.

96.   **Answer e:**

The leukemias and lymphomas involve the spleen fairly commonly, but it is distinctly unusual for any carcinoma to metastasize to the spleen.

a: Lymphocytic leukemia may metastasize to the spleen.

b: Granulocytic leukemia, as well as many other leukemias, may metastasize to the spleen.

c: Hodgkin's disease may metastasize to the spleen.

d: Lymphomas, such as non-Hodgkin's, commonly involve the spleen.

97.   **Answer e:**

A negative feedback loop exists that increases in portal venous bile salt concentration and inhibits bile salt synthesis.

a: Parasympathetic stimulation may increase bile salt secretion but has greater effects to stimulate gallbladder contraction.

b: Sympathetic stimulation will relax the gallbladder; it does not affect bile salt synthesis.

c: Cholecystokinin, as the name implies, stimulates gallbladder contraction.

d: Motilin is released from the intestinal mucosa; it stimulates gallbladder contraction.

98.   **Answer b:**

In most instances, the cystic artery arises as a branch of the right hepatic artery within the angle formed by the cystic duct and the common bile duct.

a: The cystic artery, infrequently, may arise as a branch of the left hepatic artery.

c: The left gastric artery supplies the inferior portion of the esophagus as well as the lesser curvature of the stomach.

d: The cystic artery, infrequently, may arise from the proper hepatic artery.

e: The three branches of the celiac trunk are the splenic, left gastric, and common hepatic arteries.

99.   **Answer b:**

Rationales are presented by enzyme instead of by answer choice.

1. DNA polymerase I follows DNA polymerase III, because it can digest out the RNA primer, an activity that the latter enzyme lacks.

2. DNA ligase forms the last phosphodiester bond between adjacent nucleotides of newly synthesized strands.

3. Helicase provides the single-stranded template for the primase to lay down the RNA primer.

4. Primase provides a double-stranded substrate for DNA polymerase III by synthesizing a 9-10 base primer.

5. DNA polymerase III continues synthesis from the primer until it meets the primer, which remains at the 5' end of the previous Okasaki fragment.

100.   **Answer d:**

Cleavage of the precursor 45S ribosomal RNA is done by specific endonucleases rather than spliceosomes. A 5.8S RNA is also produced.

a: Poly A is added only to the end of processed messenger RNA.

b: Spliceosomes are involved only with removal of introns from precursor messenger RNA.

c: Capping only occurs on processed messenger RNA.

e: Eukaryotic transfer RNA is not produced by processing precursor ribosomal RNA.

101.   **Answer d:**

Aminoacylation of tRNA requires ATP rather than GTP.

a: GTP forms a complex with EF-T$_u$ during binding of aminoacyl-tRNA to ribosomes.

b: GTP forms a complex with the initiation factors in the formation of 30S initiation complex.

c: GTP is required for the movement of the mRNA with the associated peptidyl tRNA from the A site to the P site.

e: The release factors require GTP to stimulate peptidyl transferase to release the peptide from tRNA at a termination codon.

102. **Answer e:**

Low serum levels of B_{12} are due to impaired intrinsic factor production.

a: The patient would have normal B_{12} levels and absorption.

b: B_{12} absorption would not be impaired.

c: The key information is low B_{12} levels.

d: If there is no problem with the absorption of the complex, a receptor-transport defect cannot be the cause.

103. **Answer e:**

Trichomoniasis is usually acquired by sexual intercourse.

a: Toxoplasmosis is usually acquired by ingestion of improperly cooked meats or by ingestion of infective oocytes from cat fecal contamination.

b: Bancroftian filariasis is acquired by the bite of a mosquito.

c: Chagas' disease is transmitted by the "kissing" bug.

d: Taeniasis is acquired by eating undercooked beef, pork, or fish.

104. **Answer b:**

Histoplasmosis is commonly associated with the excreta of bats and birds (most often starlings and chickens).

a: *Sporothrix schenckii* is usually acquired from a splinter or thorn.

c: *Coccidioides immitis* is a soil organism, usually transmitted via aerosol.

d: *Candida albicans* is part of the normal flora of humans.

e: *Aspergillus fumigatus* is common in the environment and is usually transmitted via aerosol.

105. **Answer b:**

Buspirone has no hypnotic, anticonvulsant, or muscle relaxation properties, and has minimal abuse liabilities.

a: Midazolam and phenobarbital have CNS-depressant effects and may develop cross tolerance.

c: Triazolam and ethanol have CNS-depressant effects and may develop cross tolerance.

d: Diazepam and thiopental have CNS-depressant effects and may develop cross tolerance.

e: Phenobarbital and ethanol have CNS-depressant effects and may develop cross tolerance.

106. **Answer d:**

Stomatitis, bleeding gums, tremor, and emotional depression are characteristic of mercury poisoning.

a: Exposure to phosphorous (white) would not cause stomatitis, bleeding gums, or CNS effects.

b: Elemental phosphorus may cause skin damage.

c: Nitroglycerin evokes cardiovascular symptoms.

e: Picric acid causes skin damage.

107. **Answer c:**

Type A lesions involve the ascending aorta and are the more dangerous form of this disease. They may be limited to the ascending aorta or may extend into the descending aorta as well. Type B lesions involve only the descending aorta.

108. **Answer b:**

Von Willibrand factor (VWF) is synthesized by megakaryocyte and endothelial cells. It is found in the Weibel-Palade bodies in the cytoplasm of endothelial cells. Endothelial cells release VWF into both the plasma and the subendothelial tissue.

109. **Answer d:**

The reducing equivalents from NADH are transferred to oxaloacetate to produce malate in the cytoplasm; malate is transported across the mitochondrial membrane and then oxidized producing NADH and oxaloacetate in the mitochondrial matrix. This is known as the malate-aspartate shuttle.

a: The Cori cycle describes the conversion of lactate, which is produced in exercising muscle and red blood cells, back into glucose in the liver for redistribution to the tissues. It does not involve the shuttle of NADH equivalents into the mitochondrion.

b: Diffusion of protons into the mitochondrion does occur as a part of the process of oxidative phosphorylation, but it does not contribute to the shuttle of NADH equivalents into the mitochondrion.

c: ATP is used to transport many types of molecules across membranes, especially up a concentration gradient, but not for the shuttle of NADH equivalents into the mitochondrion.

e: There is no NADH transporter protein.

110. **Answer e:**

Campylobacter jejuni rarely causes an opportunistic and fatal septicemia.

a: *Campylobacter jejuni* is one of the leading causes of enteric disease in humans.

b: All age groups are affected by *Campylobacter jejuni.*

c: Human to human fecal-oral spread does occur.

d: Contaminated milk, water, and food are common sources of infection.

111. **Answer d:**

Chlortetracycline is bound in the enamel of young children and causes discoloration.

a: Infants do not tolerate chloramphenicol as well.

b: Chlortetracycline and phenylalanine are not related.

c: Sulfonamides compete with PABA.

e: Both chlortetracycline and chloramphenicol are broad-spectrum antibiotics.

112. **Answer a:**

Monovalent anions such as perchlorate can block uptake of iodide by the thyroid gland through competitive inhibition of the iodide transport mechanism.

b: Propylthiouracil inhibits hormone synthesis by blocking organification of iodide, not through "trapping."

c: Probenecid has no effect on iodide "trapping."

d: Colchicine has no effect on iodide "trapping."

e: Estrogen has no effect on iodide "trapping."

113. **Answer d:**

NaCl reabsorption by the thick ascending limb of the loop establishes the normal high interstitial osmolality of the medulla. Urine osmolality is determined by equilibration with the medullary interstitium.

a: Aldosterone stimulates Na^+ reabsorption by the collecting duct. At normal levels of ADH, urine osmolalilty is determined by water reabsorption along an osmotic gradient into the medullary interstitium.

b: Increasing urine flow will wash out the medullary interstitial hyperosmolality and prevent an increase in urine osmolality.

c: Increasing medullary blood flow will remove solutes from the renal medulla, lowering its osmolality and therefore the osmolality of the insterstitium and the urine.

e: Angiotensin II stimulates Na^+ reabsorption directly in the proximal tubule; this reabsorption is nearly isosmotic and will have little effect on urine osmolality.

114. **Answer b:**

The hypoglossal nerve exits in the preolivary sulcus.

a: The abducens nerve exits in the pontomedullary groove.

c: The oculomotor nerve exits in the interpeduncular fossa.

d: The trochlear nerve exits from the anterior medullary velum.

e: The vagus nerve exits from the postolivary sulcus.

115. **Answer b:**

Chlamydia trachomatis may cause pneumonia in infants.

a: Both *Chlamydia trachomatis* and *Neisseria gonorrhoeae* may cause urethritis.

c: Both *Chlamydia trachomatis* and *Neisseria gonorrhoeae* may cause neonatal conjunctivitis.

d: Infection by *Chlamydia trachomatis* is not usually asymptomatic.

e: Both *Chlamydia trachomatis* and *Neisseria gonorrhoeae* may be associated with pelvic inflammatory disease.

116. **Answer c:**

Amoxapine is a metabolite of the antipsychotic drug loxapine and retains some of its antipsychotic action.

a: Trazodone is a heterocyclic antidepressant with no antipsychotic action.

b: Fluoxetine is a selective serotonin uptake inhibitor antidepressant with no antipsychotic action.

d: Amitriptyline is a tricyclic antidepressant with no antipsychotic action.

e: Imipramine is a tricyclic antidepressant with no antipsychotic action.

117. **Answer c:**

The tricyclic antidepressants do not directly influence renal functions.

a: Coma is a possible toxic effect.

b: Cardiac arrhythmias are a possible toxic effect.

d: Agitation or delirium is a possible toxic effect.

e: Respiratory depression is a possible toxic effect.

118. **Answer a:**

Postganglionic sympathetic nerve fibers form a plexus along the internal carotid artery.

b: Preganglionic sympathetic fibers destined for the head and neck synapse on postganglionic sympathetic neurons in the cervical sympathetic ganglia.

c: Preganglionic parasympathetic fibers of the head and neck do not form plexuses along the internal carotid artery.

d: Postganglionic parasympathetic fibers of the head and neck arise from neurons within the four parasympathetic ganglia and are distributed via specific nerves.

e: The nerve fibers forming a plexus along the internal carotid artery belong to the autonomic nervous system.

119. **Answer a:**

A-alpha fibers are axons of muscle spindle primaries and Golgi tendon organs and would not be found in a cutaneous nerve.

b: A-beta fibers are axons innervating the Meissner's, Pacinian, Ruffini's, and Merkel's corpuscles and would be found in a cutaneous nerve.

c: A-delta fibers are axons of mechanical and thermal nociceptors and would be found in a cutaneous nerve.

d: C fibers are axons of thermal, mechanothermal, and polymodal nociceptors and would be found in a cutaneous nerve.

e: D fibers do not exist.

120. **Answer d:**

Visual agnosia is a nonlanguage associative disorder in which objects cannot be recognized by sight alone. The patient requires input from another sense to make the identification.

a: Broca's aphasia is a disorder in which the speech is sparse, telegraphic, and nonfluent. Comprehension is relatively preserved.

b: Patients with a conduction aphasia have preserved comprehension but impaired retention.

c: Transcortical sensory aphasia is due to lesions of the angular gyrus. Patients often repeat or paraphrase the question, then discusses another topic. Often the patients are agitated and are most easily diagnosed as psychotic.

e: Patients with Wernicke's aphasia have fluent speech with intact rhythm and melody, but the speech is empty, devoid of meaningful substantive words. These patients have impaired repetition and comprehension of even their own speech.

121. **Answer d:**

Rhubarb contains oxalic acid.

a: Phenol or carbolic acid is not found in rhubarb.

b: Muscarine is not found in rhubarb.

c: Formaldehyde is not found in rhubarb.

e: Boric acid is not found in rhubarb.

122. **Answer c:**

Early in the proximal tubule the main anion reabsorbed with Na^+ is HCO_3^-. Water follows the Na^+ and HCO_3^-, raising the Cl^- concentration to create a gradient for Cl^- diffusion.

a: There is no primary Cl^- ATPase in the renal tubules.

b: Coupling of Na^+ and Cl^- for reabsorption may occur but at the luminal membrane.

d: Secondary active cotransport of $2Na^+$, $1K^+$ and $1Cl^-$ across the luminal membrane is the major mechanism for Cl^- reabsorption in the thick ascending limb of the loop of Henle.

e: A minor mechanism for Cl^- reabsorption may occur via exchange with formate; lactate is reabsorbed by cotransport with Na^+.

123. **Answer d:**

MAP = CO × TPR; for arterial pressure to increase, cardiac output must increase more than total peripheral resistance decreases.

a: Baroreceptors reset to defend the higher pressure.

b: It is the other way around: the increase in both MAP and vasodilation of muscular arterioles contribute to the increase in muscle blood flow.

c: Increased activity of the muscle pump acts to increase venous return, permitting an increase in cardiac output, but not directly influencing MAP.

e: Increased sympathetic activity during exercise increases cardiac output.

124. **Answer e:**

Deletion of the long arm of chromosome 11 causes loss of the area of the chromosome that contains the WT-1 gene, a tumor-suppresser gene. Lack of this gene is associated with an increase in the incidence of Wilm's tumors. These children also have aniridia, male genital abnormalities, and development of gonadoblastoma.

a: 47 (XY, +18) is trisomy 18. These children have micro-gnathia, congenital heart disease, horseshoe kidney, and deformed fingers.

b: 47 (XY, +21) is trisomy 21, classic Down syndrome.

c: 47 (XY, +13) is trisomy 13. These children have persistence of fetal hemoglobin, polycystic kidneys, polydactyly, congenital heart disease, and microcephaly.

d: 46 (XY, 5p−) is deletion of the short arm of chromosome 5, *Cri du chat* syndrome. These children have low birth weight, a strange cat-like cry, microcephaly, epicanthic folds, congenital heart disease, and abnormalities of the hands and feet.

125. **Answer c:**

Haploid sperm cells (spermatids) have completed the second meiotic division and thus can not undergo further division either by mitosis or meiosis.

a: The Golgi phase is first stage of spermiogenesis.

b: The cap phase is the second stage of spermiogenesis.

d: The acrosome phase is the third stage of spermiogenesis.

e: The maturation phase is the final stage of spermiogenesis.

126. **Answer b:**

When a skeletal muscle cell relaxes, the I band increases in width.

a: When a skeletal muscle cell relaxes, the A band remains the same width.

c: When a skeletal muscle cell relaxes, the Z band remains the same width.

d: When a skeletal muscle cell relaxes, the H band increases in width.

e: When a skeletal muscle cell relaxes, the sarcomere increases in width.

127. **Answer c:**

Hypotonia is not exhibited by patients with Parkinson's disease.

a: Bradykinesia (slowness of movement) is common in patients with Parkinson's disease.

b: Cogwheel rigidity is common in patients with Parkinson's disease.

d: Resting tremor is common in patients with Parkinson's disease..

e: Shuffling gait is common in patients with Parkinson's disease.

128. **Answer d:**

The superior colliculus sends visual information to the upper cervical cord through the crossed tectospinal tract.

a: The central caudal nucleus innervates the levator palpebrae superioris muscle.

b: The medial geniculate nucleus is a relay nucleus in the auditory pathway.

c: The red nucleus gives rise to the crossed rubrospinal tract and the uncrossed rubroolivary tract.

e: The trochlear nucleus gives rise to the trochlear nerve, which innervates the superior oblique muscle.

129. **Answer e:**

The sphincter ani internus muscle is composed of smooth muscle fibers and is under involuntary or autonomic control.

a: The levator ani muscle is formed of skeletal muscle fibers and is under voluntary control.

b: The bulbospongiosus muscle of the male and female is composed of skeletal muscle fibers and is under voluntary control.

c: The ischiocavernosus muscles of the male and female are composed of skeletal muscle fibers and are under voluntary control.

d: The superficial transverse perinei muscles are small striated muscles and are under voluntary control.

130. **Answer d:**

The single characteristic finding in any stage of syphilis infection is obliterative endarteritis and a chronic inflammatory infiltrate that is especially rich in plasma cells. The organisms are often very difficult to demonstrate and generally require the use of special silver stains.

a: Acute inflammation with liquifactive necrosis is not associated with syphilis.

b: Tuberculoid granuloma is not associated with syphilis.

c: Diffuse lymphatic infiltrate within the lesion is not an indication of syphilis.

e: Large colonies of visible organisms within the lesion is not an indication of syphilis.

131. **Answer d:**

An increase in stroke volume with no change in end-diastolic volume means ejection fraction is increased (i.e., cardiac contractility is increased).

a: Starling's law of the heart would predict that an increase in stroke volume is related to an increase in end-diastolic volume.

b: The effect described is an increase in contractility opposite to the parasympathetic effects on the heart.

c: The effect described is an increase in contractility. Decreased sympathetic activity would decrease contractility.

e: The effect described is an increase in contractility.

132. **Answer c:**

The hepatic veins arise within the substance of the liver and drain into the inferior vena cava.

a: The portal vein returns venous blood from the portal circulation to the liver. Blood in the portal vein will eventually reach the hepatic veins within the liver.

b: The inferior mesenteric vein is a tributary of the hepatic portal vein.

d: The azygos vein returns venous blood to the superior vena cava.

e: The middle colic vein is a tributary of the superior mesenteric vein.

133. **Answer e:**

The usual pathologic lesions in delayed-type hypersensitivity are perivascular cellular infiltrates and edema.

a: True. The onset following antigen challenge is usually 24-28 hours.

b: True. The effector cells are CD4$^+$ T cells and/or macrophages.

c: True. The effector molecules are cytokines.

d: True. Delayed-type hypersensitivity may be transferred to animals by lymphocytes.

134. **Answer d:**

The inferior rectal nerves arise as branches of the pudendal nerves within the ischioanal fossa.

a: Spinal cord segments S2-S4 contain the preganglionic parasympathetic cell bodies, whose axons travel in the pelvic splanchnic nerves.

b: Preganglionic parasympathetic fibers within the pelvic splanchnic nerves are destined for the rectum, sigmoid colon, descending colon, and terminal portion of the transverse colon.

c: General visceral efferent (preganglionic parasympathetic) fibers of the pelvic splanchnic nerves will synapse on postganglionic neurons in the wall of the sigmoid colon.

e: The pelvic splanchnic nerves also carry afferent fibers to the CNS, e.g., pain fibers from the wall of the urinary bladder.

135. **Answer a:**

The atrioventricular pressure difference will be greatest early in diastole, so most filling occurs in the first third of diastole.

a: Later in diastole the pressure difference between atria and ventricle will be lessened, compared to earlier in diastole.

c: During isovolumetric contraction, the A-V valves are closed and no filling occurs.

d: During isovolumetric relaxation, the A-V valves are closed and no filling occurs.

e: The A-V valves are closed during ejection, and blood is exiting through the aorta and pulmonary artery.

136. **Answer e:**

Chronic lymphocytic leukemia is not associated with hepatic vein thrombosis. The common thread among the other conditions mentioned is either a tendency toward thrombosis (polycythemia, pregnancy, oral contraceptives) or slowed blood flow (hepatocellular carcinoma). On the other hand, about one third of cases have no discernible antecedent cause.

a: With polycythemia, there is a tendency toward thrombosis which can lead to Budd-Chiari syndrome.

b: In pregnancy, there is a tendency toward thrombosis which can lead to Budd-Chiari syndrome.

c: Use of oral contraceptives can cause thrombosis which can lead to Budd-Chiari syndrome.

d: With hepatocellular carcinoma, blood flow is slowed. This can lead to Budd-Chiari syndrome.

137. **Answer e:**

Richter's syndrome is a large cell immunoblastic lymphoma that develops as a complication of B cell chronic lymphocytic leukemia in about 5% of cases.

a: The peripheral white count may be normal in acute myelogenous leukemia.

b: Acute myelogenous leukemia can be fatal in less than 2 months.

c: Major clinical problems of acute myelogenous leukemia include neutropenia, anemia, and thrombocytopenia.

d: Discrete tumor masses may form in bones, soft tissues and lymph nodes.

138. **Answer b:**

Transduction requires bacteriophages as mediators of gene transfer.

a: Conjugation requires physical contact between "mating" bacteria in order for gene transfer to take place.

c: Transfection is the infection of a cell with purified viral nucleic acid, which results in replication of the virus.

d: Transformation is the transfer of free nucleic acid between bacterial cells and does not require a vector.

e: Lysogeny is the integration of viral nucleic acid into the bacterial chromosome.

139. **Answer b:**

Increased, not decreased, osmotic pressure causes thirst.

a: Decreased extracellular fluid volume causes thirst.

c: Lesions of the supraoptic nucleus destroy the neurons that make antidiuretic hormone. This lesions leads to diabetes insipidus and unbearable thirst.

d: Heavy salt intake causes thirst.

e: Loss of blood causes thirst.

140. **Answer a:**

Alpha motor neurons innervating the hand would be in the most lateral portion of the anterior horn at these levels.

b: These are the correct spinal levels but the wrong horn.

c: Lissauer's tract contains axons entering the cord that carries sensory information.

d: Nucleus proprius is in the dorsal horn.

e: The substantia gelatinosa is also in the dorsal horn.

141. **Answer b:**

The flexor hallucis longus tendon is the most posterior structure located deep to the flexor retinaculum.

a: The flexor digitorum longus tendon lies between the tendon of the tibialis posterior and the posterior tibial artery in this location.

c: The posterior tibial artery lies between the tendon of the flexor digitorum longus and the tibial nerve in this location.

d: The tibial nerve lies between the posterior tibial artery and the tendon of the flexor hallucis longus in this location.

e: The tendon of the tibialis posterior muscle is the most anterior structure located deep to the flexor retinaculum.

142. **Answer c:**

The ECA demonstrated that one out of three American adults had experienced a psychiatric disorder at some time in their life and 20% had an active disorder at the time of the assessment. The most common disorders were phobias and alcohol abuse with 14.3% of adults having had a phobia at some point in their life (9% within the year of assessment) and 13.8% having abused alcohol during the life span (6% in the current year).

a: The ECA estimates the lifetime occurrence of dysthymia as 3.3% and somatization as 0.1%

b: The prevalence of schizophrenia and mania were estimated at 1.5% and 0.8% respectively.

d: Although drug abuse (6.2%) was a common problem, it occurred significantly less frequently than alcohol abuse. Antisocial personality disorder was estimated at 2.6%

e: Common problems in primary care settings, major depression (6.4%) and panic (1.6%), were still less frequent than phobia and alcohol abuse.

143. **Answer d:**

Propranolol is a beta blocker and therefore decreases the force of the contraction of the muscle of the heart.

a: Because propranolol is a beta blocker, it is useful in treating ventricular arrythmias.

b: Propranolol, a beta blocker, does depress cardiac pacemaker activity.

c: Propranolol blocks catecholamine-induced bronchial dilation.

e: Propranolol reduces the incidence of catecholamine-induced hyperglycemia.

144. **Answer d:**

Prostatic hyperplasia usually occurs in a different anatomic location in the prostate than does adenocarcinoma. It is virtually a universal finding in older males, and other than both diseases being found in males who are beyond middle age, there is no convincing statistical evidence that the two disease are related.

a: True. Nodular hyperplasia does occur in the preprostatic region, proximal to the vena montanum.
b: True. Nodular hyperplasia is thought to be mediated by dihydrotestosterone.
c: True. Nodular hyperplasia does not occur in eunuchs.
e: True. Nodular hyperplasia is a virtually universal finding is older males.

145. **Answer d:**

Wuchereria bancrofti is not found in the United States. It is found in central Africa, many parts of Asia, the Philippines, Central and South America, Trinidad, Surinam, and Panama.

a: *Necator americanus* is found in southern parts of the United States.
b: *Enterobius vermicularis* is the most common helminth infection in North America.
c: *Trichuris trichiura* is found world-wide.
e: *Trichinella spiralis* is found world-wide and is very common in the United States.

146. **Answer b:**

When left ventricular pressure exceeds aortic pressure, the pressure gradient favors opening of the aortic valve.

a: The isovolumetric relaxation period occurs at the beginning of diastole, before the atrioventricular valve opens.
c: As left ventricular pressure decreases below left atrial pressure, the atrioventricular valve opens and the ventricle begins to fill.
d: The right ventricle begins to fill at the beginning of diastole, and the aortic valve opens early in systole.
e: If aortic diastolic arterial pressure exceeds left ventricular pressure, the aortic valve will be closed.

147. **Answer c:**

This choice describes how an increase in activity of the sympathetic nerves increases heart rate (in concert with a decrease in parasympathetic activity).

a: Increased sympathetic nervous activity decreases the duration of systole by increasing the rate of the Ca^{2+} reuptake by the sarcoplasmic reticulum.

b: Increased sympathetic nervous activity generally causes vasoconstriction.
d: Increased sympathetic nervous activity increases ventricular contractility.
e: Increased sympathetic nervous activity stimulates renin secretion from the juxtaglomerular cells.

148. **Answer d:**

Squamous cell carcinoma in sun-damaged skin is a remarkably indolent tumor. Less than 2% will metastasize to the regional lymph nodes. Squamous cell carcinoma, which arises in foci of deep scarring such as burn scars or sinus tracts, has a much higher incidence of metastasis.

a: True. Squamous cell carcinoma in sun-exposed skin does tend to be raised lesions with rolled pearly edges.
b: Squamous cell carcinoma in sun-exposed skin does tend to be histologically well differentiated.
c: Squamous cell carcinoma in sun-exposed skin does readily metastasize to lymph nodes.
e: Squamous cell carcinoma in sun-exposed skin is rare in black-skinned people.

149. **Answer b:**

Opening slow Ca^{2+} channels allows diffusion of Ca^{2+} into the microtubules, initiating release of Ca^{2+} from the sarcoplasmic reticulum.

a: Norepinephrine activates adenylyl cyclase.
c: Norepinephrine stimulates Ca^{2+} uptake into the sarcoplasmic reticulum.
d: There is no direct effect of epinephrine on actin synthesis, and actin synthesis is not directly related to cardiac contractility.
e: Increasing the rate of depolarization increases heart rate but not contractility.

150. **Answer a:**

Drug A's effect is practically reversed after drug B and abolished after drugs B and C together, thus drug A should act on two distinctive receptors. The only drug on the list that stimulates two receptors is epinephrine (alpha and beta).

b: Drug A's effect is practically reversed after drug B and abolished after drugs B and C together, thus drug A should act on two distinctive receptors. Isoproterenol stimulates only beta receptors, and its initial action would decrease blood pressure.
c: Drug A's effect is practically reversed after drug B and abolished after drug B and C together, thus drug A should act on two distinctive receptors. Phenylephrine stimulates only alpha receptors.

d: Drug A's effect is practically reversed after drug B and abolished after drugs B and C together, thus drug A should act on two distinctive receptors. Terbutaline stimulates only beta$_2$ receptors.

e: Drug A's effect is practically reversed after drug B and abolished after drugs B and C together, thus drug A should act on two distinctive receptors. Clonidine stimulates only alpha (alpha$_2$) receptors.

151. **Answer a:**

Drug A's effect is practically reversed after drug B, thus drug B should be an alpha receptor inhibitor. The only one on the list is phentolamine.

b: Drug A's effect is practically reversed after drug B, thus drug B should be an alpha receptor inhibitor. Scopolamine is a muscarinic antagonist.

c: Drug A's effect is practically reversed after drug B, thus drug B should be an alpha receptor inhibitor. Propranolol is a beta blocker.

d: Drug A's effect is practically reversed after drug B, thus drug B should be an alpha receptor inhibitor. Hexamethonium is a ganglionic blocker.

e: Drug A's effect is practically reversed after drug B, thus drug B should be an alpha receptor inhibitor. Timolol is a beta blocker.

152. **Answer d:**

Drug A's effect is practically reversed after drug B, and completely abolished after C (B and C together) thus drug C should be a beta receptor inhibitor. The only one on the list is timolol.

a: Drug A's effect is practically reversed after drug B, and completely abolished after C (B and C together) thus drug C should be a beta receptor inhibitor. Acetylcholine is a cholinergic antagonist.

b: Drug A's effect is practically reversed after drug B, and completely abolished after C (B and C together) thus drug C should be a beta receptor inhibitor. Prazosin is an alpha$_1$ blocker.

c: Drug A's effect is practically reversed after drug B, and completely abolished after C (B and C together) thus drug C should be a beta receptor inhibitor. Phenylephrine is an alpha agonist.

e: Drug A's effect is practically reversed after drug B, and completely abolished after C (B and C together) thus drug C should be a beta receptor inhibitor. Phentolamine is an alpha blocker.

153. **Answer e:**

Drug A's effect is practically reversed after drug B and completely abolished after C (B and C together) thus drug C should be a beta receptor inhibitor. Nonselective beta blockers, as well as selective beta$_1$ blockers, may exert negative inotropic effect.

154. **Answer c:**

The peroneus longus muscle belongs to the lateral compartment of the leg and functions to plantarflex and evert the foot.

a: The extensor digitorum longus is a muscle of the anterior compartment of the leg that dorsiflexes the foot.

b: The extensor hallucis longus is a muscle of the anterior compartment that extends the great toe and aids in dorsiflexion of the foot.

d: The peroneus tertius muscle belongs to the anterior compartment of the leg and inserts on the base of the fifth and fourth metatarsals. It aids in eversion and dorsiflexion of the foot.

e: Contraction of the tibialis anterior muscle of the anterior compartment of the leg results in dorsiflexion and inversion of the foot.

155. **Answer b:**

Chief cells secrete pepsinogen, an inactive precursor of the proteolytic enzyme, pepsin.

a: Serous cells in the lacrimal gland synthesize and secrete lysozyme.

c: Serous cells in the submandibular gland synthesize and secrete lysozyme.

d: Paneth cells, most of which are located in the small intestine, synthesize and secrete lysozyme.

e: Neutrophils synthesize and secrete lysozyme.

156. **Answer a:**

Auditory input is not directly used to regulated normal posture.

b: Muscle and joint receptor input from the limbs is important in posture.

c: Receptors in cervical ligaments and neck muscles are important in posture.

d: The vestibular system is very important in postural mechanisms.

e: The visual system is an important source of information in regulating posture.

157. **Answer e:**

Hyperlipidemia, hypertension, diabetes, and smoking are all firmly established risk factors for the development of atherosclerosis. Mönckeberg's arteriosclerosis is the deposition of calcium within the media of medium to small arteries. It does not cause narrowing of the arterial lumen and is thought to be of little clinical significance.

a: Hyperlipidemia is a known risk factor for the development of atherosclerosis.

b: Hypertension is a known risk factor for the development of atherosclerosis.

c: Diabetes is a known risk factor for the development of atherosclerosis.

d: Cigarette smoking is a known risk factor for the development of atherosclerosis.

158. **Answer d:**

The oculomotor nerve usually exits between the superior cerebellar and posterior cerebral arteries.

a: The abducens nerve exits in the groove between the medulla and pons.

b: The facial nerve exits in the cerebello-medullo pontine angle.

c: The glossopharyngeal nerve exits in the postolivary sulcus.

e: The trochlear nerve exits dorsally from the brainstem.

159. **Answer d:**

Diffusion of a cation into the cell will depolarize the membrane potential, making it less negative.

a: The permeability to K^+ is the highest of these three ions, which explains why the resting membrane potential is close to the Nernst potential for K^+.

b: Diffusion of an anion into the cell would make the potential more negative; the electrical gradient will oppose diffusion of Cl^- into the cell.

c: K^+ is transported actively into the cell.

e: There is not pacemaker potential in skeletal muscle.

160. **Answer b:**

The fact that creatinine clearance before cimetidine was greater than inulin clearance indicates net secretion of creatinine; the most likely explanation for the decrease in creatinine clearance is then competition for transport.

a: This is by definition an increase in creatinine clearance.

c: This process might occur but would not account for the change in creatinine clearance.

d: An increase in blood flow would not result in a decrease in clearance for a solute (creatinine) that undergoes tubular secretion.

e: An increase in glomerular capillary hydrostatic pressure would increase the glomerular filtration rate, increasing creatinine clearance.

161. **Answer e:**

There are many signs that this patient has increased secretion of growth hormone (coarse skin, enlargement of the bones of the face and hands). The bitemporal hemianopsia, along with gradual worsening of the visual impairment and the headache, would indicate that this is a tumor impinging on the optic chiasm.

a: Patients with diabetes insipidus would have complaints about constant thirst and very frequent voiding.

b: The patient's signs and symptoms are not consistent with a gonadotrophin-secreting tumor.

c: The patient's signs and symptoms are not consistent with hyperthyroidism.

d: The patient's signs and symptoms are not consistent with primary hypothyroidism.

162. **Answer a:**

The internal pudendal artery and vein are closely related to the ischial spine and are at risk when sutures are placed in the sacrospinous ligament. Sutures placed as such must be located a safe distance from the ischial spine, to which the ligament is attached.

b: The superior gluteal vessels are located too far superiorly to be at risk in this procedure.

c: The obturator vessels are located too far laterally to be at risk in this procedure.

d: The lateral sacral vessels are located too far posteromedially to be at risk in this procedure.

e: The uterine vessels arise too far anteriorly to be a risk during this procedure.

163. **Answer b:**

Peptides that bind to Class II molecules are processed in acidic endosomes or lysosomes, not in the cytoplasm.

a, c, d, e: These are the recognized steps in Class II MHC-associated antigen presentation. Prior to step E, there is expression of peptide-MHC complexes on the cell surface.

164. **Answer b:**

Normal conversational speech in a noisy office or restaurant is 60 to 70 decibels.

a: 10 to 20 decibels is the range for whispers in a quiet dwelling.

c: 100 to 110 decibels is the range for hearing discomfort.

d: 140 to 150 decibels is the threshold for pain.

e: 180 to 200 decibels can cause permanent hearing loss.

165. **Answer c:**

Many of the axons of the ascending reticular activating system terminate in the intralaminar nuclei, e.g, centromedian and centrolateral nuclei.

a: The anterior nucleus is part of the limbic pathway and receives its major input from the mammillary bodies.

b: The dorsomedial nucleus receives its major input from the amygdala, olfactory, and hypothalamic areas.

d: The nucleus basalis of Meynert is not involved.

e: The septal nuclei are not involved.

166. **Answer d:**

The lymphatic drainage of the ascending colon is to the superior mesenteric lymph nodes.

a: The lymphatic drainage of the ureters is to the lumbar (lateral aortic) lymph nodes.

b: The lymphatic drainage of the testes is to the lumbar (lateral aortic) lymph nodes.

c: The lymphatic drainage of the descending colon is to the lumbar (lateral aortic) lymph nodes.

e: The lymphatic drainage of the uterine tubes follows that of the ovaries to the lumbar (lateral aortic) lymph nodes.

167. **Answer e:**

Cancers of the left colon may be symptomatic, because they cause obstruction fairly early in the course of the disease. This is mainly due to a combination of the small caliber of the left colon and the stool becoming more solid as it progresses through the length of the colon.

a: True. Adenocarcinomas do arise largely from adenomatous polyps.

b: True. Diet is a significant risk factor in colorectal carcinoma.

c: True. Loss of multiple suppressor genes is required to develop colon cancer.

d: True. Chronic ulcerative colitis is a predisposing condition for colon cancer.

168. **Answer b:**

In Whipple's disease the lamina propria mucosa of the gut contains large numbers of macrophages. The macrophages are stuffed with PAS-positive bacilliary forms. Similar findings are seen in mesenteric lymph nodes and occasionally in synovial membranes, the brain, and the cardiac valves. Recently, using molecular biologic methods, the bacillary forms have been identified as an actinomycete, *Tropheryma whippelii*. Patient's with Whipple's disease characteristically have malabsorption with diarrhea and weight loss. On occasion they may have polyarthritis and ill-defined CNS complaints. Remarkably, despite the numbers of organisms present, inflammation is virtually absent.

a: Tropical sprue is not associated with large numbers of macrophages containing masses and PAS positive bacilli in the lamina propria.

c: Non-tropical sprue is not associated with large number of macrophages containing masses of PAS positive bacilli in the lamina propria.

d: Protein losing enteropathy is not associated with large numbers of macrophages containing masses of PAS positive bacilli in the lamina propria.

e: Bacterial overgrowth syndrome is not associated with large numbers of macrophages containing masses of PAS positive bacilli in the lamina propria.

169. **Answer a:**

The polyenes bind firmly to ergosterol in the fungal cell membrane and form pores that result in the loss of cellular macromolecules and ions.

b: Imidazole derivatives inhibit the synthesis of fungal lipids.

c: Imidazole derivatives inhibit the synthesis of fungal lipids.

d: Flucytstosine inhibits thymidylate synthetase.

e: Griseofulvin probably interferes with microtubule function.

170. **Answer d:**

Parasympathetic stimulation is the most powerful mechanism for stimulating salivary secretion, including secretion of amylase and mucin.

a: Blood flow is stimulated by parasympathetic stimulation.

b: HCO_3^- secretion is enhanced by parasympathetic stimulation.

c: Na$^+$ reabsorption from saliva is inhibited by parasympathetic stimulation.

e: Parasympathetic stimulation is the most powerful mechanism for stimulating salivary secretion.

171. **Answer c:**

Chloracne is a characteristic symptom following exposure to polychlorinated biphenyls and related compounds (e.g., dioxin).

a: Chloracne is not characteristic of exposure to chlordecone.

b: Chloracne is not characteristic of exposure to chlordane.

d: Chloracne is not characteristic of exposure to chloramphenical.

e: Chloracne is not characteristic of exposure to methylmercuric chloride.

172. **Answer d:**

Although patients with rheumatoid arthritis have circulating IgM antibodies to their own IgG molecules, there is no evidence that these antibodies cause the formation of harmful immune complexes or are contributory to joint lesions.

a: Myasthenia gravis is mediated by antibodies against the acetylcholine receptor.

b: Goodpasture's syndrome is mediated by antibodies to type IV collagen in basement membranes of kidney glomeruli and lung alveoli.

c: Grave's disease is mediated by antibodies to thyroid-stimulating hormone receptors on thyroid follicular epithelial cells.

e: Insulin-resistant diabetes mellitus is mediated by antibodies against the insulin receptor.

173. **Answer a:**

The lingula is a "tongue-like" projection of the anteroinferior portion of the upper lobe of the left lung, immediately inferior to the cardiac notch.

b: Each lung possesses an oblique fissure.

c: The most superior portion of each lung is known as the apex and lies superiorly to the middle third of the clavicle.

d: The horizontal fissure is a characteristic feature of the right lung.

e: The right lung has an upper, middle, and lower lobe, whereas the left has only an upper and lower lobe.

174. **Answer d:**

The alpha-beta or gamma-delta heterodimer (a.) contains both a constant region and a variable region (b.). There is a single T cell receptor that specifically recognizes MHC-associated antigen (c.). The T cell receptor has both transmembrane and cytoplasmic domains (e.).

a: True. The T cell receptor contains both an alpha and beta chain or a gamma and delta chain.

b: True. The polypeptides and the T cell receptor contain both a constant (C) region and a variable (V) region.

c: True. The single T cell receptor confers specificity for both antigen and MHC.

e: True. T cell receptors contain both transmembrane and cytoplasmic domains.

175. **Answer c:**

Second order axons carrying pain information from the body decussate in the anterior white commissure.

a: The anterior commissure connects the two temporal lobes and has decussating axons carrying olfactory information.

b: The anterior medullary velum contains the decussating axons of the trochlear nerve.

d: The decussation of the medial lemniscus has crossing axons carrying fine two-point discrimination and vibration sense.

e: The posterior commissure contains crossing axons from the pretectal areas.

176. **Answer e:**

Many times the point mutation will also correlate with a change in function for the protein, as well as altering the restriction site.

a: Restriction enzymes are only produced by bacterial and not by eukaryotic cells.

b: Although restriction fragments of different lengths result from point mutations, they result from the destruction of restriction sites, not their creation.

c: The different length of restriction fragments is due to point mutations, which prevent cleavage of the DNA helix, producing one longer fragment in place of two shorter ones.

d: Southern blotting, which uses labeled DNA probes, is the method used for detecting the fragments produced from a restriction digest. Western blotting uses antibodies to detect specific proteins which, like the restriction diet, are separated by electrophoresis.

177. **Answer c:**

Thiazide diuretics have the most remarkable anti-hypertensive action followed by the loop diuretics. Potassium sparing diuretics have a weaker action with fewer untoward effects.

178. **Answer b:**

The structure of the active site, like the overall structure of the enzyme, is flexible and can be induced to change its shape in the presence of substrate. The change in shape is designed to bring amino acid side chains in the active site into proper alignment to bind the substrate and to help it to form the transition state.

a: The induced fit model refers only to the binding of substrate to the active site and does not refer to inhibitors or other ligands. Ligands that bind to allosteric sites are called effectors and are usually metabolites, whereas inhibitors are usually drugs or poisons.

c: Enzymes do not change the shape of optically active isomers in order to permit binding. Although the enzyme is flexible and can change its shape, the induced fit remains highly specific for the correct stereoisomer. Interestingly, some optical isomers are close enough in their fit into the active site to serve as excellent competitive inhibitors.

d: While cooperativity does require multiple subunits and does involve conformational change, it does not refer to changes in the active site. Cooperativity refers to changes induced in the overall enzyme that affect the accessibility of the active site to substrate on other subunits of the enzyme.

e: The transition state is adopted by the substrate *after* binding to the active site.

Matching answers 179 and 180

179. **Answer e:**

Niemann-Pick disease results from a deficiency in sphingomyelinase, causing an accumulation of sphingomyelin. This produces symptoms including liver and spleen enlargement, in addition to mental retardation.

180. **Answer d:**

McArdle's disease results from a deficiency in muscle (not including liver) phosphorylase resulting in the loss of an immediate source of glucose to support muscle contraction. If the patient persists with exercise, the cramps will disappear, due to the mobilization and utilization of free fatty acids as an energy source. Normal muscular activity is adequately supported by glucose uptake from the serum.

a: Metachromatic leukodystrophy results from a deficiency of arylsulfatase A, causing accumulation of a sulfate containing ceramide. Demyelination of nerve cells and mental retardation are symptoms.

b: Gaucher's disease results from a deficiency of beta-glucosidase, causing accumulation of ceramide with a glucose moiety attached. This is the most frequent form of sphingolipidoses.

c: Tay-Sachs disease results from a deficiency of beta-hexosaminodase A, resulting in the accumulation of GM_2 ganglioside. The related Tay-Sachs variant, or Sandhoff's disease, is due to a deficiency of both beta-hexosaminodase A and B. The symptoms of mental retardation and blindness of Tay-Sachs are the same, but progress more rapidly.

Matching answers 181 and 182

181. **Answer f:**

Activated mast cells convert arachidonic acid, by the action of 5-lipoxygenase and other enzymes, into the three main leukotrienes, LTC_4, LTD_4, and LTE_4.

182. **Answer g:**

Epithelial cells of organs, such as the intestine, express F_c receptors for dimeric forms of IgA molecules. This receptor is commonly called the secretory component.

Matching answers 183 and 184

183. **Answer d:**

Lepore hemoglobin is a beta thalassemia variant produced by unequal crossing over between the 5′ end of the delta globin gene and the 3′ end of the beta globin gene. The result is that the normal beta globin in the adult is replaced by a delta-beta hybrid globin, which has a normal function in oxygen transport, but is only produced at the low rate characteristic of delta globin.

184. **Answer e:**

Bart's hemoglobin is composed of $gamma_4$ tetramers and appears during fetal development in the patients with a deletion in all four alpha globin genes. The condition is called hydrops faetalis and is fatal.

a: Hemoglobin H is composed entirely of $beta_4$ tetramers as a result of beta globin excess because of alpha globin deficiency in alpha thalassemia.

b: Hemoglobin A_2 is a normal minor form of adult hemoglobin (2% to 3% of total) containing delta globins in place of beta globins.

c: Fetal hemoglobin has the composition of alpha$_2$ gamma$_2$ tetramers. The gamma globins impart to these tetramers a greater affinity for oxygen than the adult form, because of weaker binding of 2,3-bisphosphoglycerate.

Matching answers 185 and 186

185. **Answer a:**

The development of object permanence, a child's gained understanding that an object continues to exist even when not in view, is a critical cognitive task that occurs prior to age 2 (i.e., in the sensorimotor stage).

186. **Answer c:**

Conservation, the ability to understand that changing the form of an object does not necessarily change its essential qualities, is a cognitive task associated with the concrete operations phase (ages 7 to 11).

b: During the preoperational thought phase (ages 2 to 7), a child learns to use language but typically remains unable to use logic to explain the causal relationships between events.

d: Piaget's stage of formal operations (age 11 through adolescence) corresponds with the developing child's grasp of abstract reasoning, use of deductive and inductive reasoning, and full understanding of symbolic representations. Not all individuals obtain a formal operations level of cognitive capacity.

e: Deductive reasoning refers to the ability to reason from generalities to particular situations. This type of reasoning is associated with the formal operations stage.

Matching answers 187 through 189

187. **Answer d:**

Chlamydia trachomatis is the only obligate intracellular bacterium from the above list, and it is a leading cause of sexually transmitted disease.

188. **Answer a:**

Neisseria gonorrhoeae is a gram-negative diplococcus that is the leading cause of pelvic inflammatory disease.

189. **Answer e:**

Haemophilus influenzae is the most common cause of meningitis in unimmunized children under 5 years of age.

Matching answers 190 through 194

190, 193. **Answer a:**

T_3 is the primary biologically active form of thyroid hormone (Question 193); T_3 and T_4 enter cells where T_4 is converted to T_3. To initiate a biological effect, T_3 then binds to a receptor on chromatin to induce protein synthesis (Question 190).

191, 192. **Answer d:**

Thyroid-stimulating hormone is produced by thyrotropes in the anterior pituitary gland and acts on the thyroid.

194. **Answer e:**

Thyroglobin is a high molecular weight (660,000) protein that acts as a storage form for thyroid hormones and is the main component of thyroid colloid.

b: Thyroxine (T_4) is less potent than T_3; it was not used as a choice in this question set.

c: Thyroxine-binding globulin carries both T_3 and T_4 in the blood; it was not used as a choice in this question set.

Matching answers 195 and 196

195. **Answer e:**

Glycerol kinase is not present in adipose tissue, limiting the source for glycerol phosphate to the glycolytic pathway. Thus, when blood levels are low (and thus insulin levels), little or no precursor is available for triacylglycerol synthesis. Instead, when blood glucose levels are low, free fatty acids are released from the adipose tissue to serve as an energy source for gluconeogenesis in the liver and kidney.

196. **Answer c:**

Citrate lyase helps to shuttle acetyl CoA from the mitochondria to the cytosol by cleaving citrate into oxaloacetate (the carrier) and acetyl CoA, reversing their condensation catalyzed by the citrate synthase reaction. The oxaloacetate is converted to pyruvate before returning to the mitochondrial matrix.

a: Fatty acyl CoAs are the precursors for attachment to glycerol phosphate in the synthesis of triacylglycerols, and they are synthesized from free fatty acids in the cytoplasm by fatty acyl CoA synthetase. They are present in adipose tissue as well as the liver and the intestinal mucosa.

b: The malate shuttle does not function in fat synthesis. Its purpose is to shuttle reducing equivalents from NADH into the mitochondrial matrix from the cytosol.

d: Acetyl CoA carboxylase is present in adipose tissue and the liver to initiate the synthesis of fatty acids from acetyl CoA produced during carbohydrate (and protein) catabolism.

Matching answers 197 and 198

197. **Answer d:**

The Lesch-Nyhan syndrome is due to a genetic deficiency in hypoxanthine-guanine phosphoribosyltransferase, which prevents the salvage of both hypoxanthine and guanine. The blocked salvage steps simultaneously result in a decrease in IMP and GMP concentrations (feedback inhibitors of the first step in purine synthesis) and a buildup of PRPP (the limiting substrate for the first step in purine synthesis).

198. **Answer c:**

Adenosine deaminase deficiency leads to extremely large buildups of dATP, which inhibits ribonucleotide reductase. This causes an impairment in both T-cell and B-cell function, thus the name severe combined immune deficiency (SCID).

a: Orotic aciduria is due to a deficiency in the enzymes that convert orotate into uridine 5′-monophosphate. The buildup of orotic acid leads to abnormal growth and megaloblastic anemia and is successfully treated with a diet rich in uridine.

b: Purine nucleoside phosphorylase deficiency results in an accumulation of dGTP and dATP, both of which inhibit ribonucleotide reductase. This causes impairment of T-cell function but not B-cell function.

e: Gout is caused by deposition of uric acid crystals in the joints, a result of hyperuricemia. This is caused by one of several unusual genetic diseases all of which result in an increase in PRPP synthetase and of purine overproduction (and overexcretion).

Matching answers 199 and 200

199. **Answer a:**

Blocking is defined as an abrupt halting of speech in which the patient does not regain the goal of the previous statement being made.

200. **Answer b:**

Circumstantiality refers to the presentation of details which are seen as irrelevant to the current topic. Although patients displaying circumstantiality provide excessive information, ultimately a response is made which addresses the question asked or content of the conversation.

c: Perseveration is the repetition of speech or motor behaviors.

d: Flight of ideas is a term describing a patient's rapid transition from one idea to another often resulting in fragmented ideas. When a patient displays a flight of ideas a degree of coherency is present.

e: When a patient displays mutism, verbal responses do not occur, although the patient has the ability to demonstrate an awareness of the environment.

Mosby's Reviews Series
Copyright © 1996,
Mosby-Year Book, Inc.

How to install this program—Windows users

1. Place the disk in Drive A: (or B:)
2. From Program Manager, select File, then Run, then enter:
   A:SETUP (or B:SETUP if your disk drive is B:)
3. Follow the instructions on screen.

How to run this program—Windows users

Open the MOSBY Program Group and select the ACE program.

How to install this program—Macintosh users

1. Insert the disk into the disk drive. Double click on the disk icon.
2. Double click on the Install icon. The program will be saved to your hard drive.

How to run this program—Macintosh users

Open the MOSBY folder and select the ACE program.

For complete instructions on using the program, please read the "How to use this Program" file.

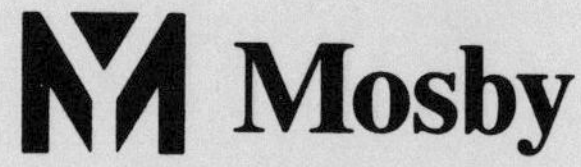 **Mosby**

Dedicated to Publishing Excellence

WE WANT TO HEAR FROM YOU!

To help us publish the most useful materials for students, we would appreciate your comments on this book. Please take a few moments to complete the form below, and then tear it out and mail to us. Thank you for your input.

Mosby's reviews: BASIC SCIENCES

1. What courses are you using this book for?

__medical school
__pharmacy school
__physician assistant program
__nursing school
__dental school
__osteopathic school
__undergrad
__other _____________________________

__1st year
__2nd year
__3rd year
__4th year
__other

2. Was this book useful for your course? Why or why not?

__yes __no____
____
____

3. What features of textbooks are important to you? (*check all that apply*)

__color figures
__summary tables and boxes
__summaries
__self-assessment questions
__price
__other ____

4. What influenced your decision to buy this text? (*check all that apply*)

__required/recommended by instructor
__recommendation by student
__bookstore display
__other ____

5. What other instructional materials did/would you find useful in this course?

__computer-assisted instruction
__lab time   __slides
__case studies book
__other ____

Are you interested in doing in-depth reviews of our basic science textbooks? If so please fill out the information below.

NAME:____

ADDRESS:____

____

TELEPHONE:____

THANK YOU!

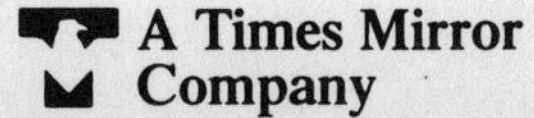 **A Times Mirror Company**

BUSINESS REPLY MAIL

FIRST CLASS MAIL   PERMIT No. 135   St. Louis, MO.

POSTAGE WILL BE PAID BY ADDRESSEE

CHRIS REID
MEDICAL EDITORIAL
MOSBY–YEAR BOOK, INC.
11830 WESTLINE INDUSTRIAL DRIVE
ST.LOUIS, MO 63146-9987